CLINICAL BEHAVIORAL SCIENCE

CLINICAL BEHAVIORAL SCIENCE

Edited by
Frederick Sierles
University of Health Sciences
The Chicago Medical School
North Chicago, Illinois

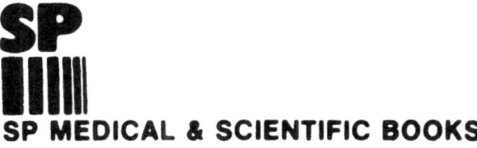

SP MEDICAL & SCIENTIFIC BOOKS

New York

SPECTRUM PUBLICATIONS, INC.
175-20 Wexford Terrace, Jamaica, N.Y. 11432

Library of Congress Cataloging in Publication Data
Main entry unter title:

Clinical behavioral science.

Includes index.
1. Medicine and psychology. 2. Human behavior.
3. Social medicine. I. Sierles, Frederick. [DNLM:
1. Behavioral sciences. 2. Psychopathology. WM100
C6386]
R726.5.C55   616.89   80-36786
ISBN 978-94-011-7975-1   ISBN 978-94-011-7973-7 (eBook)
DOI 10.1007/978-94-011-7973-7

To Laurene
and my parents

Acknowledgments

I wish to thank the following individuals for their constructive criticism of portions of the book: Michael Taylor, Ingrid Hendrickx, Richard Abrams, Julian Berman, Hazim Zakko, Joseph Ryan, Georgeda Buchbinder, Hilliard Foster, Morton Miller, Hagop Akiskal, John Halversen, and Harvey Strassman. I am most grateful to Charlotte Hughes and Georgia Gunn for countless hours of typing the manuscript, to Erna Braun for her illustrations, to Jack DeBruin and Joseph Nadakapadam for their photographs, and to Laurene Sierles for indexing. Hannah and Joshua Sierles deserve special mention for tolerating my unavailability during the writing of this book. Finally, I wish to thank my parents for their gift of intellectual curiosity.

Some of the funds for the writing of the book came from National Institute of Mental Health Grant MH05-984-25.

Contributors

RICHARD ABRAMS, M.D.
Professor and Vice Chairman
Department of Psychiatry
University of Health Sciences
The Chicago Medical School
North Chicago, Illinois

BERNHARD E. BLOM, Ph.D.
Assistant Professor
Department of Psychology
University of Health Sciences
The Chicago Medical School
North Chicago, Illinois

GEORGEDA BUCHBINDER, Ph.D.
Research Associate
Department of Anthropology
Queens College
The City University of New York
New York, New York

MICHAEL EGGER, M.D.
Private Practice of Psychiatry
Council Bluffs, Iowa

CHARLES HILLENBRAND, M.D.
Assistant Professor
Department of Psychiatry
Stritch School of Medicine
Loyola University
Maywood, Illinois

P.S.B. SARMA, M.D.
Associate Professor and Chief
Division of Child Psychiatry
University of Health Sciences
The Chicago Medical School
North Chicago, Illinois

WILLIARD SHANKEN, M.D.
Private Practice of Psychiatry
Lansdale, Pennsylvania

FREDERICK SIERLES, M.D.
Associate Professor and Director
Medical Student Education in Psychiatry
University of Health Sciences
The Chicago Medical School
North Chicago, Illinois

MICHAEL ALAN TAYLOR, M.D.
Professor and Chairman
Department of Psychiatry
University of Health Sciences
The Chicago Medical School
North Chicago, Illinois

EDWARD TYLER, M.D.
Clinical Professor
Department of Psychiatry
University of Louisville School of Medicine
Louisville, Kentucky

Preface

This short text is designed to present those aspects of the behavioral sciences that are clinically relevant to physicians in all branches of medicine. It should also be helpful to medical students studying for the behavioral sciences section of Part 1 of the national boards, to physicians taking the behavioral sciences portion of the FLEX exam, and to psychiatrists preparing for their American Board of Psychiatry certifying exam.

Behavior is a product of brain function and is manifested by actions in response to sitmuli. It is fundamental to the maintenance of health, and plays a role in causing and intensifying many illnesses. Abnormal behaviors can reveal to us, and even allow us to localize, brain dysfunction and disease. And they can cause, for patients, their families, and friends, considerable suffering. On an intellectual level, trying to comprehend the behavior of our patients (and our own behavior as well), contributes to making medicine a truly intriguing profession.

Behavioral science is not, as you might suspect, synonymous with psychiatry. When I began teaching behavioral sciences 7 years ago, I was struck by how little I knew about behavior and behavioral sciences. The scope of the behavioral sciences is so vast that the field, as well as the disciplines of which it is composed, is unmasterable. Entire books, and entire careers in research, could be devoted to subjects that are merely touched upon in this book. Thus, for any individual subject this brief book cannot properly convey the depth or sophistication of a high-quality monograph or years of clinical experience. Nevertheless, there is merit in brevity, for clinicians and medical students are busy people who appreciate a book that gets to the point: *Clinical Behavioral Science* is certainly an attempt to pare down subjects to their essentials.

It begins with the biological sciences as they pertain to behavior, moves to areas that are on the interface between the biological and the social sciences, and concludes with social sciences and social issues. The reader must realize, of course, that the dichotomy between the biological and social sciences is an arbitrary one—biological and social influences are usually interwined.

As a teacher of medical students and physicians, and as a practicing psychiatrist, I rely heavily upon the information contained in this text. I hope the reader finds it an equally helpful companion.

Frederick Sierles

Contents

CLINICAL
BEHAVIORAL
SCIENCE

Part I

The Biological Sciences and Behavior

1

The Genetics of Behavior

MICHAEL ALAN TAYLOR

INTRODUCTION

All body functions are genetic in the sense that gene patterns determine species, sex, physical characteristics, functional capacities of organs, and vulnerability of organs to disease. This premise applies equally to all organ systems, including the nervous system. Thus, the brain's anatomy and physiology, and the brain's functional manifestation, behavior, can be seen as being determined by genetic endowment. Of course, in comparison with that of other species, the genetic "substrate" of our brain development is particularly sensitive to influence by environmental factors.

SERIOUS PSYCHIATRIC ILLNESSES

Investigations of major psychiatric disorders demonstrate significant genetic liability. For example, it has been shown that relatives of people with affective disorders [1-3], schizophrenia [1], and sociopathy [4,5] are at greater risk for affective disorders, schizophrenia, and sociopathy, respectively, than the general population. [1,6]. Studies of the concordance for illness in monozygotic twins compared with dizygotic twins [1,7-10], and comparisons of morbidity risks for the biological and adoptive parents of psychiatrically ill adoptees [11,14], also support the hypothesis of a strong genetic liability for these three disorders (see Table 1).

Table 1   Summary of Genetic Studies of the Major Psychoses

Type of study	Schizophrenia	Affective disorder
General population frequency	0.6-1.0%	1-4%
First-degree relative mordibity risk	10-15% (pre-1970 studies) 2-3% (post-1970 studies)	10-24%
Monozygotic twin concordance	10-69% (pre-1970 studies) (Mean: 27%—post-1961 studies)	33-96% (Mean: 57%)
Dizygotic twin concordance	0-19% (pre-1970 studies) (Mean: 10% post-1961 studies)	9-67% (Mean: 14%)
Adoption studies	Conflicting	Two positive studies

NORMAL AND DEVIANT BEHAVIORS

Normal and deviant behavior patterns arise from multiple genetic and environmental causes. Our ability to separate genetic from environment determinants is imperfect, but certain generalizations are possible. In "normal" people, the genetic contribution to personality has been assessed by combining standard personality inventories with monozygotic-dizygotic twin concordance comparisons [15,16]. Significant concordance has been demonstrated for the following behavior patterns:

Social introversion	Sociability (extroversion)
Social apprehension	Socialization
Shyness	Communality
Passivity	Self-confidence
Aloofness	Activism (high drive and energy)
Coldness and lack of emotionality	Emotional overresponsibility
Low drive and energy	Moodiness and pessimism
Orderliness	Compulsivity

Combining the Minnesota Multiphasic Personality Inventory (MMPI), one of the standardized personality inventories, with monozygotic-dizygotic twin comparisons, has demonstrated that social introversion, sociopathic deviation, moodiness and pessimism, cheerfulness and optimism, and low drive and energy all exhibit heavy genetic liability [17,18]. Similar studies of parents and siblings [19,20], although difficult to interpret, show similar patterns of genetic loading.

Studies comparing monozygotic and dizygotic twins separated early in life [21-24] confirm the above findings, and further analysis [19] to determine degree of heritability show that the main determinant of these personality patterns (particularly forcefulness, energy and drive, and introversion and extroversion) is genetic.

Genetic contributions to deviant personality traits and certain behavioral disorders have also been evaluated. Monozygotic-dizygotic twin comparisons, again the major research strategy, have demonstrated strong concordance and heavy genetic liability for "global neuroticism" [25], anxiety traits and anxiety neurosis [26-28], obsessional neurosis [27,29-31], "hysterical" traits and Briquet's syndrome [28,32-34], sociopathy [4,5], criminality [34], and male homosexuality [35,36].

SOCIOBIOLOGY AND BEHAVIOR

Our behavior can also be examined in the broader context of evolutionary theory [37,38]. This approach accepts the basic premises that evolution by natural selection is the primary force responsible for the genetic makeup of all organisms, that genetic makeup in turn determines neuronal organization, and that neuronal organization is vital to instinctive and acquired behavior. Modern evolutionary theory [39,40] posits that there is a differential in reproductive success among individuals within a species, and that this differential is transmitted from individuals in one generation to their offspring in the next. Thus, it is the individual, not the species, that is primarily affected by selective processes. However, over many generations this process produces a gradual change in the makeup of the species.

Behavior, whatever its precise origins, can be viewed as the phenotype that results from this evolutionary process. In all species, genotype plus environment determines the mature phenotype. The sensitivity of the genotype to external factors (its plasticity), and the relative influence of environment upon it, increase proportionately with the "ascending" by the species of the phylogenetic tree [41,42]. But, although we are genotypically the most plastic of species, our genetic endowment surely must be carefully studied. For example, our repertoire of behaviors includes aggression, adultery, altruism, courtship, homosexuality, parenting, rape, territoriality, transexualism, and sociality, all of which have been observed in a variety of nonhuman species, and each of which, when it occurs in a nonhuman species, has been explained in terms of how the behavior enhances the ability of the animal to transmit its genes into the genetic pool of the next generation. [43]. An understanding of these behaviors in other animals may in turn help us to understand these and other social behaviors in ourselves: Socio-environmental explanations alone logically cannot suffice.

Sociobiologists distinguish between *proximate* and *ultimate* explanations for biological events. Proximate explanations answer questions like "What makes some birds migrate?" Ultimate explanations answer questions like "What are the evolutionary consequences of migration, as compared with no migration, for this species?" The first approach tells us *how* it's done; the second approach, *why* it's done.

The pineal-hypothalamic axis of migratory birds appears to be sensitive to total daily sunlight. As days become longer, sex hormone levels increase, body fat is burned, and spring migration occurs. As days become shorter, sex hormone levels decrease, body fat is accumulated, and fall migration occurs. This is a proximate explanation, the "how" of migration. The ultimate explanation of migration must include the effect of migration on the likelihood of individuals of one generation transmitting their genes to the genetic pool of the next generation. In species where environmental conditions favor the migratory individual as the transmitter of genetic material, the species, in time, will become migratory. Phrased differently, the migratory individual's migratory capacities will be progressively better represented in successive generations [43].

There are also proximate and ultimate explanations of brain function. Neurochemical, neurophysiological, and neuropsychological mechanisms of brain function are proximate explanations. Ultimate explanations of behaviors, prominently including those offered by sociobiologists, focus upon the evolutionary consequences, but these explanations have understandably aroused massive controversy, for they challenge strongly held positions. For example, altruism, group sociality, parenting, and mate selection in humans are traditionally considered learned behaviors reflecting cultural patterns. But studies of these behaviors in nonhuman species [37,44-48] have shown they may actually be products of evolutionary processes, enhancing the fitness of the individual's genes entering the next generation, and making the individual more fit in evolutionary terms [49,50].

For example, when danger is perceived, prairie dogs sound an alarm [43], an act which brings attention and danger to the alarm-sounder. But the alarm increases the chances that individuals nearby who possess the alarm-sounder's genes will survive, thus increasing the *evolutionary* fitness of the alarm-sounder.

Worker bees, pinnacles of altruism, forego reproduction to care for the colony. But their efforts are not even-handed, for they provide more food for their sisters (with whom they share three-quarters of their genes) than for their brothers (with whom they share one-quarter of their genes). If they reproduced, they would share only half their genes with their offspring. Thus, for the worker bee, altruism pays off in increasing survival of its own genes, and thus in its own evolutionary fitness. In humans, similar behaviors, such as altruism and group sociality, may be analogous to those in nonhuman species, and may not entirely be the product of learning.

From all evidence [51-56], the human brain is a product of evolution, which retains, anatomically and functionally, its nonhuman heritage. Behaviors characteristic of reptilian, paleomammalian, and primate brains are part of the human repertoire (Table 2). But what about uniquely human characteristics? For example, what about cerebral lateralization with speech, language, complex motor functions, and analytic and sequential data-processing localized in the "dominant" hemisphere, and spatial integration, gestaltic, visual, and parallel processing found in the "nondominant" hemisphere? The answer which comes from anatomic, physiological, and genetic studies is that this lateralization of function is determined genetically, as are the dextrality of function (right-handedness) of human populations and the development of langauge.

CLINICAL USEFULNESS

The clinical usefulness of information about the genetic determinants of behavior is limited, as exact modes of transmission are not yet known, and

Table 2   Brain Evolution and Behavior

Phylogenic level	Functional system	Anatomic development	Behavior patterns
Reptilian	Sensori-motor	Reticular activating system, midbrain, basal ganglia, thalamus, rudimentary cortex	Territoriality, hunting, homing, mating, rearing young, primitive consciousness, perception of body parts in space, axial movements
Paleo-mammalian	Limbic	Hypothalamus, anterior thalamic nucleus, hippocampus, Papez circuit, cingulate gyrus, orbito-frontal/pyriform/insular cortex	Emotion, appetitive states, sexual and motivational behaviors, learning, arousal, flight/fight emotions
Neo-mammalian	Neocortex (symmetrical)	Cerebral hemispheres (primary and secondary cortex)	Complex motor behavior; mnestic, gnostic, praxic functions
Human	Asymmetrical neocortex	Frontal lobes, inferior parietal lobule, temporal lobes (tertiary cortex) function; complex motor	Speech and language; abstract thinking; higher mnestic, gnostic, and praxic behavior

Source: From Ref. 52, with permission.

environmental influences upon human behavior are so great, yet so poorly studied. Nevertheless, an understanding of the data can facilitate clinical practice. For example, the knowledge that affective disorder is familial will be a signal to the diagnostician that the presence of affective disorder in a patient's family member increases the probability that the patient also suffers from that condition. This may be particularly helpful in "atypical cases." Armed with the information of genetic determinants of behavior, genetic counseling for psychiatric patients and their families becomes an additional therapeutic tool [57]. The clinician can inform patients and their families about estimated risks among different family members, dispel mistaken notions, and help develop plans for coping with potential morbidity.

CONCLUSION

Each of our modes of integrating incoming information (cerebral lateralization), speech and langauge (dominant cerebral hemisphere), basic emotional traits (limbic system), and patterns of personality has a fundamental genetic origin. Our genotypic plasticity, however, provides us with a unique ability to influence our own behavior patterns. Therefore, comprehensive understanding of human behavior must take into account human evolution and basic brain structure and function, and the interaction of these with the environment.

REFERENCES

1. Slater, E., and Cowie, J. *The Genetics of Mental Disorders.* Oxford, London (1971).
2. Winokur, G., Clayton, P., and Reich, T. *Manic-Depressive Illness.* Mosby, St. Louis (1969).
3. Abrams, R., and Taylor, M.: A Comparison of Unipolar and Bipolar Depressive Illness. *Am. J. Psychiatry* 137:1084-1087, 1980.
4. Guze, S., Wolfman, E., McKinney, J., and Cantwell, D. Psychiatric illness in the families of convicted criminals. A study of 519 first-degree relatives. *Dis. Nerv. Syst.* 28:651-659 (1973).
5. Cloninger, C., and Guze, S. Psychiatric illness in the families of female criminals. A study of 288 first-degree relatives. *Br. J. Psychiatry* 122:697-703 (1973).
6. Weissman, M., Myers, J., and Harding, P. Psychiatric disorders in a U.S. urban community. *Am. J. Psychiatry* 135:459-462 (1978).
7. Zerbin-Rudin, E. Our genitik der depressiven erkrankungen, in *Das Depressive Syndrom.* H. Hippius and H. Sellbach, ed. Urban and Schwarlzenberg. Munich (1969).
8. Allen, M. Twin studies of affective illness. *Arch. Gen. Psychiatry* 33:147-148 (1976).
9. Bertelsen, A., Harold, B., and Hauge, M. A Danish twin study of manic disorders. *Br. J. Psychiatry* 130:330-351 (1977).
10. Christiansen, K. Crime in a Danish twin population. *Acta Genet. Med. Gemellol.* 19:323-326 (1970).

11. Mendlewicz, J., and Rainer, J. Adoption study supporting genetic transmission in manic-depressive illness. *Nature (Lond.)* 268:327-329 (1977).

12. Cadoret, R. Evidence for genetic inheritance of primary affective disorder in adoptees. *Am. J. Psychiatry* 135:463-466 (1978).

13. Rosenthal, D., Wender, P., Kety, S., Welner, J., and Schulsinger, F. The adopted-away offspring of schizophrenics. *Am. J. Psychiatry* 128:307-311 (1971).

14. Crowe, R. The adopted offspring of women criminal offenders. *Arch. Gen. Psychiatry* 27:600-603 (1972).

15. Shields, J. Heredity and psychological abnormality, in *Handbook of Abnormal Psychology*; 2nd ed., H. Eysenck, ed. Knapp, San Diego (1973).

16. Vanderberg, S. Hereditary factors in normal personality traits (as measured by inventories), in *Recent Advances in Biological Psychiatry*, Vol. 9. J. Wortes, ed. Plenum, New York (1967).

17. Gottesman, I. Differential inheritance of the psychoneuroses. *Eugenics Q.* 9:223-227 (1962).

18. Gottesman, I. Heritability of personality. A demonstration, in *Psychological Monographs #572*. G. Gimble, ed. Vol. 77, No. 9:1-21 (1963).

19. Cattell, R., Stice, G., and Kristy, N. A first approximation of nature-nurture ratios for eleven primary personality factors in objective tests. *J. Abnorm. Soc. Psychol.* 54:143-159 (1957).

20. Elston, R., and Gottesman, I. The analysis of quantitative inheritance simultaneously from twin and family data. *Am. J. Hum. Genet.* 20:512-521 (1968).

21. Fuller, J., and Thompson, W. *Behavior Genetics.* Wiley, New York (1960).

22. Newman, H., Freeman, F., and Holzinger, K. *Twins: A study of heredity and environment.* Univ. Chicago Press, Chicago (1937).

23. Shields, J. *Monozygotic Twins Brought Up Apart and Brought Up Together.* Oxford, London (1962).

24. Jueo-Nielson, N. Individual and environment. A psychiatric psychological investigation of monozygotic twins reared apart. *Acta Psychiatr. Scand. (Suppl.) 183* (1965).

25. Shields, J. Personality differences and neurotic traits in normal twin school children. *Eugenics Rev.* 45:213-246 (1954).

26. Slater, E., and Shields, J. Genetical aspects of anxiety, in *Studies of Anxiety: British Journal of Psychiatry*, Spec. Publ. No. 3. M. Lader, ed. Headley Bros., Ashford, England (1969).

27. Brown, F. Heredity in the psychoneuroses. *Proc. R. Soc. Med.* 35:785-790 (1942).

28. Cohen, M., Badol, D., Kilpatrick, A., Reed, E., and White, P. The high familial prevalence of neuro-circulatory asthenia (anxiety neurosis, effort syndrome). *Am. J. Hum. Genet.* 3:126-158 (1951).

29. Inouye, E. Similar and dissimilar manifestations of obsessive-compulsive neurosis in monozygotic twins. *Am. J. Psychiatry* 121:1171-1175 (1965).

30. Rosenberg, C. Familial aspects of obsessional neurosis. *Br. J. Psychiatry* 113:405-413 (1967).

31. Marks, I., Crowe, M., Drewe, E., Young, J., and Dewhurst, W. Obsessive-compulsive neurosis in identical twins. *Br. J. Psychiatry* 45:991-998 (1969).

32. Arkonac, O., and Guze, S. A family study of hysteria. *N. Engl. J. Med.* 268:239-242 (1963).

33. Woerner, P., and Guze, S. A family study and marital study of hysteria. *Br. J. Psychiatry* 114:161-168 (1968).

34. Guze, S. *Criminality and Psychiatric Disorders.* Oxford, New York (1976).

35. Kallmann, F. Comparative twin study on the genetic aspects of male homosexuality. *J. Nerv. Ment. Dis.* 115:283-298 (1952).

36. Heston, L., and Shields, J. Homosexuality in twins. A family study and a registry study. *Arch. Gen. Psychiatry* 18:146-160 (1968).

37. Wilson, E. *Sociobiology: The new synthesis.* Belknap, Harvard, Cambridge (1975).

38. Wilson, E. *On Human Nature*. Harvard, Cambridge (1978).
39. Mayer, E. Evolution. *Sci. Am.* 239:47-55 (1978).
40. Ayala, F. The mechanisms of evolution. *Sci. Am.* 239:56-59 (1978).
41. Hinde, R. *Animal Behavior: A synthesis of ethology and comparative psychology*. McGraw-Hill, New York (1970).
42. Lehrmen, D. Semantic and conceptual issues in the nature-nurture problem, in *Developmental and Evolution of Behavior*. L. Aronson, D. Lehrman, J. Rosenblatt and E. Tobach, eds. Freeman, San Francisco (1970).
43. Barash, D. *Sociobiology and Behavior*. Elsevier, New York (1977).
44. Greene, P., and Barash, D. Genetic bases of behavior — especially of altruism. *Am. Psychol.* 31:359-361 (1976).
45. Chance, M., and Mead, A. Social behavior and primate evolution. *Symp. Soc. Exp. Biol.* 7:395-439 (1953).
46. Barash, D. Social behavior of the hoary marmot (marmoto Calegate). *Anim. Behav.* 22:257-262 (1974).
47. Barash, D. Some evolutional aspects of parental behavior in animals and man. *Am. J. Psychol.* 89:195-217 (1976).
48. Burton, M. *Animal Courtship*. Praeger, New York (1954).
49. Hamilton, D. The genetical theory of social behavior I and II. *J. Theoret. Biol.* 7:1-52 (1964).
50. Maynard-Smith, J. Group selection and kin selection. *Nature (Lond.)* 201:1145-1147 (1964).
51. Holloway, R. The costs of fossil (animal) brains, in *Biological Anthropology: Readings from Scientific American*. Freeman, San Francisco (1975).
52. McLean, P. Man's reptilian and limbic inheritance, in *A Triune Concept of the Brain and Behavior: Hinchs memorial lectures*. T. Boag and D. Campbell, eds. Univ. of Toronto, Toronto (1973).
53. Dimond, S., and Blizard, D. (eds.). *Evolution and Lateralization of the Brain*. N.Y. Acad. Sci., New York (1977).
54. Geschwind, N. Language and the brain, in *Biological Anthropology: Readings from Scientific American*. Freeman, San Francisco (1975).
55. Dimond, S., and Beaumont, J. (eds.). *Hemisphere Function in the Human Brain*. Halsted, New York (1974).
56. Harnad, S., Doty, R., Goldstein, L., Jaynes, J., and Krauthammer, G. (eds.). *Lateralization in the Nervous System*. Academic, New York (1977).
57. Tsuang, M. Genetic counseling for psychiatric patients and their families. *Am. J. Psychiatry* 135:1465-1475 (1978).

2

The Behavioral Neurological Examination

MICHAEL ALAN TAYLOR

INTRODUCTION

All behavior (normal, deviant, and pathological) reflects brain function. Behavioral neurology deals with brain diseases and disorders that manifest themselves as behavioral changes rather than as motor (e.g., paralysis of a limb) or sensory (e.g., homonymous hemianopsia) changes [1]. Psychiatrists traditionally focus on behavioral abnormalties due to subtle brain dysfunctions without structural damage or obvious metabolic disorders, while neurologists traditionally emphasize motor, sensory, and behevioral changes due to nervous system disease associated with structural damage or obvious metabolic disorder. In behaviorial neurology, these specialties overlap in the study of relationships between higher cortical functions (e.g., mnestic, gnostic, praxic, and language functions and dysfunctions) and brain anatomy, particularly the anatomy of the neocortex. The basic science of this field is termed *neuropsychology,* and it deals with both normal and pathological neocortical functioning [2,3].

Until the early 19th century, the brain was thought to be functionally *equipotential;* that is, it was believed that there was no localization of higher cortical processes, as each brain region could and did assume all these functions. The brain was conceived of, functionally, as a "bowl of jello" [4]. In 1861, Paul Broca reported on a series of patients who manifested labored dysarthric speech in which small words and word endings were omitted (motor aphasia), and who had lesions of the left posterior inferior precentral frontal gyrus. In 1874, Carl Wernicke reported on a series of patients who demonstrated fluent but jargon-filled speech with word approximations and/or newly coined words (receptive aphasia) and who had lesions in the left-posterior superior temporal gyrus. The era of localization had begun, and by the first quarter of the 20th century, the jello brain had been replaced by a "bean" brain; that is, a "bag of beans" in which each bean had its own locus and function. Modern data support neither concept; today's neuropsychologists view the brain as regionalized, anatomically and functionally, but think of it more in terms of systems and complex organizations than in terms of small discrete functional units [2,3].

BASIC CONCEPTS

1. Cerebral Lateralization

The left and right hemispheres of most people differ in the facility with which each hemisphere processes qualitatively different stimuli. One of the hemispheres is organized to handle symbolic and language stimuli by decoding, classifying, reorganizing and synthesizing the stimuli [2,5-8]. The other hemisphere is organized to handle nonsymbolic, motor-perceptual and spatial stimuli [2,5-8]. Although each hemisphere is dominant over the other in its specialized "areas of expertise," by convention the hemisphere organized for symbolic and language function is called *dominant* and the other hemisphere is called *nondominant*. Approximately 97% of individuals have a left hemisphere that is dominant for language function. The remaining 3% have right cerebral hemisphere dominance for language, or "mixed" dominance. Thus, the left hemisphere is the dominant hemisphere for 97% of the population.

2. Handedness

Handedness refers to the fact that humans have a preferred hand. Approximately 90% of the population is right-handed (dextral) and approximately 10% is left-handed (sinistral) or ambidextrous. For a given patient, cerebral dominance for language cannot be inferred by handedness alone. Most right-handers *and* most left-handers are left-brain-dominant. The identification and localization of brain lesions often requires knowing which of the patient's hemispheres is dominant. If the examiner always said left, he would have a 3% error [5,8-11], a margin of error which a neurosurgeon cannot afford. Although there are elaborate methods for identifying the dominant hemisphere, they have medical risks [8]. A fairly simple, noninvasive, and reliable method is to ask the patient to write his name on a line you have drawn. When the preferred hand, the hand with which the patient writes, is held in a "hook" position above the line, this strongly suggests that the dominant hemisphere is on the same side as (ipsilateral to) the preferred hand. When the preferred hand is held below the line, this strongly suggests that the dominant hemisphere is on the side opposite (contralateral) to the preferred hand [12].

3. Primary, Secondary, and Tertiary Cortex

Primary cortex refers to cortical areas which receive initial incoming (afferent) sensory (e.g., auditory, visual) stimuli. The *secondary cortex* organizes information (e.g., sound patterns, light patterns) received by the primary cortex into perceptions (e.g., human voice, moving objects). The *tertiary cortex* interprets these perceptions (e.g., "lovely melodic voice," "red car making a fast turn") via complex associations, and integrates perceptions from several secondary sensory areas. Thus, the tertiary cortex acts as an associational area for associational areas (secondary cortex). Higher cortical functions are functions of tertiary cortical areas, and of all species, humans have the most highly developed tertiary cortex. Large parts of the parietooccipital area, the temporal lobes, and most of the frontal lobes rostral to the precential gyrus, are part of the tertiary cortex; however, a complete examination of cortical functioning involves the testing of primary, secondary, and tertiary regions. [2].

4. Soft Neurological Signs

"Soft" neurological signs are behaviors that indicate central nervous system dysfunction, but which do not permit localization of the dysfunction. "Hard" signs (e.g., constructional dyspraxia, extensor plantar reflex, and unilateral limb paralysis) are findings that indicate central nervous system dysfunction which often do permit localization of the dysfunction. To the behavioral neurologist "soft" signs are important manifestations of cerebral dysfunction and, when properly demonstrated, are both reliable (reproducible) and valid in identifying brain disease [13,14]. Table 1 shows some of the more common soft signs.

TESTING OF COGNITIVE (HIGHER CORTICAL) FUNCTION

1. The Frontal Lobe

The frontal lobes comprise 25% of adult brain weight. The portion of the frontal lobes rostral to the motor areas has executive function over other cortical areas, and is considered by many to be the tertiary cortex for the limbic system. Except for language, frontal lobe functions cannot be separated clear-

Table 1   Soft Neurological Signs

Sign	Task/Behavior	Abnormal Response
Palmomental Reflex	Repeated scratching of base of thumb	Slight downward movement of the mouth and jaw which does *not* extinguish
Grasp Reflex	Pressure (examiner's fingers) exerted on palm	Subject's fingers close about examiner's (grasps them)
Gegenhalten	Passive movement of subject's limbs	Subject resists with equal pressure to that of examiner's
Snout/Rooting Reflex	Stroking corner of subject's mouth	Subject's lips purse and move towards stimulation
Motor Impersistence	Subject makes a fist, closes eyes tightly, protrudes tongue, looks away while examiner manipulates opposite limb	Unable to maintain each of these behaviors for 20 seconds
Adventitious Motor Overflow	Rhythmic and rapid tapping with fingers. Each hand separately	Movements also seen in inactive hand (chorea also an overflow movement)
Double Simultaneous Discrimination (Face Hand Test)	Examiner simultaneously lightly touches cheeks and hands in sequence	Tendency to not perceive the touch on the hands

ly into dominant and nondominant categories [2]. Table 2 lists the frontal lobe functions that can be evaluated in a clinical examination, and the tasks which test those functions. [2].

Global orientation refers to awareness of place, person, and time. In the presence of clear consciousness, global disorientation reflects frontal lobe dysfunction. This is also true for *concentration*. Serial 7s (subtracting 7 from 100 and then subtracting 7 from each subsequent answer, all within 90 sec with no errors), and spelling a five-letter word (e.g., earth) backwards, are tests of concentration [15].

The frontal lobes *regulate motor behavior* [2]. Hyperactivity, hypoactivity, and all catatonic motor phenomena can be manifestations of frontal lobe dysfunction. The ability to sustain a voluntary movement is also under the direction of the frontal lobes. A patient should be able to tap rapidly with his fingers, make a fist, protrude his tongue, or keep his eyes closed, each for 20 sec. Failure to do so is termed *motor impersistence* and suggests frontal dysfunction. The inability to stop a motor act *(motor perseveration)* is also a "frontal sign" of motor dysregulation. One test for motor perseveration is to ask the patient to draw a circle. Figure 1 is an example of a perseverated circle.

Table 2   Frontal Lobe Function

Function	Task	Abnormal Response
Global Orientation	Name the day of the week, month, year, location	Any error
Concentration	Spell "earth" backwards, serial sevens	any improper letter sequence, one or more errors or longer than 90 seconds
Regulation of motor behavior	Drawing circle, finger-tapping, maintaining motor tasks (making a fist, holding arms out, closing eyes), tests of stimulus bound motor phenomena	drawing multiple lines, slow awkward taps, unable to persist for more than 20 seconds Gegenhalten, Echopraxia
Language	Repeat: "no ifs, ands, or buts," "Methodist Episcopal," "Massachusetts Avenue"	missed words or syllables; repetition of internal syllables; dropping of word endings Broca's aphasia
Active Perception	Identification of upside down objects	turning of head to identify, unable to identify until objects turned right side up
Judgment	Comments about real life problems	unrealistic or foolish solutions and plans
Abstract thinking	Identifying similarities, problem solving	any error

The frontal lobes are also responsible for initiating activities in other brain areas; thus, the inability to begin simple tasks *(inertia)* is a sign of frontal dysfunction.

Motor (Broca's) aphasia is associated with lesions of the dominant frontal lobe. It is characterized by slow, labored, dysarthric speech lacking in fluency. Often, small words and word endings are omitted, so speech is also "telegraphic." Patients with motor aphasia have difficulty repeating phrases

DRAW A CIRCLE: Normal   Abnormal

   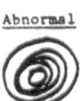

FIG. 1.   Motor perseveration.

such as "No ifs, ands, or buts," "Methodist Episcopal," and "Massachusetts Avenue" [16,17].

Judgement and *abstract thinking* are also frontal lobe functions. Judgment is best tested by asking the patient about problems in his life and how he plans to deal with them. Abstract thinking is tested by asking him to explain the similarity between an orange and a pear, a bicycle and an airplane, and a fly and a tree [2,18].

2. The Parietal Lobes

Touch, pain, and temperature senses are represented in primary cortex in the posterior central gyrus, which is located in the anterior portion of the parietal lobe opposite (contralateral) to the side of the body where the sensation is being tested. Proprioception, stereognosis, and graphesthesia are functions represented in secondary cortex in the contralateral parietal lobe, just caudal to the posterior central gyrus.

The largest part of each parietal lobe is tertiary cortex [2,19]. The nondominant parietal lobe coordinates motor, sensory and spatial perception. Its functions include the awareness of one's body in space, the recognition of faces, and the ability to copy the outline of simple objects (e.g., Greek cross, key).

The dominant parietal lobe coordinates visual and language functions, which include reading (lexic function) and writing (graphic function). The ability to do simple math, to identify one's fingers (e.g., thumb, ring finger, flipping a coin), to spell, to know right from left, and to identify relationships (e.g., "my father's brother is my uncle") are also functions of the dominant parietal lobe. Tests of dominant and nondominant parietal functions are shown in Table 3 [2,16,19-26].

3. Occipital Lobes

The primary occipital cortex in each hemisphere receives visual stimuli from the opposite visual field. The two occipital lobes work in unison, so visual perception is essentially a bilateral phenomenon. Thus, lesions in secondary or teritiary cortex cannot be lateralized by routine procedures. It is also difficult to separate functionally the tertiary occipital cortex from the tertiary parietal cortex. [2]. Visual acuity is a test of peripheral visual and nervous function, and of the primary occipital cortex. The ability to recognize background from foreground, and to recognize objects visually, are tests of secondary occipital cortex. The ability to identify visually objects that are partially obscured (Fig. 2) is a function of the tertiary occipital cortex. There are more elaborate tests of tertiary occipital cortex; these include the testing

Table 3   Tests of Parietal Lobe Functions

Dominant	Non-dominant
1. Calculations: Acalculia	1. Copy outline of simple objects (Greek cross, key): construction apraxia
2. Right/left orientation: Right/left disorientation	2. Recognition of Faces: Prosopagnosia
3. Writing: Agraphia	3. Awareness of body parts in space: spatial neglect
4. Identification of fingers: Finger agnosia	4. Contralateral proprioception, stereoagnosis, graphesthesia, sensation, copying examiner's hand movement (Kinesthetic Apraxia)
5. Reading: Dyslexia	
6. Demonstrate use of simple objects: Ideomotor apraxia	
7. To Categorize: "Who is your brother's father," "Who is your father's brother?"	
8. Contralateral proprioception, stereoagnosis, graphasthesia, sensation, copying examiner's hand movements (Kinesthetic Apraxia)	

of visual memory, the identification and matching of complex visual patterns, and the presentation of visual stimuli to one hemisphere at a time, by means of a special projection system called a tachistoscope [2,3].

4.   Testing of the Temporal Lobe

The nondominant temporal lobe, usually the right, is a relatively "silent" cortical area. The perception of rhythms, tones, and musical notes occurs here. Testing for dysfunction may require the use of elaborate or cum-

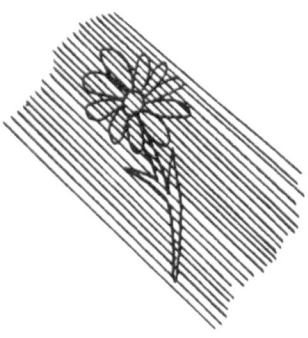

FIG. 2.   Obscured object.

bersome audio equipment. Asking the patient to repeat simple tapped rhythms or to distinguish high and low tones are crude tests of this cortical area [2].

The testing of the dominant temporal lobe is essentially the testing of receptive language function. The left posterior superior temporal gyrus (Wernicke's area) is the tertiary auditory cortex. Dysfunction here produces fluent aphasia characterized by paraphasic speech (work approximations, neologisms), jargon, and circumlocutory speech. Word deafness (inability to understand spoken speech) and anomia (inability to name objects) can also occur. Table 4 shows tests of language function [2,3,16,17].

5. Testing of Verbal Memory

Memory testing is part of the complete examination of brain function. Memory is not a single, holistic function—*long-term memory* (months and years), *recent memory* (days and weeks), *short-term memory* (minutes and hours) and *immediate recall* (right away) can all be selectively impaired. Except for severe bilateral hippocampal dysfunction, altered consciousness, or extreme inattention (poor concentration), immediate recall is rarely, if ever, impaired. Short-term memory is often disturbed, particularly in patients suffering from

Table 4   Test of Language Function

Task	Dysfunction	Abnormal Responses
Repeat: "No ifs, ands, or buts," "The President lives in Washington," "Methodist Episcopal," "Massachusetts Avenue"	Expressive language	Missed words or syllables; repetition of internal syllables; dropping of word endings
Name common objects (e.g., key, watch, button, etc.)	Anomia	Cannot name: word approximations; describes functions rather than word
Conversion during examination	Receptive language	Word approximations, neologisms, word salad, stock words, tangential speech
Write a sentence	Dysgraphia	No longer able to write cursively; loss of sentence structure; loss of word structure; abnormally formed letters
In individual steps, copy sentence, read it, and do what it says ("Put the paper in your pocket")	Dysgraphia, dyslexia comprehension	No longer able to write cursively; loss of sentence structure; loss of word structure; abnormally formed letters

psychomotor epilepsy, intoxications, and other acute coarse brain disease (disease with clear structural damage or obvious metabolic disorder). Recent memory can be disturbed in both acute and chronic coarse disease. In chronic coarse disease, the most established memory patterns may be spared; thus, long-term memory is often the last to be disturbed by illness.

Memory testing is not valid if the patient is in an altered state of consciousness. If concentration is severely impaired, verbal memory can be tested by asking the patient to remember a pair or series of words. Immediate repetition is a test of immediate recall. Repetition after 10 min is a test of short-term memory. Recent and long-term memory can be tested only by obtaining detailed information about the patient's past life. Poor verbal memory suggests dysfunction in the dominant hippocampus and other deep limbic system structures.

Amnesia refers to the inability to recall past events. Global amnesia exists in hysterics and in the movies. The inability to recall events prior to a point in time is called *retrograde* amnesia. It is common following head trauma, but it usually extends back in time only a few seconds or minutes. *Antrograde amnesia* refers to the inability to recall events occurring after a point in time. This type of amnesia results from faulty registration of new material because of continuing brain dysfunction; the loss of certain specific memories is usually permanent, but the amnesia-causing process is limited in duration. The longer the period of antrograde amnesia, the more severe the brain dysfunction [2,3,18,27-29].

REFERENCES

1. Pincus, J.H., and Tucker, G.J. *Behavioral Neurology,* 2nd ed. Oxford, New York, (1978).
2. Luria, A.R. *The Working Brain: An introduction to neuropsychology* B. Hough, transl. Basic Books, New York (1973).
3. Golden, C.J. *Diagnosis and Rehabilitation in Clinical Neuropsychology* Thomas, Springfield, Ill. (1978).
4. Krech, D. Cortical localization of function, in *Psychology in the Making,* L.L. Postman, ed. Knopf, New York, (1962).
5. Levy, J. The origins of lateral asymmetry, in *Lateralization in the Nervous System.* S. Harnard, R. Doty and L. Goldstein, J. Jaynes, and G. Krauthammer, eds. Academic, New York (1977), pp. 195-209.
6. Levy, J. Psychobiological implications of bilateral asymmetry, in *Hemispheric Function in the Human Brain.* S.F. Dimond and J.G. Beaumont, eds. Halsted, New York (1974), pp. 121-183.
7. Seaman, J.G. Coding and retrieval processes and the hemispheres of the brain, in *Hemisphere Function in the Human Brain.* S.F. Dimond and J.G. Beaumont, eds. Halsted, New York (1977), pp. 184-203.
8. Wada, J., and Rasmussen, T. Intra-carotid injection of sodium amytal for the lateralization of cerebral speech dominance. *J. Neurosurg.* 17:266-282 (1960).

9. Geschwind, N. The anatomical basis of hemisphere differentration, *Hemisphere Function in the Human Brain*. S.F. Dimond and J.G. Beaumont, eds. Halsted, New York (1977), pp. 7-24.

10. Rubens, A.B. Anatomical asymmetries and human cerebral cortex, in *Lateralization in the Nervous System*. S. Harnard, R. Doty, L. Goldstein, J. Jaynes, and G. Krauthammer, eds. Academic, New York (1977), pp. 503-516.

11. Kocel, K.M. Cognitive abilities: Handedness, familial sinistrality, and sex, in *Evolution and Lateralization of the Brain*. S.F. Dimond and J.G. Beaumont, eds. N.Y. Acad. Sci., New York (1977), pp. 233-243.

12. Levy, J., and Reid, M. Variations in writing posture and cerebral organization. *Science* 194:337-339 (1976).

13. Cox, S.M., and Ludburg, A.M. Neurological soft signs and psychopathology. 1. Findings in schizophrenia. *J. Nerv. Ment. Dis.* 167:161-165 (1979).

14. Quitkin, F., Rifkin, A., and Klein, D.F. Neurologic soft signs in schizophrenia and character disorders. *Arch. Gen. Psychiatry* 33:845-853 (1979).

15. Spear, F.G., and Green, R.: Inability to concentrate. *Br. J. Psychiatry* 112:913-915 (1966).

16. Brown, J.W. *Aphasia, Apraxia and Agnosia: Clinical and theoretical aspects*. Thomas, Springfield, Ill. (1972).

17. Brown, J.W. *Mind, Brain, and Consciousness: The neuropsychology of cognition*. Academic, New York (1977).

18. Matarazzo, J.D. *Wechsler's Measurements and Appraisal of Adult Intelligence*, 5th ed. Oxford, New York (1972).

19. Critchley, M. *The Parietal Lobes*, Hafner, New York (1953).

20. Gerstmann, J. Some notes on the Gerstmann syndrome. *Neurology* 7:866-869 (1957).

21. Nelson, J. Gerstmann's syndrome. Finger agnosia, apraphia, comparison of right and left and acalculia. *Arch. Neurolog. Psychiatry* 39:536 (1938).

22. Strub, R., and Geschwind, N. Gerstmann syndrome without aphasia. *Cortex* 10:378-387 (1974).

23. Denny-Brown, D. The nature of apraxia. *J. Nerv. Ment. Dis.* 126:9-32 (1958).

24. Geschwind, N. The apraxias: Neural mechanisms of disorders of learned movement. 63:188-195 (1975).

25. Geschwind, N. Disconnection in animals and man, part II. *Brain* 88:585-644 (1965).

26. Benson, D.F., and Barton, M. Disturbance of constructional ability. *Cortex* 6:19-46 (1970).

27. Barbizet, J. *Human Memory and Its Pathology*. D.K. Jardine, transl. W.H. Freeman, San Francisco (1970).

28. Bleuler, M. Acute mental concomtants of physical diseases, in *Psychomatic Aspects of Neurological Disease*. D.F. Benson and D. Dlumer, eds. Grune & Stratton, New York (1975), pp. 37-61.

29. Wechsler, D. A standardized memory scale for clinical use. *J. Psychol.* 19:87-95 (1945).

3

The Aphasia Screening Test and the Minimental State Examination

FREDERICK SIERLES

INTRODUCTION

It is crucial for physicians to identify and localize brain dysfunction. The standard neurological examination, while relatively easy to perform, and necessary as well, emphasizes motor and sensory functions and deemphasizes cognitive functions. This limits the sites in the brain that can be tested, and misses several secondary and tertiary cortical areas.

The Reitan-Indiana Aphasia Screening Test [1], named after Dr. Ralph Reitan who designed it, and the Minimental State Examination [2] of Folstein, Folstein, and McHugh, are easily administered, brief, noninvasive tests designed to identify, localize, and lateralize brain dysfunction, and can be employed by any medical student or physician. Each test can be done in 4 or 5 min if the patient is alert and cooperative, and in 8-20 min if the patient is not fully alert and cooperative. In general, the less cooperative the patient, the greater the likelihood of brain dysfunction, so the extra minutes are worth the examiner's time. These tests are performed towards the end of the initial medical interview, although they can be performed at any point in the course of a patient's treatment.

Comparing the results of Aphasia Screening Tests with the results of neurosurgical procedures performed on the tested patients, Reitan and Heimburger [1] demonstrated the concurrent validity of the Aphasia Screening Test in terms of its capacity to lateralize lesions. Comparing the results of Minimental State Exams with clinical diagnoses and WAIS results on the same patients, Folstein, Folstein, and McHugh [2] demonstrated the concurrent validity of the Minimental State Examination in terms of its capacity to distinguish diffuse cortical dysfunction from normal cortical function or focal cortical dysfunction. Tsai and Tsuang [3] demonstrated concurrent validity of this test by comparing its results to computerized tomographic scan results. Employing 24-h retests with one tester, 24-h retest with two testers, and 28-day retests with clinically stable patients, Folstein, Folstein, and McHugh demonstrated the high reliability of the Minimental State Examination.

To perform both tests together, the examiner needs a pen or pencil, 11 blank unlined pieces of paper, an Aphasia Screening Test booklet, and a well-lit room with a table on which the patient and examiner can write. The Aphasia Screening Test booklet can be obtained from Dr. Ralph Reitan* at the University of Arizona. Bear in mind that if the patient is not fluent in English, is uneducated, or is a child, test results will be harder to interpret.

THE APHASIA SCREENING TEST [1]

When you and the patient are comfortable, tell the patient something like "I'd like to ask you some questions from a little blue book." After pausing for a response, add "When I ask you to copy the outline of a drawing, please copy the outline only, copy it in the same size as the original drawing, and don't take you pen (or pencil) off the paper." Then take out the aphasia screening booklet, which consists of 18 cards for presentation to the patient, and 18 sets of instructions for the examiner. These cards are pictured in Figure 2. As you can see, the examiner need not memorize the questions, for the instructions appearing on each card are in full view of the examiner. The booklet should be placed flat on the table and visible to both patient and examiner, with the instruction card facing the examiner. The examiner presents one card at a time to the patient. (I have never run into a problem resulting from the patient knowing that I was reading the instructions from the instruction card.)

You need to know not only whether the patient performs a task proficiently, but also whether he has the capacity to perform the task at all. If he performs poorly at his first attempt at the task, he should be told something like "Are you sure that's right?" or "Try that again; I think you can do better," and encouraged to try again. Any errors should be noted, whether on the first or the second try. Your instructions must be clear, as any error may be significant. To minimize distraction, a separate blank unlined sheet of

---

*Mailing address: Ralph M. Reitan, Ph.D., Department of Psychology, University of Arizona, Tucson, Arizona 85721

paper should be presented to the patient for each task which requires that the patient write or draw. Patients with frontal lobe dysfunction can be distracted by slight imperfections in the test booklet or on their paper; for example, a patient copied the outline of an ink smudge which appeared accidentally on a card on which he was asked to copy the outline of a square. Frontal lobe dysfunction, particularly perseveration and impaired concentration, can also produce errors on tests of functions of other lobes of the brain; for example, a perseverated square could be confused for a dyspraxic Greek cross.

Now let's proceed to the individual cards pictured in Figure 2. In cards 1-3, the patient is asked first to "Copy the shape," then to "Name it," and finally to "Spell it." Copying the shape requires the skill called constructional praxis, and the inability to do this properly is called constructional dyspraxia, which is usually the result of nondominant (usually right-sided) parietal lobe dysfunction. In rare instances, constructional dyspraxia can also result from interhemispheric dysconnection: If the patient copies the shape poorly with his preferred hand, ask him to copy the shape with his nonpreferred hand. This covers the rare occasion where the poor performance with the preferred hand was due to interhemispheric dysconnection. If the dyspraxia was due to nondominant parietal dysfunction, the patient will also copy poorly with his nonpreferred hand. If the dyspraxia was due to interhemispheric dysconnection, the patient will copy correctly with his nonpreferred hand after having copied incorrectly with his preferred hand.

Two dyspraxic drawings are portrayed in Figure 1. Please note that the drawing on the left represents contructional dyspraxia of particular kind,

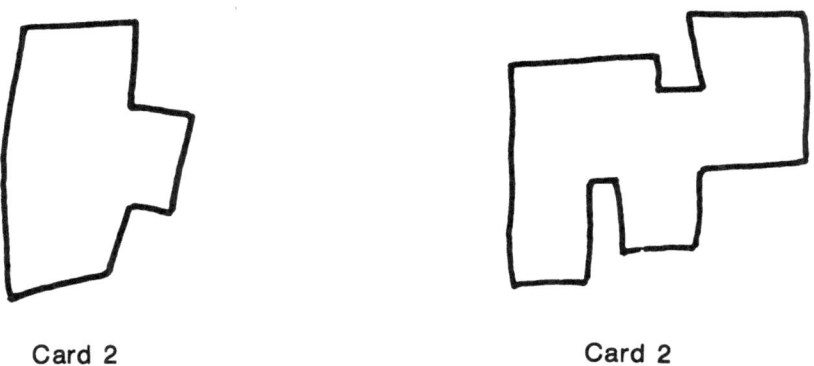

Card 2   Card 2

FIG. 1.   Constructional dysparaxia.

revealing left spatial neglect in a patient who, interestingly, did not shave the left side of his face. Naming the shape is simply called naming, which is a function of the dominant (usually the left) temporoparietal area. The inability to name familiar objects is called dysnomia. The ability to spell the name of the shape is called spelling praxis, which is also a function of the dominant temporoparietal area. The inability to spell common words is called spelling dyspraxia.

With card 4, you ask the patient to "Name that" or "Tell me what that is." The only acceptable answer is "baby," a word everyone knows. "Kid," "child," and "boy" are unacceptable, so the patient may have to be asked "Can you name another word?" if he does not say baby the first time. This tests the ability to name, which is a dominant temporoparietal function, but more importantly, it tests for active perception, which is a frontal lobe function. Active perception is the ability to mentally rotate an object without turning one's head. If the patient cannot name the baby, you then turn the card on its side so that the baby appears upright. If the patient says "It's a baby" only after you rotate the card, the dysfunction was in the frontal lobe. If the patient still cannot say baby after the card is rotated, the dysfunction is in the dominant temporoparietal area.

On card 5, you ask the patient to "*Write* what *that* is." You do not tell him it is a clock, and he may or may not say clock before writing it. Although this tests the ability to name, more importantly it tests the ability to write. The inability to write is called dysgraphia, which points to dysfunction in the dominant temporoparietal region. If the patient prints "CLOCK," this is acceptable, but also ask him to "Write it in script." This may identify a more subtle dysfunction, since script-writing is learned later in childhood and is a more highly developed skill.

For card 6, ask the patient to "Name it." I have already discussed naming. On card 7, ask the patient to "Read this." The ability to read numbers (e.g., 7 and 2) is called "number gnosis," and the inability to do this is called number agnosia, which points to dysfunction of the dominant temporoparietal region. The capacity to read full words (such as SIX) is, logically, called reading. Reading disability is called dyslexia, and is associated with dominant temporoparietal dysfunction. Sometimes patients with left spatial neglect due to nondominant parietal dysfunction will read the card as "SIX 2," leaving out the 7.

On card 8, ask the patient to "Read this." The skill is called letter gnosis, and the dysfunction is called letter agnosia, which localizes to the dominent temporoparietal area. For each of cards 9 and 10, ask the patient to "Read this."

On card 11, ask the patient to "Write this." As before, although printing is acceptable, the examiner should ask the patient to "Write it in script." On card 12, ask the patient to "Read this." I have already discussed writing and reading.

On card 13, ask the patient to "Compute this" or "Figure this out." If he starts writing, ask him to "Try it first in your head." If he can't do it in his head, he may do it with pen and paper. Calculation is a dominant parietal function, and impaired calculation is called dyscalculia.

On card 14, first ask the patient to "Name this" or "Tell me what this is," which again tests naming. Then tell him, "With your hand, show me how you would use it." If he has trouble understanding this instruction, you may hold out a hand and say "If this key was in your right hand like this, how would you use it to get the door open?" The patient must be able to extend his forearm and twist his wrist in a clockwise fashion. This ability to perform an action from memory on command is called ideomotor or ideokinetic praxis, which is a function of the dominant parietal lobe. The inability to do this is called ideomotor (ideokinetic) dyspraxia. Finally, you ask the patient to copy the outline of this key, again testing for constructional praxis.

On card 15, you begin by asking the patient to "Read this." This again tests reading. After he has read it, you then ask him to "do it." Patients aren't used to being asked to touch one extremity to the other side of the body, and frequently touch their left hand to their left ear rather automatically. If the patient does this, he should be asked something like "Did you do that right?" or "Are you sure you touched your *left* hand to your *right* ear?" and instructed to "Try again." If he still does it incorrectly, he should be asked to perform other two-stage tasks testing right-left orientation. In testing right-left orientation, it is important to have the patient perform a two-stage task, because there is a 50-50 (1 in 2) chance of his guessing correctly on a one-stage task (such as "Show me your left hand"), but only a 1 in 4 chance of guessing correctly in a two-stage task such as "Touch your right hand to your left eye." Right-left orientation is a function of the dominant parietal lobe. The inability to distinguish right from left is called right-left disorientation.

THE MINIMENTAL STATE EXAMINATION [2]

This test, in addition to providing data which may help to lateralize and localize brain dysfunction, helps distinguish between diffuse brain dysfunction on the one hand, and no dysfunction or focal brain dysfunction on the other.

Most psychiatrists define dementia as a syndrome caused by diffuse coarse brain disease which produces diffuse intellectual dysfunctioning and where the patient's condition tends to deteriorate. In their discussion of the Minimental State Exam, Folstein, Folstein, and McHugh define dementia as any coarse brain disease producing diffuse intellectual dysfunction with the patient in a state of clear consciousness, regardless of etiology and regardless of whether the patient's condition is expected to deteriorate or improve.

The maximum score is 30. In various series, the range of scores for patients defined by Folstein, Folstein, and McHugh [2] as demented is 0-22 with a range of means of 6.6 to 9.6. The range of scores of elderly patients with endogenous depression with cognitive impairment (sometimes called pseudopseudodementia) is 9-27, with a range of means of 13-27. The range of scores of people with all psychiatric syndromes other than dementia and pseudopseudodementia is 8-30 with a range of means of 8-30. The range of scores for normals is 24-30 with a mean of 27.6. Thus, a score of 0-7 bespeaks dementia, a score of 0-23 speaks for at least some degree of brain dysfunction and demands an explanation, and a score of 24-30 rules out dementia.

When both you and the patient are comfortable, tell him that there is another series of questions you would like to ask. Keep "score" on a piece of paper as you ask the questions. The questions, and the points given for each question, are listed in Table 1 at the end of this chapter.

Begin by asking "What is the day, date, and season?" Then ask specifically for the parts omitted, being sure that you have covered the *year, season, date, day,* and *month,* each of which is worth 1 point towards a *total of 5 points.* Then ask the patient "Where are we now?" or "What is the name of this place and where is it located?" After the patient responds, ask specifically for the parts omitted, being sure that you have covered the *state, county, town, hospital,* and *floor,* each of which is worth 1 point towards a *total of 5 points.* Orientation to time and place are examples of global orientation, a frontal lobe function, if tested in a patient with clear consciousness. An abnormality would be described as impairment of global orientation or impairment of orientation to time or place. Global orientation must be distinguished from left-right orientation and east-west orientation, which are dominant parietal lobe functions, and spatial orientation, which is a nondominant parietal function. You should bear in mind, of course, that the function of memory plays a part in the process of orientation. If you need to distinguish between the memory and orientation components of these tests of orientation, you can ask the patient "What *kind* of place is this?", "What *part* of the day is this?", or "What *kind* of work do I do?", and note his response to your question about the season.

Then ask the patient to repeat the names of *three unrelated objects,* such as book, house, and candle, which you proceed to present to him. After he repeats these objects, tell him you are going to ask him to repeat these three words from memory in about 5 min. The immediate repetition of the three objects is a test of registration (immediate recall), which is a frontal lobe function, and which is scored as 1 point for each object towards a *total of 3.*

After proceeding with the rest of the test for about 5 min, you ask the patient "Now what were those three words I asked you to remember several minutes back?" This is a test of short-term memory, which is a dominant hippocampal function, and which is scored as 1 point for each object remembered correctly, again towards a *total of 3 points.* The examiner should use the same three objects for all patients he sees, to guarantee that he, the examiner, recall them himself without effort, and to develop a reliable sense of typical responses to the identical question.

Then say to the patient, "Starting with 100, subtract 7, and then continue to subtract 7 from each remainder." Alternatively, you could ask the patient "How much is 100 minus seven?" and when he answers, you would say "And how much is that (e.g., 93) minus 7?" Proceed until the patient has made *five serial subtractions of 7* (e.g., 93, 86, 79, 72, 65), *from 100,* each of which is worth 1 point towards a *total of 5 points.* Although this is a test of calculating ability, it is predominantly a test of concentration, which is a frontal lobe function. If the patient cannot or will not perform this task, ask him to spell the word "world," and if he does it correctly, ask him to "Spell the word world backwards." Each letter correctly placed in backwards order is worth 1 point to a *total of 5 points.* Although having the patient spell the word world is a test of spelling praxis, the spelling of the word backwards is again a test of concentration. If the patient has been on your ward before, and has likely been asked previously to "Spell the word world backwards," you may ask him to spell the word earth, or any other five-letter word, backwards, as long as it is not likely that the patient will know from memory the spelling of that word backwards.

Then point to your *wristwatch* and ask him "What is this?" or "Name this." After he has done so, point to your *pen or pencil* and ask him to name it. These are tests of naming, which I have discussed earlier, and each is worth 1 point towards a *total of 2 points.*

Then say to him "Repeat after me: No ifs, and, or buts," which is worth *1 point.* It is a test for Broca's area (dominant frontal) function, and an abnormality is called Broca's aphasia. Broca's aphasia is characterized by slow, labored "telegraphic" speech distinguished by the absence of small words like prepositions, as in the telegram message "don't call send money." A typical aphasic response to the above questions would be "no ifs" or "no ifs and buts" instead of "no ifs, ands, or buts."

Give the patient a piece of paper and say to him *"Take this paper in your right hand, fold it in half, and put it on the floor."* Each of the three stages of this three-stage command is worth 1 point towards a *total of 3 points.* Performance of a three-stage command is a frontal lobe function. Follow this by giving the patient a piece of paper on which you have printed the words *"CLOSE YOUR EYES,"* and say to him "Read this and then do it." If he closes his eyes, he

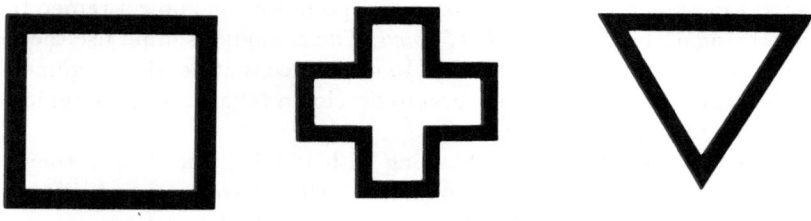

1. Copy
   (Construction apraxia).
2. Name
   (Anomia).
3. Spell
   (Spelling apraxia).

4. Copy
   (Construction apraxia).
5. Name
   (Anomia).
6. Spell
   (Spelling apraxia).

7. Copy
   (Construction apraxia).
8. Name
   (Anomia).
9. Spell
   (Spelling apraxia).

Card 1
Localizations:
1. Nondominant
   parietal.
2. Dominant
   temporoparietal.
3. Dominant
   temporoparietal.

Card 2
Localizations:
4. Nondominant
   parietal.
5. Dominant
   temporoparietal.
6. Dominant
   temporoparietal.

Card 3
Localizations:
7. Nondominant
   parietal.
8. Dominant
   temporoparietal.
9. Dominant
   temporoparietal.

FIG. 2.   The Reitan-Indiana Aphasia Screening Test*

Source: From Ref. 1, with permission. Please note that for each of the 15 cards, the instructions are right-side-up for the examiner and the portion shown to the patient is inverted for the examiner. Also note that instructions 18, 19, 20, 22, 23, 24, 26, 32, 33, and 34 on cards 10, 11, 12, 13, and 15 are not routinely presented.

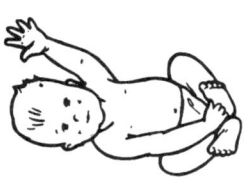
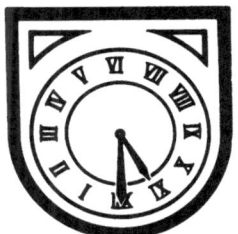
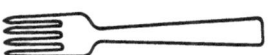

10. **Name** (**Anomia**).	11. **Write** (**Agraphia**).	12. **Name** (**Anomia**).

Card 4	Card 5	Card 6
Localization:	Localization:	Localization:
10. Frontal and dominant temporoparietal.	11. Dominant temporoparietal.	12. Dominant temporoparietal

FIG. 2.   *(continued)*

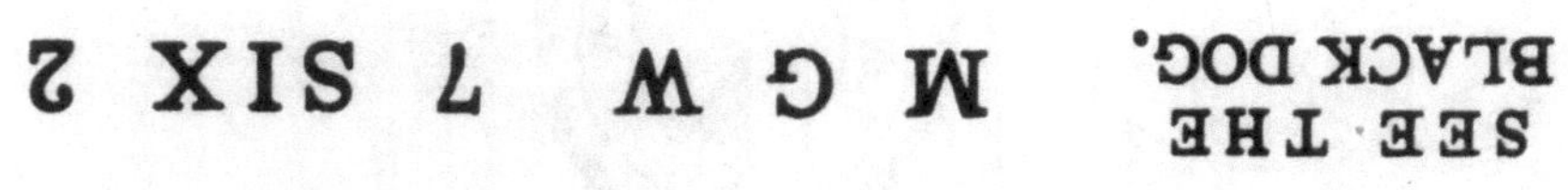

2 XIS 7 W G M   BLACK DOG.
                 SEE THE

13. Read
    (Letter and number   14. Read   15. Read
    agnosia and alexia).   (Letter agnosia).   (Alexia).

            Card 7   Card 8   Card 9
    Localization: Localization: Localization:
    13. Dominant   14. Dominant   15. Dominant
        temporoparietal.   temporoparietal.   temporoparietal.

FIG. 2.   *(continued)*

WINNER OF DOG SHOWS.
ANIMAL, A FAMOUS
HE IS A FRIENDLY

SQUARE

SEVEN

16. Read
    (Alexia).

18. Repeat "Triangle"
    (Central dysarthria).
19. Repeat "Massachusetts"
    (Central dysarthria).

20. Repeat "Methodist
    Episcopal"
    (Central dysarthria).
21. Write
    (Agraphia).

22a. Read
22. Repeat
    (Auditory verbal
    agnosia).
23. HE SHOUTED THE
    WARNING.
    Repeat; explain
    (Auditory verbal
    agnosia; central
    dysarthria).
24. Write
    (Agraphia).

Card 10
Localization:
16. Dominant
    temporoparietal.

Card 11
Localization:
21. Dominant
    temporoparietal.

Card 12
Localization:
22a. Dominant
    temporoparietal.

FIG. 2. *(continued)*

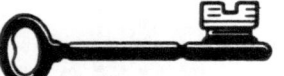

= 72 - 58

PLACE
LEFT HAND
TO RIGHT EAR.

25. Compute
    (Acalculia).
26. Compute "17 X 3"
    (Acalculia).

27. Name
    (Anomia).
28. Demonstrate use
    (Ideo-kinetic apraxia).
29. Draw
    (Construction apraxia).

30. Read
    (Alexia).
31. Place
    (Right-left disorienta-
    tion; body agnosia).
32. Place left hand to
    left elbow
    (Auditory verbal
    agnosia; right-left
    disorientation;
    body agnosia).
33. Test for visual, aud-
    itory, and tactile
    suppression.
34. Extend and vary above
    items as necessary.

Card 13
Localization:
25. Dominant
    parietal.

Card 14
Localizations:
27. Dominant
    temporoparietal.
28. Dominant
    parietal.
29. Nondominant
    parietal.

Card 15
Localizations:
30. Dominant
    temporoparietal.
31. Dominant
    parietal.

FIG. 2.   *(continued)*

Table 1. The Minimental State Examination of Folstein, Folstein, and McHugh

Specific Test	Function and Area Tested	Points	Score
1. What is the year/season/day/ date/month?	Orientation (frontal)	5	
2. What is the state/county/town/ hospital/floor?	Orientation (frontal)	5	
3. Repeat three items.	Registration (frontal)	3	
4. Serial subtraction of sevens *or* spell "world" backwards.	Concentration (frontal)	5	
5. Name wristwatch and pen.	Naming (dominant temporoparietal)	2	
6. Say "No ifs, ands, or buts."	Expressive speech (dominant frontal)	1	
7. Take this paper in your right hand, fold it in half, and put it on the table.	Three-stage command (frontal)	3	
8. Read "close your eyes" and do it.	Reading (dominant temporoparietal)	1	
9. Remember the three items from part 3.	Short-term memory (dominant hippocampal)	3	
10. Write a sentence.	Writing (dominant temporoparietal)	1	
11. Copy intersecting pentagons.	"Construction" (nondominant parietal)	1	

Source: From Ref. 2.

gets *1 point*. This is a test of reading, a dominant temporoparietal function.

Give the patient another piece of paper and ask him to "*Write me a simple short sentence. It can be about anything.*" It is a test of writing (dominant temporoparietal function) and is scored *1 point* if the sentence is understandable and has a subject and predicate. Usually, the patient writes something personally revealing and pertinent to the interview (like in a projective test) but this has absolutely no bearing on the scoring of the test. For example, a patient wrote "Thank you for interviewing me," which although pleasing, was merely given the 1 point it deserved. Finally, on still another blank sheet of paper draw *intersecting pentagons* and say to the patient "Copy that shape." The ability to draw each pentagon separately is called constructional praxis which, as we stated earlier, measures nondominant parietal functioning, but the ability to intersect the pentagons properly requires intact frontal lobe function as well.

CONCLUSION

As we stated before, these are efficient, valid, and reliable screening tests for localizing and lateralizing brain dysfunction, tests which can be employed by any medical student or physician in almost any medical setting. One weakness of the screening tests is that they do not sufficiently test occipital lobe and nondominant temporal lobe functioning, but this is easily remedied. The nondominant temporal lobe can be tested by asking the patient to repeat several rhythms you tap on a table, or to sing a familiar song. The occipital lobe can be tested by having the patient name an object in a picture in which there are visual distractions, or having the patient remember the location of a point on a line drawn several moments before.

REFERENCES

1. Heimburger, R., and Reitan, R. Easily administrated test for lateralizing brain lesions. *J. Neurosurg.* 18:301-312 (1961).
2. Folstein, M., Folstein, S., and McHugh, P. Minimental state. *J. Psychiatr. Res.* Pergamon, New York 12:189-198 (1975)
3. Tsai, L., and Tsuang, M. The mini-mental state test and computerized tomography. *Am. J. Psychiatry*, April 1979, 136(4A):436-438.

4
Psychological Testing
FREDERICK SIERLES

INTRODUCTION

Psychological tests are clinical measures of aspects of a person's behavior. Physicians should be familiar with psychological assessment procedures because they may want to request that such tests be performed, will receive test results, and should learn to administer a few of the less complex and comprehensive instruments. But except for the screening tests for coarse brain disease, and for the Minnesota Multiphasic Personality Inventory (MMPI), administration and interpretation of psychometrics is the province of psychologists. A physician interested in learning more about these tests should refer to the test manual, to Buros' *Mental Measurements Yearbook* [1], or to a standard text such as Anastasi's *Psychological Testing*. [2].

The American Psychological Association, in its *Standards for Educational and Psychological Tests* [3], stipulates that data about the reliability and validity of the test should be included in the test manual. There are many categories of psychological tests, which include intelligence tests, tests of creativity, occupational skills tests, tests for cognitive dysfunction, personality inventories, tests of interests and values, and projective tests [2]. In this chapter, I will discuss intelligence tests, tests for coarse brain disease, self-report personality inventories, and projective tests.

INTELLIGENCE TESTS

Intelligence is the ability to solve problems by reasoning, and is a general concept which subsumes abilities like abstract reasoning, pattern recognition, vocabulary, and arithmetic. A person could be highly intelligent but weak in a few of these areas, or of modest intelligence and excel in a few areas. Thus, a presentation of intelligence test results should discuss specific strengths and weaknesses as well as global intelligence. Intelligence is measured by intelligence tests; this has led some psychologists to joke with some degree of truth that "intelligence is what intelligence tests measure." Some authors have tried to separate "biological" from "culturally influenced" intelligence, between "general" and "specific" intelligence, and between "crystallized" and "fluid" intelligence, but this is beyond the scope of this chapter. Table 1 specifies intelligence tests most popularly used at each age range. Note the use of the Denver Developmental Scale, discussed in Chapter 20, for children under 4 years.

The Wechsler scales consist of subtests grouped under the general categories "verbal" and "performance." The WAIS [4] subtests are listed in Table 2.

Verbal and performance subtest scores are combined into a full-scale intelligence quotient (IQ). IQ distributions were originally established by using a bell-shaped curve with 6% of the population (beyond two standard deviations from the mean) in the standardization (normative) sample considered a priori either very superior (the top 3%) or retarded (the bottom 3%). Table 3 lists the terms associated with the various IQ ranges.

The Wechsler scales, as well as the Stanford-Binet Intelligence Scale which antedated them, are very reliable [2].

Their concurrent and predictive validity are also high. The scales correlate strongly with the Adaptive Behavior Scales for the mentally retarded, years of education eventually completed, high school and college grade-point averages, prestige of occupation, and socioeconomic status [5]. Of course, none of these correlations are perfect. The correlation between IQ and effectiveness at work, while positive and significant, is not high. These data indicate that while intelligence is an important factor, other influences also strongly affect performance at work and at school.

Skilled laborers score higher on performance than on verbal subtests,

Table 1 Intelligence Tests Most Commonly Used at Each Age Range

Age range (years)	Name of test	Professional usually capable of administration and interpretations
0-4	Denver Developmental Scale Scale	Pediatrician, child psychologist, child psychiatrist
4 1/2-6 1/2	Wechsler Preschool and Primary Intelligence Scale (WPPSI)	Psychologists
6-16 years, 11 1/2 months	Wechsler Intelligence Scale for Children—Revised (WISC-R)	Psychologists
16 and over	Wechsler Adult Intelligence Scale (WAIS)	Psychologists

Table 2 Subtests of the WAIS

Name	Examples
Verbal Subtests	
General information	1. How many wings does a bird have?
	2. What is pepper?
General comprehension	1. What is the advantage of keeping money in a bank?
	2. Why is copper often used in electrical wires?
Arithmetic	1. Three men divided 18 golf balls equally among themselves. How many golf balls did each man receive?
Similarities	1. In what way are a lion and tiger alike?
	2. In what way are a circle and a triangle alike?
Vocabulary	1. What does "farce" mean?
Performance Subtests	
Digit symbol	The subject is presented with a coding key in which each number is associated with a specific symbol (e.g., 1 and symbol X). Then he is presented with a long series of numbers with adjacent blank spaces, and asked to fill in the appropriate symbols in the adjacent blank spaces as rapidly as possible.
Picture completion	The subject is given a series of pictures in which a portion of the picture is missing, and asked to name that missing portion (e.g., a picture of a girl without a nose).
Block design	The subject is given a series of cubes with different colors and patterns on each surface of the cube. Then, one at a time, he is given pictures of specific designs which he is to construct by rearrangement of the cubes.
Picture arrangement	The subject is presented with groups of pictures that are out of sequence and which, when rearranged correctly, tell a story in logical sequence, as in a comic strip.
Object assembly	The subject is presented with a few portions of a picture, as in a jigsaw puzzle, and asked to assemble the portions into a completed picture.

Note: For the WISC-R, the subtests are similar to those of the WAIS, with some modifications. For the WPPSI, four subtests (digit span, picture arrangement, digit symbol, and object assembly) are replaced by four others (sentences, animal house, mazes, and geometric designs).

and white-collar employees do better on verbal than on performance subtests [2]. People with dominant hemisphere lesions score worse on verbal than on performance subtests, and people with nondominant hemisphere

Table 3   IQ Levels and Associated Terms

IQ	Associated Term
130 and above	Very superior
120-129	Superior
110-119	Bright normal
90-109	Average
80-89	Dull normal
69-79	Borderline
0-68	Mental retardation

pathology score worse on performance than on verbal subtests [2,5]. Since the dominant hemisphere by definition is the primary hemisphere for language, and the nondominant hemisphere has a regulatory role in visual-spatial and motor functions, these data also demonstrate concurrent validity of the Wechsler tests.

IQ tests have a number of practical functions. A diagnosis of mental retardation requires documentation by a developmental scale or IQ test [and by a social quotient (SQ) on the Vineland Social Maturity Scale]. IQs are used by some agencies in screening for occupations requiring considerable intelligence; for example, American astronauts are required to have an IQ of at least 130 [6]. Intelligence tests may help identify coarse brain disease, and possibly to localize it to one hemisphere.

Intelligence test performance tends to be stable over the elementary, high school, and college period [2]. Nevertheless, for a given individual, this certainly may not be the case [2,7]. Factors affecting scores include examiner-related effects such as poor administration of the test, and subject-related effects such as genetic makeup, intrauterine influences, environmental stimulation and parental availability, amount of prior schooling, health, coaching for the test, having taken the test previously, and mood and motivation during the test.

Heated controversies have developed over comparisons of mean IQs of different ethnic groups. Such comparisons were not the purpose of these tests; however, truly culture-free tests probably do not exist [2].

Despite the many factors contributing to IQ scores, there is solid evidence that genetic makeup is the principal influence. This is shown by studies which take into account degrees of genetic relatedness (e.g., IQ differences between monozygotic and dizygotic twins or siblings) and of environmental influence (e.g., IQ similarities of siblings reared together as compared with siblings reared apart) [8,9]. Figure 1 portrays composite data from 52 studies accounting for the influence of genetics and environment.

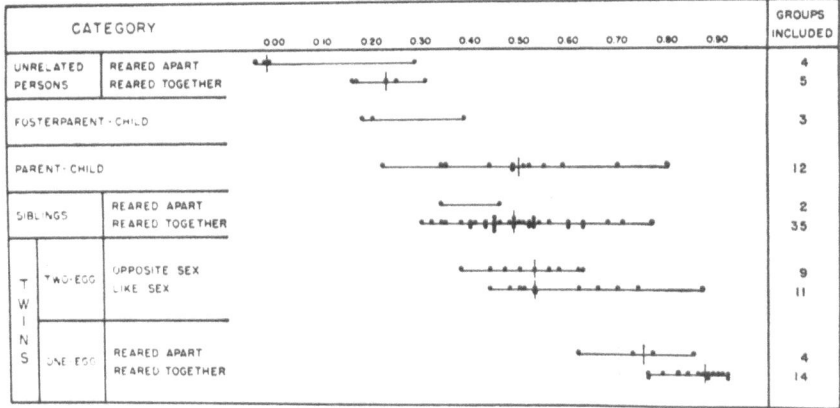

FIG. 1. Correlation coefficients for "intelligence" test scores from 52 studies. Some studies reported data for more than one relationship category; some included more than one sample per category, giving a total of 99 groups. Over two-thirds of the correlation coefficients were derived from IQs, the remainder from special tests (for example, Primary Mental Abilities). Mid-parent-child correlation was used when available; otherwise, mother-child correlation. Individual correlation coefficients obtained in each study are indicated by *circles*; medians are shown by *vertical lines* intersecting the *horizontal lines* that represent the ranges. (From L. Erlenmeyer-Kimling and L. Jarvik. Genetics and intelligence. A review. *Science* 142:1477-1479, 1953, with permission.)

TEST FOR COARSE BRAIN DISEASE AND COGNITIVE DYSFUNCTION

An important use of psychological tests in clinical medicine is in identification and localization of coarse brain disease and cognitive dysfunction. Tests used primarily for this purpose include three screening tests and two test batteries. The screening tests are the Reitan-Indiana Aphasia Screening Test, the Minimental State Examination of Folstein, Folstein, and McHugh, and the Bender-Gestalt; the test batteries are the Luria Battery and the Halstead-Reitan Battery. Because I am suggesting that all physicians master the Aphasia Screening and Minimental State tests, a separate chapter has been devoted to them (see Chap. 3).

The Bender-Gestalt

This screening test, more properly called the Bender Visual Motor Gestalt Test, was developed by L. Bender, who selected a group of nine designs from a larger group of designs used by M. Wertheimer. The Bender-Gestalt designs are presented in Figure 2.

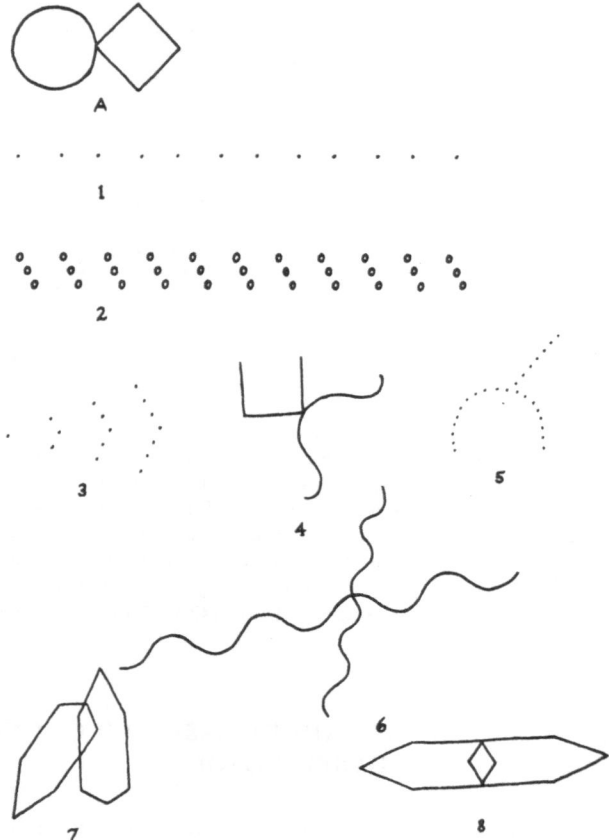

FIG. 2.   The Bender-Gestalt test. *Source* Bender, L. The Bender Gestalt Test. American Ortho-psychiatric Association, 1938, with permission.

The subject is shown these nine designs, one at a time on separate cards, and asked to copy them on a piece of unlined blank paper. In a second version of the test, the subject is also asked to reproduce from memory as many of these designs as possible. Scoring systems for this test have been devised [10,11].

The test-retest reliability of the Bender-Gestalt is high [2]. It can distinguish between patients with coarse brain disease, controls, and psychiatric patients [12]. It has a high positive correlation with IQ for children between 5 and 10 years.

However, because of its brevity, it has a weakness—it measures one function of each of three lobes of the brain, the nondominant parietal lobe (constructional praxis), the frontal lobe (the interdigitation of geometric shapes), and the occipital lobe (visual memory). For this reason, I prefer the Aphasia Screening Test and the Minimental State Examination to the Bender-Gestalt.

The Luria Battery

This test was designed by A. Luria [13], and a formal scoring system developed by Golden, Hammeke, and Purisch [14]. The battery consists of tests of functions listed in Table 4.

The concurrent validity of the Luria battery is outstanding. Golden and co-workers [14] compared 50 hospitalized control patients with 50 matched neurological patients with a clinical diagnosis of coarse brain disease. They reported: "tests were run between the control and neurologic group on all 285 scores generated by the test. Of the 285 comparisons made, 253 were signifiant at the .05 level (df = 98). In all cases, the neurologic group performed

Table 4 The Luria Battery with South Dakota Scoring Modification

Functions tested	*Examples*
Motor functions	"Do as I do." (Place right hand under chin with fingers bent.)
Rhythm (acousticomotor functions)	"You will now hear a rhythm on the tape. When I tell you that the rhythm is over, I want you to tap with your hand the rhythm you heard on the tape." (Play three rhythms. Score as right or wrong.)
Cutaneous and kinesthetic functions (tactile)	"Feel this object and tell me exactly what it is." (Instruct the subject to hold his right palm up and place object on the fingers. Objects include quarter, key, eraser, and paper clip.)
Visual functions	(Show clock faces.) "Tell me what time these clock faces show."
Impressive speech	"Which boy is shorter if John is taller than Peter?"
Expressive speech	"Repeat after me: Hairbrush . . . screwdriver . . . laborious."
Reading and writing	"Write these words (dictate): wren . . . knife."
Arithematic skills	"Add these numbers in your head: 5 . . . 9 . . . 7."
Mnestic (memory)	"I am going to show you a card, and I want you to look at it carefully. When I remove the card, I want you to draw as much from it as you can remember." (Present card for 7 sec.)
Intellectual processes	"What has the same relation to good as high to low?"

Source: From Golden, C., Hammeke, T., and Purisch, A. Diagnostic validity of a standardized neuropsychological battery derived from Luria's neuropsychological tests. *J. Consult. Clin. Psychol.* (American Psychological Association) 32:338-354 (1976), with permission.

less effectively (a higher score) than the control group . . . It was (also) found that a weighted, linear combination of 30 variables was sufficient to separate the groups with 100% accuracy" [14].

The Halstead-Reitan Battery

This battery is a modification, by Reitan, of an examination developed by Halstead for the investigation of behavior in brain-damaged and normal people. It takes longer (6-8 hr) to administer than does the Luria battery, but more psychologists are currently able to administer it than the Luria battery. It contains 10 subtests, including the MMPI (a self-report personality inventory to be discussed later), the WAIS and the Reitan-Indiana Aphasia Screening Test. In addition to identifying and localizing brain dysfunction, it is useful in providing feedback for vocational rehabilitation and other rehabilitation programs.

Matarazzo et al. [15] demonstrated high test-retest reliability for this battery. The validity of the battery is also high [16]; Halstead was able to distinguish, to a highly significant degree, between controls, people with frontal lobe lesions, and people with lesions elsewhere in the brain [17]. Vega and Parsons could distinguish between controls and people with demonstrated brain dysfunction [18], as could Wheeler, Burke, and Reitan, who were able to make this distinction 90.7% of the time [19].

SELF-REPORT PERSONALITY INVENTORIES

In these, the subject is asked a long series of true-false questions, each of which tests for a personality characteristic such as introversion or hypochondriasis. Their principal use is to delineate attributes of personality for both normal and ill individuals.

The most popular of the personality inventories is the Minnesota Multiphasic Personality Inventory (MMPI), which consists of 550 statements to which the subject replies "true," "false," or "cannot say." It is easy to administer and the results are easy to record, but meaningful clinical interpretation is difficult. Questions resemble the following:

"I do not always act honestly."
"My mind sometimes leaves my head."
"I am an outgoing person."
"My skills are better than ever."

After tabulating the number of affirmative responses in each category, a profile (see Fig. 3) is made, and interpretation of the meaning of the profile is made by a psychologist, a computer, or both.

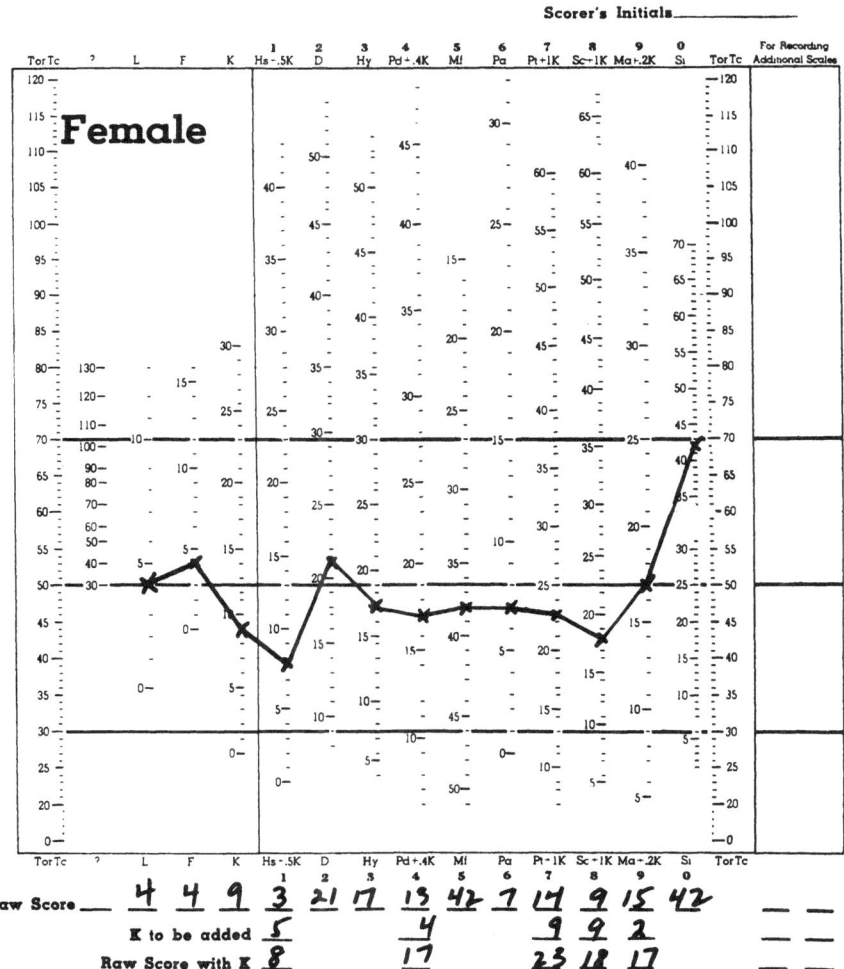

FIG. 3.   MMPI profile of a 20-year old college student.

The abbreviations in the scale apply to the following:

L	= lie score	Mf	= masculinity-femininity
F	= validity score	Pa	= paranoia
K	= correction score	Pt	= psychasthenia
Hs	= hypochondriasis	Sc	= schizophrenia
D	= depression	Ma	= hypomania
H	= hysteria		
Pd	= psychopathic deviant		

The L, F, and K scales are calculated from questions designed to test whether the patient is trying to make himself appear in a favorable light (high score on L scale), or in an unfavorable light (low score on K scale), or if he is being careless (high score on F scale). High scores on certain scales do not necessarily mean that the subject has a certain psychiatric illness; for example, a high score on the Sc (schizophrenia) scale corresponds to severe psychiatric illness, not necessarily to schizophrenia itself. The utility of the test in making a specific diagnosis is poor [20]. Interpretation of the total profile is considered more useful than a "glance" at the graph alone; studies of retest and split-half reliabilities have yielded variable results.

PROJECTIVE TESTS

In projective tests, the subject is presented with ambiguous stimuli such as inkblots (the Rorschach), drawings of people (Thematic Apperception Test/TAT), uncompleted sentences (sentence completion test), and blank pieces of paper (draw a person) and asked to produce specific, tangible responses. The theory is that since the stimuli are vague, responses must be a product of fantasy and imagination, which are influenced by covert or unconscious aspects of personality. It is easy to see that "in their theoretical framework, most projective techniques reflect the influence of psychoanalytic concepts" [2]. Projective tests are used by psychoanalytically oriented psychiatrists to delineate unconscious influences on behavior and to assist in making diagnoses. Studies of the reliability of the projective tests yield conflicting results [21,22].

The Rorschach test [23], designed by H. Rorschach, is the best-known projective test. It consists of 10 standard inkblots, shown one by one to the patient. Card 1 is pictured in Figure 4. Practicioners who employ the Rorschach reach diagnostic conclusions based upon the form, content, color, and movement of patient responses.

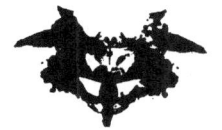

FIG. 4. Card 1 of the Rorschach test. (Reproduced by permission of Verlag Hans Huber, Bern, Switzerland.)

REFERENCES

1. Buros, O. *Mental Measurements Yearbook.* Gryphan, Highland Park, N.J. (1979).
2. Anastasi, A. *Psychological Testing.* Macmillan, New York (1976).
3. Joint Committee of the American Psychological Association, American Educational Research Association, and National Council on Measurement in Education, F. Davis, Chair. *Standards for Educational and Psychological Tests.* Am. Psychol. Assoc., Washington, D.C. (1974).
4. Wechsler, D. *The Measurement of Adult Intelligence.* Williams and Wilkins, Baltimore (1944).
5. Matarazzo, J. *Wechsler's Measurement and Appraisal of Adult Intelligence.* Oxford, New York (1972).
6. Collins, M. *Carrying the Fire.* Farrar, Straus and Giroux, New York (1974).
7. Honzik, M., MacFarlan, J., and Allen, L. The stability of mental test performance between two and eighteen years. *J. Exp. Ed.,* 17:309-324 (1948).
8. Erlenmeyer-Kimling, L., and Jarvik, L. Genetics and intelligence. A review. *Science* 142:1477-9 (1953).
9. Burks, B. The relative influence of nature and nurture upon mental development. *National Society for the Study of Education, 27th Yearbook, Part 1,* Bloomington, Ind. (1928).
10. Pascal, G., and Suttell, B. *The Bender-Gestalt Test: Quantification and validity for adults.* Grune & Stratton, New York (1951).
11. Koppitz, E. *The Bender-Gestalt Test for Young Children: research and application.* Grune & Stratton, New York (1975).
12. Tolor, A., and Schulberg, H. *An Evaluation of the Bender-Gestalt Test.* Thomas, Springfield, Ill. (1963).
13. Luria, A. *The Working Brain.* Basic Books, New York (1973).
14. Golden, C., Hammeke, T., and Purisch, A. Diagnostic validity of a standardized neuropsychological battery derived from Luria's neuropsychological tests. *J. Consult. Clin. Psychol.* 46:1258-1265 (1978).
15. Matarazzo, J., Matarazzo, R., Wrens, A., and Gallo, A. Retest reliability of the Halstead impairment index in a normal, a schizophrenic and two samples of organic patients. *J. Clin. Psychol.* 32:338-354 (1976).
16. Klove, H. Validation studies in adult clinical neuropsychology, in *Clinical Neuropsychology: Current status and applications.* R. Reitan and L. Davison, eds. Winston, Washington, D.C. (1974).
17. Halstead, W. *Brain and Intelligence: A quantitiative study of the frontal lobes.* Univ. Chicago, Chicago (1947).
18. Vega, A., and Parsons, O. Cross-validation of the Halstead-Reitan tests for brain damage. *J. Consult. Psychol.* 31:619-625 (1967).

19. Wheeler, L., Burke, C., and Reitan, R. An application of discriminant functions to the problem of predicting brain damage using behavioral variables. *Percept. Mot. Skills* 16:417-440 (1963).

20. Chapman, L., and Chapman, J. Psychological tests and psychodiagnosis, in *Critical Issues in Psychiatric Diagnosis*. R. Spitzer and D. Klein, eds. Raven, New York (1978).

21. Goldfried, M., Stricker, G., and Weiner, I. *Rorschach Handbook of Clinical and Research Applications*. Prentice-Hall, Englewood Cliffs, N.J. (1971).

22. Baughman, E. Rorschach scores as a function of examiner difference. *J. Proj. Tech.* 15:243-249 (1951).

23. Rorschach, H. *Psychodiagnostics*. Verlag Hans Huber, Bern, Switzerland (1942).

5

Brain Biochemistry and Its Relevance to Behavior

FREDERICK SIERLES

INTRODUCTION

Almost by definition, brain biochemistry plays an integral role in brain functioning and behavior. Unfortunately, direct studies of brain biochemistry in living humans are not currently feasible, so many conclusions must be reached by indirect studies of blood, urine, and cerebrospinal fluid and direct studies of cadaver brains, or of living animals.

Some clinically important syndromes, such as delirium and dementia, are produced by readily identifiable biochemical abnormalities. Thus, when one of these syndromes is diagnosed, a well-defined battery of laboratory tests is available. And it goes without saying that proper diet, and replacement therapy in deficit syndromes, can prevent the development of some biochemical abnormalities in the brain.

Research in brain biochemistry may lead to discoveries about the causes and treatment of some of the major psychiatric conditions. Some findings have already provided us with useful clues. Others have provided useful first steps in the development of routine laboratory tests for major psychiatric syndromes. Nevertheless, much of what is already known is not immediately applicable clinically, many of the hypotheses are gross oversimplifications, and some are subjects of considerable controversy. Also, in many studies rigorous diagnostic criteria were not used, so the reliability of their findings is open to question.

SPECIFIC SUBSTANCES AND SYNDROMES

Oxygen

The brain is a very active user of oxygen, and is very sensitive to hypoxia. The globus pallidus, cerebellum, and cerebral white matter (particularly the frontal cortex) are most vulnerable to hypoxia, and the brain stem is least vulnerable [1]. When the oxygen saturation of arterial blood falls below 90% due to impairment of the respiratory process at any level, the patient is susceptible to anxiety, irritability, emotional lability, and delirium. Delirium is characterized by diffuse intellectual impairment with fluctuation in state of consciousness, confusion, tachycardia, pallor, hallucinations and illusions, muttering, and suggestibility.

Complete lack of a blood supply to the brain (associated naturally with anoxia) for over 5 min, which occurs during untreated cardiac arrest, produces irreversible brain damage and sometimes brain death, a syndrome characterized by lack of responsiveness and reflexes, and a flat electroencephalogram in the presence of a continued heartbeat. Carbon monoxide, deliberately or accidentally inhaled in large quantities, competes successfully with oxygen for sites on the hemoglobin molecule, and has the same effect as hypoxia. Carbon monoxide poisoning is recognized by history, skin coloration, and blood carbon monoxide levels, and is treated by oxygen inhalation, ideally in a hyperbaric chamber. Under surgical hypothermia with a temperature of 15°C and consequently its greatly diminished metabolic requirement, the brain can tolerate complete anoxia for 45 min. [2].

Glucose

The brain utilizes glucose almost exclusively as a source of energy, although in severe, prolonged hypoglycemia it uses other sources. Glucose and oxygen are "almost the exclusive metabolic substrates of the brain" [1]. The symptoms of hypoglycemia are almost identical with those of hypoxia, the only difference being that in hypoglycemia onset of symptoms is delayed 30-45 min because the brain has some stored glucose. When blood glucose falls below 70 for more than an hour, the patient may become delirious. If the hypoglycemia is prolonged, permanent brain damage (including dementia, a syndrome characterized by diffuse intellectual dysfunctioning with a tendency to deteriorate) or death may result. The treatment of hypoglycemia is glucose given orally or intavenously depending on the urgency of the situation.

Amino Acids, Peptides, and Proteins

Amino acids (free, in polypeptides, and in proteins) make up almost half of the brain's dry weight. Memory has been associated with the process of protein synthesis. There are numerous inherited disorders, usually auto-somal-recessive, of amino acid metabolism. Many of these conditions are listed in Table 1 [3]. Typical findings in many of these conditions include mental retardation, seizures, ataxia, and speech disturbances. Mental re-tardation is discussed at length in Chapter 20. Of these inborn errors, the se-quelae of phenylketonuria and maple syrup urine disease are preventable if diagnosed early and treated with special diets.

The discovery of endorphins by Hughes [4,5] was fairly recent. Endor-phins are peptides that occur naturally in the brain, and which have mor-phine-like activity. Specific opiate receptor sites have been identified in the brain, and these bind endorphins (some of which are called enkephalins) as well as opiates. One of the endorphins, β-endorphin, is found in the same large protein molecule (called "big ACTH") as the pituitary corticotropin substance and adrenocorticotropic hormone (ACTH). The periaqueductal gray matter in the brain, an area with a role in processing pain sensations, also has high concentrations of endorphins.

Electrolytes

Water, acid-base and electrolyte balance are also crucial in brain func-tioning. Alkalosis (arterial blood pH $>$ 7.42) and acidosis (arterial blood pH $<$ 7.37), hypernatremia (serum sodium $>$ 143 mEq/liter) and hypo-natremia (serum sodium $<$ 133 mEq/liter), hypercalcemia (serum calcium $>$ 11 mg/100 ml) and hypocalcemia (serum calcium $<$ 9 mg/100 ml), hypermagnesemia (serum magnesium $>$ 3.6 mg/100 ml) and hypomagnes-emia (serum magnesium $<$ 1.8 mg/100 ml), and diminished levels of zinc and manganese can call cause behavioral changes, the most common of which is delirium. The primary treatment of behavioral changes in these in-stances is to correct the underlying biochemical imbalances.

Lipids

Lipids also play an important role in brain function. They are a major constituent of myelin. After water, cholesterol is the most abundant com-pound in the brain. The lipidoses are inborn errors of metabolism associated

Table 1 Inherited Disorders of Amino Acid Metabolism

Amino acid classification	Disorder	Clinical findings	Laboratory findings	Available leukocyte assay	Enzymatic defect
Urea cycle	Hyperammonemia	Feeding difficulty, vomiting, lethargy,	Respiratory alkalosis, hyperammonemia	No	Ornithine transcarbamylase
	Citrullinemia	Feeding difficulty, vomiting, coma	Respiratory alkalosis, hyperammonemia, elevated blood, and urine citrulline	No	Argininosuccinate synthetase
	Argininosuccinicaciduria	Ataxia, seizures	Hyperammonemia, argininosuccinicacidemia and -uria	Yes	Argininosuccinate lyase
	Argininemia	Spastic diplegia, seizures	Hyperammonemia, elevated blood and urine arginine	No	Arginase
sulfur-containing	Methionine malabsorption (oasthouse-syndrome)	Hypotonia, seizures. musty urine odor	α-Hydroxybutyricaciduria, elevated urine methionine (?)	No	Gut transport of methionine
	Sulfituria and thiosulfaturia	Pyramidal tract signs, blindness, dislocated lenses	Elevated urine sulfite, thiosulfate, and S-sulfo-cysteine	No	Sulfite oxidase
Glycine	Hyperglycinemia (nonketotic)	Development failure, seizures	Elevated blood and urine glycine	No	Glycine decarboxylase (?)
Aromatic	Tyrosinemia	Cirrhosis, rickets, Fanconi syndrome	Hypophosphatemia, tyrosinemia and tyrosyluria, generalized aminoaciduria	No	p-Hydroxyphenylpyruvic acid oxidase (?)
β-Amino	β-Alaninemia	Lethargy, seizures	Elevated blood and urine β-alanine, γ-aminobutyricaciduria	No	β-Alanine: α-ketoglutarate transaminase (?)
Dipeptide	Carnosinemia	Seizures	Elevated blood and urine carnosine	No	Carnosinase
Branched-chain	Branched-chain ketoaciduria (maple syrup urine disease)	Feeding difficulty, lethargy, coma, maple syrup-like odor	Metabolic acidosis, hypoglycemia, elevated blood and urine leucine, isoleucine and valine, branched-chain ketoaciduria	Yes	Branched-chain ketoacid decarboxylase

Table 1   Inherited Disorders of Amino Acid Metabolism (continued)

Amino acid classification	Disorder	Clinical findings	Laboratory findings	Available leukocyle assay	Enzymatic defect
	Valinemia	Feeding difficulty, vomiting, lethargy	Elevated blood and urine valine	Yes	Valine: α-ketoglutarate transaminase
	Isovalericacidemia	Progressive neurological dysfunction, odor of "sweaty feet"	Metabolic acidosis, elevated blood and urine isovaleric acid	Yes	Isovaleryl-CoA dehydrogenase
	β-Hydroxyiso-valericaciduria	Feeding difficulty, acrid urine odor	Urinary excretion of β-hydroxy-isovaleric acid and β-methyl-crotonylglycine	No	β-Methylcrotonyl-CoA carboxylase (?)
	Propionicacidemia (ketotic hyperglycinemia)	Feeding difficulty, vomiting, lethargy, seizures	Metabolic ketacidosis, hypoglycemia, hyperammonemia, hypercinemia and -uria, long-chain ketonuria, elevated blood and urine propionate	Yes	Propionyl-CoA carboxylase (?)
	Methylmalonic-aciduria (B_{12}-unresponsive)	Feeding difficulty, vomiting, lethargy	Metabolic ketoacidosis, hypogly-cemia, hyperammonemia, hyper-glycinemia and -uria, long-chain ketonuria, methylmalonicacidemia and -uria	Yes	Methylmalonyl-CoA mutase
	Methylmalonic-aciduria (B_{12}-unresponsive)	Feeding difficulty, vomiting, lethargy	(see B_{12}-unresponsive form)	Yes	Detective conversion of vitamin B_{12} to deoxyadenosyl-B_{12}
	Methylmalonic-aciduria and homocystinuria	Feeding difficulty, lethargy, coma	Methylmalonicaciduria, cystathioninemia, homocystin-uria, hypomethioninemia	Yes	Detective conversion of vitamin B_{12} to deoxyadenosyl-B_{12} and methyl-B_{12}

Source: From C. Scriver and L. Rosenberg. Amino Acid Metabolism and Its Disorders. Saunders, Philadelphia, 1973, with permission (Ref. 3).

with enzyme deficits, which in turn cause accumulation of normal and abnormal lipids in the brain and other organs. Many of these conditions listed in Table 2 [6] are characterized by mental retardation and seizures; some are fatal.

Monoamines

Brain monoamines, which include dopamine, norepinephrine, epinephrine, serotonin, and phenylethylamine, probably have important neurotransmission roles in brain functioning. The synthesis of dopamine and norepinephrine from the amino acid tyrosine is portrayed in Figure 1.

The pathway taken in the metabolism of norepinephrine depends upon the site where it is acted upon. If it is acted upon at the postsynaptic receptor neuron, it is catalyzed by the enzyme catechol-O-methyltransferase (COMT) to normetanephrine, some of which is excreted in the urine. If the norepinephrine in the cytoplasm of the presynaptic noradrenergic neuron "leaks" into the mitochondria of the same presynaptic neuron, and is acted upon in the mitochondria, the monoamine oxidase in the mitochondria degrades the norepinephrine to dihydroxymandelic acid and dihydroxyphenylglycol, which are probably methylated to form 3-methoxy-4-hydroxymandelic acid (VMA) and 3-methoxy-4-hydroxyphenylglycol (MHPG). The chemical structures of the metabolites of norepinephine are protrayed in Figure 2. The clinical significance of the metabolism of norepinephrine is discussed later in this chapter.

The synthesis of 5-hydroxytryptamine from the amino acid tryptophan is portrayed in Figure 3. Monoamine oxidase plays a role in this process as well, resulting in the transformation of serotonin into 5-hydroxyindoleacetic acid (5-HIAA). Serotonin in the median raphe nucleus is thought to play a role in slow-wave sleep, and L-tryptophan (a serotonin precursor) has been used as a hypnotic agent. Possible additional clinical significance of indoleamine metabolism is discussed later in this chapter.

Another interesting group of brain monoamines is the phenylethylamines. 2-Phenylethylamine is derived from phenylalanine (as are the catecholamines) and metabolized by monoamine oxidase (MAO) (as is also the case with the catecholamines), as portrayed in Figure 4 [7]. Phenylethylamine is known to cause the release of catecholamines, and this may produce a direct stimulating effect on the brain much like that of the amphetamines.

Table 2   Inherited Disorders of Lipid Metabolism

Designation	Clinical features	Product stored	Enzyme deficiency
Gaucher's Infantile (cerebrovisceral)	Normal at birth; death by age 2; severe cerebral involvement with hyperextension of head, strabismus, retraction of lips. Hepatosplenomegaly, Gaucher cells in marrow.	Glucocerebroside	β-Glucosidase deficiency
Adult (visceral)	Chronic nonneuronopathic; no cerebral involvement. Hepatosplenomegaly; episodic bone pain with involvement of hip and long bones. Gaucher cells in marrow; lymphadenopathy. Spectrum of benign to more malignant course.	Glucocerebroside	Diminished pH, 4.0; β-glucosidase activity (?)
Juvenile	Heterogeneous group; hepatosplenomegaly and neurological abnormalities; Gaucher cells.	? Glucocerebroside	
Niemann-Pick cerbrovisceral	Onset in infancy; death by age 3; progressive rapid neurological deterioration. Hepatosplenomegaly; cachexia; 30% with cherry red spot in macula; foam cells in marrow stain for lipid and phosphorus.	Sphingomyelin + cholesterol (neural and visceral)	Sphingomyelinase (no artificial subtrate)
Visceral	Older onset; visceral involvement only. Pulmonary infections; hepatosplenomegaly; normal intelligence.	Sphingomyelin + cholesterol (visceral)	Sphingomyelinase
Visceral-cerebral	Moderate course; lesser visceral involvement and late onset of CNS involvement. May have cherry red spot. Death between 5-15. Older onset (2-6 years).	Sphingomyelin + cholesterol (visceral and neural)	Sphingomyelinase (?)
Visceral-cerebral	Nova Scotia variant. Ataxia and dyskinesia; early jaundice with hepatosplenomegaly. Protracted degenerative course.	Sphingomyelin + cholesterol (primary cholesterol)	(?) Diminished or sphingomyelinase
Farber's disease (lipogranulomatosis)	Childhood onset; progressive arthropathy. Subcutaneous nodules, nutritional failure, and psychomotor retardation.	Ceramide	Ceramidase

(Continued)

Table 2 Inherited Disorders of Lipid Metabolism (continued)

Designation	Clinical features	Product stored	Enzyme deficiency
Generalized gangliosidosis (gangliosidosis GM_1)	Acute infantile cerebral disorder; onset at birth; - death by age 2 with decerebrate rigidity; similar to Hurler's coarsening of facial features, bone changes, hirsutism, hepatosplenomegaly. Lipids in liver, spleen, marrow, kidney, and blood cells.	Ganglioside GM, and asialo derivative in brain) visceral storage of mucopolysaccharide	β-Galactosidase (GM_1, β-galactosidase)
Juvenile gangliosidosis GM_1	Onset age 1; locomotor ataxia, frequent falling, internal strabismus, progressing to decerebrate rigidity by age 3. No hepatosplenomegaly. Mild bony abnormalities.	Same as above	β-Galactosidase (GM_1 β-galactosidase)
Gangliosidosis GM_2 Type I: Tay-Sachs	Normal at birth; onset 4-6 months; weakness, progressive mental and motor deterioration, blindness, macrocephaly, hyperacusis, paralysis, and dementia. Cherry red spot in macula. Jewish parentage.	GM_2 ganglioside	N-acetyl hexosaminidase A
Type II: Sandhoff	Clinically indistinguishable from above. Non-Jewish parentage.	GM_2 ganglioside and globoside in viscera	N-acetyl hexosaminidase A and B
Type III: Juvenile gangliosidosis GM_2	Onset 2-6 years; locomotor ataxia, loss of speech progressive spasticity, and weakness progressing to decerebrate rigidity and blindness. Death by age 5-15. No cherry red spots.	GM_2 ganglioside	Partial deficiency hexosaminidase A and B
Fabry's disease	Males have crises of severe incapacitating burning pain in extremities, fever, characteristic skin lesion, angiokeratoma corporis diffusum universale, corneal opacities, anhidrosis, multiple system involvement: renal impairment, hypertension, cardiac failure. Heterozygous females may have limited disease. X-linked inherited.	Ceramide trihexoside widespread deposition; blood vessels, nerve cells, RES, myocardia, kidney	α-Galactosidase

(Continued)

Table 2 Inherited Disorders of Lipid Metabolism (continued)

Designation	Clinical features	Product stored	Enzyme deficiency
Lactosyl ceramidosis	Childhood onset. Slowly progressive CNS impairment. Hepatosplenomegaly, foam cells. Macrocytic anemia, leukopenia, and thrombocytopenia (one case).	Lactosyl ceramide	β-Galactoside (?)
Krabbe's globoid cell leukodystrophy	Rapidly fatal infantile neurological disorder. Globoid cells in brain tissue.	No overt accumulation of galactocerebroside	β-Galactosidase galactocerebrosidase; psychosine β-galactosidase
Metachromatic keukodystrophy (sulfatide lipidoses) Late infantile	Onset 1-4 years; gait disturbance, incoordination, leading to dementia; macular changes. Vegetative state by 5 years. Nerve biopsy: metachromasia.	Galactosyl (SO_4) ceramide	Aryl sulfatase A
Juvenile	As above, but later onset. Sometimes seen in same kindred as above.		Aryl sulfatase A; levels higher than in infantile
Adult	Rare; onset in adult life with psychosis and dementia; motor signs much later (up to 30 years).	Galactosyl (SO_4) ceramide	Aryl sulfatase A diminished but not absent
Variant (Austin type)	Rare; onset 1-3 years. Dysostosis multiplex, hepatosplenomegaly with generalized CNS involvement; early death. Nerve biopsy: metachromasia.	Galactosyl (SO_4) ceramide and sulfated mucopolysaccharides, steroid sulfates	Aryl sulfatases A, B, and C; steroid sulfatase deficiencies

Source: From R. Hirschhorn and G. Weissman. Genetic disorders of lysosomes, in *Progress in Medical Genetics.* Saunders, Philadelphia, 1976, with permission (Ref. 6).

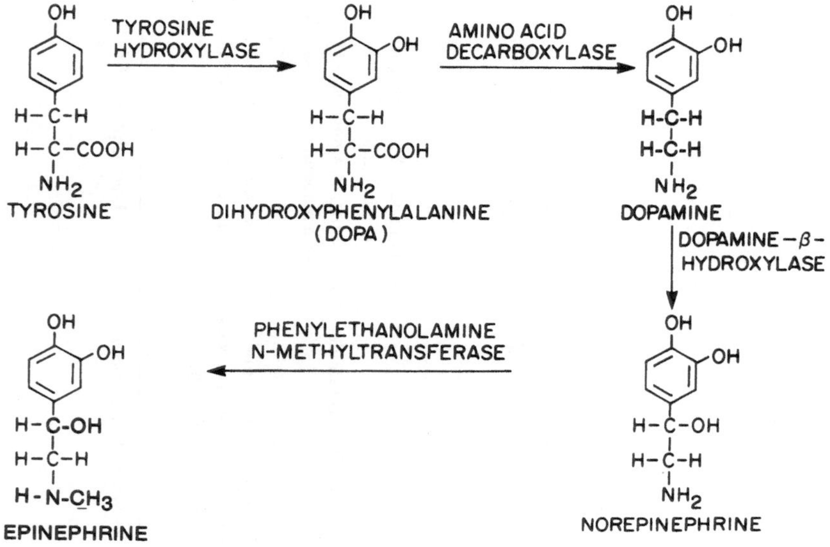

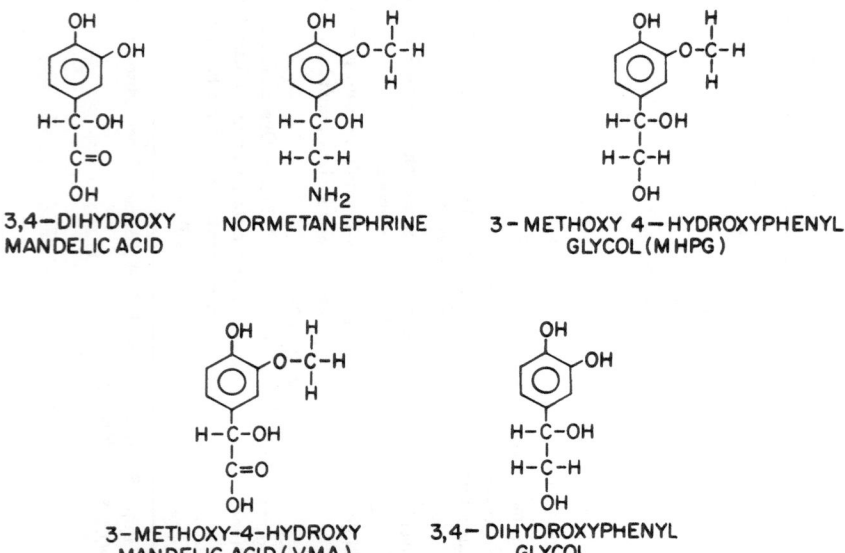

FIG. 1.   Synthesis of dopamine and norepinephrine from the amino acid tyrosine.

FIG. 2.   Metabolites of norepinephrine.

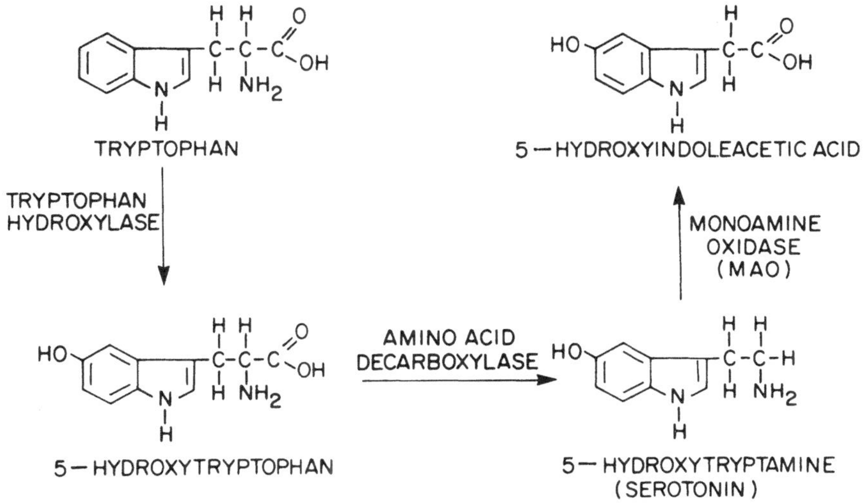

FIG. 3.   Synthesis of 5-hydroxytryptamine (serotonin) from the amino acid tryptophan.

BIOCHEMICAL THEORIES OF AFFECTIVE DISORDERS AND SCHIZOPHRENIA

Affective Disorders

There are two major affective disorder syndromes, major depression and mania. According to Taylor and Abrams [8], in major depression the patient has a sad or anxious affect and at least three of the following six: (1) anorexia with a 5-lb weight loss in the past 3 weeks, (2) early morning awakening (terminal insomnia), (3) diurnal mood variation with a severely sad mood early in the morning tending to "lighten" as the day progresses, (4) psychomotor retardation or agitation, (5) suicidal ideation; and (6) feelings of guilt or worthlessness. In mania, the patient typically manifests motor hyperactivity, rapid or pressured speech, and euphoric or irritable mood. Major depressions not due to coarse brain disease are best treated with electorconvulsive therapy, although tricyclic antidepressants or lithium may also be effective. Mania not due to coarse brain disease is best treated with lithium carbonate, although electroconvulsive therapy or neuroleptics may also be effective.

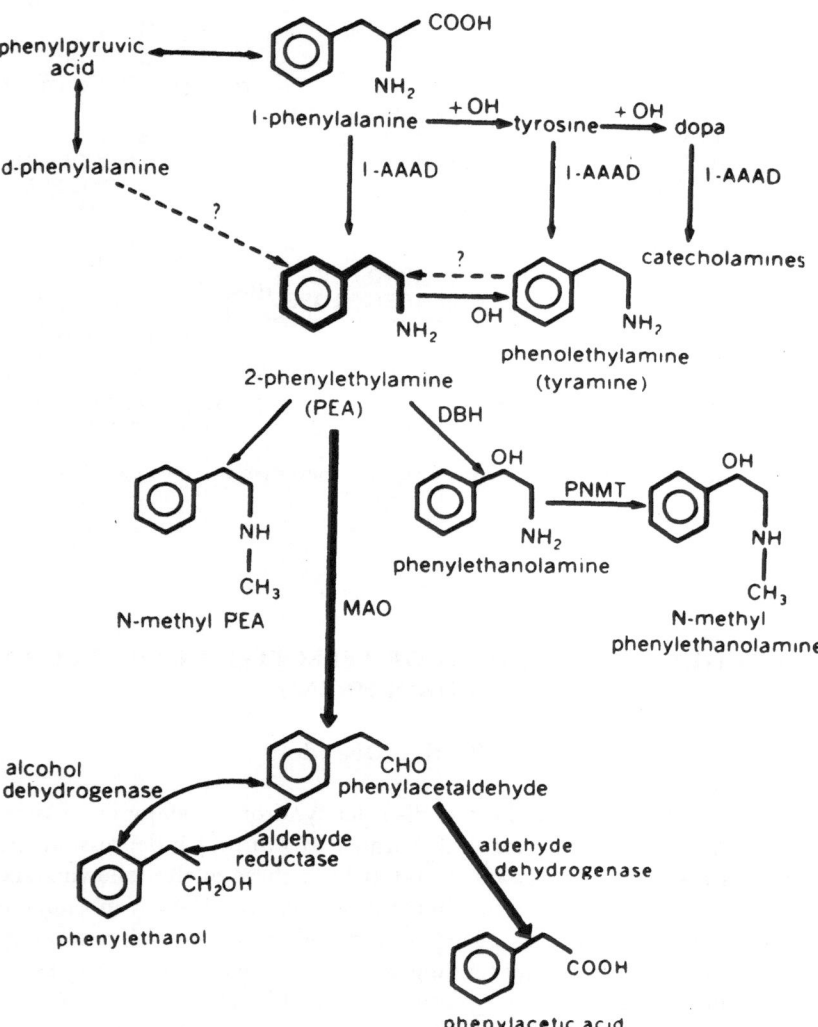

FIG. 4. Synthesis of 2-phenylethylamine and its metabolism. (From H. Sabelli and A. Mosnaim, The phenylethylamine hypothesis of affective behavior. *The American Journal of Psychiatry*, Vol. 131, p 697, 1974. Copyright © 1974, The American Psychiatric Association. Reprinted by permission.

Catecholamine Hypothesis of Major Depression

This theory holds that in major depressions, there is a deficiency of nor-epinephrine at receptor sites on postsynaptic receptor neurons in the brain. The following data, much of which comes from animal studies, are in keeping with this hypothesis. Reserpine (Serpasil), an antihypertensive agent known to produce depression as a side effect in humans, has been shown to cause intracellular deamination of norepinephrine (as well as of dopamine and serotonin) in the presynaptic neuron. Tricyclic antidepressants, used in the treatment of major depression, have been shown to interfere with the re-uptake of norepinephrine by the presynaptic noradrenergic neuron, as well as to interfere with the deamination of norepinephrine in the presynaptic neuron by mitochondrial monoamine oxidase. Amphetamines, which can have a transient (although not curative) euphoriant and stimulant effect, cause the release of norepinephrine and dopamine from presynaptic nor-adrenergic neurons, and impede both the deamination and reuptake of nor-epinephrine. Monoamine oxidase inhibitors, useful in anxiety states and certain atypical depressions, impede the deamination of norepinephrine and serotonin by monoamine oxidase in the presynaptic noradrenergic neuron. Electroconvulsive therapy, the best treatment of major depression, increases the turnover (the utilization and metabolism) of norepinephrine, dopamine, and serotonin in the brain.

It must be reemphasized that many of these findings are from animal studies, and that there is no proof that these processes occur in human brains. And even if these processes do occur in human brains, there is no proof that the relationship is causal. The catecholamine hypothesis is also an oversimplification, for catecholamine metabolism is intimately related to other metabolic pathways.

The 3-Methoxy-4-Hydroxyphenylglycol (MHPG) Hypothesis

A variation on the catecholamine hypothesis is the 3-methoxy-4-hydroxyphenylglycol hypothesis. MHPG is the major metabolite of norepinephrine in several nonhuman species, and Schildkraut [9] suggests that it may be the major metabolite of norepinephrine in humans as well. Several studies have shown that for patients with both manic and depressive episodes, levels of urinary MHPG are lower during depression and higher during mania. Also, patients with manic and depressive episodes have less MHPG in their urine than patients with chronic character depressions, suggesting a possible diagnostic utility of urinary MHPG. Also, depressed patients with high urinary levels of MHPG are more likely to respond to amitryptilline (Elavil) than to imipramine (Tofranil) or its metabolites, while depressed patients with low urinary levels of MHPG are more likely to respond to imipramine and its metabolites than to amitryptilline [9].

Permissive Hypothesis of Affective Disorders

Prange et al. [10] hypothesized that several metabolic pathways are simultaneously involved in the genesis of major depression and mania. They write: "a deficit in central indoleaminergic transmission *permits* (italics mine) affective disorder, but is insufficient for its cause; and changes in central catecholaminergic transmission, when they occur in the context of a deficit in indoleaminergic transmission, act as a proximate cause for affective disorders and determine their quality, catecholaminergic transmission being elevated in mania and diminished in depression."

Indoleamine (Serotonin) Hypothesis of Affective Disorder

Coppen and Noguera [11] reviewed studies of cerebrospinal fluid levels of 5-hydroxyindoleacetic acid (5-HIAA), the major metabolite of serotonin, in depressed and manic patients. They noted that most studies revealed a decreased level of 5-HIAA in both depressed and manic patients and that the low levels persist after recovery. They hypothesized a constitutional factor common to both major depression and mania. The fact that monoamine oxidase inhibitors, which increase serotonin as well as catecholamine and phenylethylamine levels, are useful in certain atypical depressions supports this hypothesis. Treatment of major depressions with tryptophan, a serotonin precursor, has yielded conflicting results in a number of studies, and there is a degree of oversimplification in this hypothesis as well.

ACTH, Adrenal Corticosteroids, Electrolytes, and Depression [12]

Numerous studies have demonstrated increased cortisol secretion and sodium retention in major depression. In normal subjects, there is a drop in cortisol secretion in the late evening and early morning; in patients with major depression, cortisol levels remain high. This may be related to dysfunction in the hypothalamus/pituitary axis. In normal subjects, the secretion of ACTH and the consequent secretion of cortisol are suppressed by the synthetic steroid dexamethasone, just as endogenous adrenal steroids decrease ACTH levels by a well-known feedback mechanism. In patients with major depressions dexamethasone suppression does occur, but the decrease in cortisol lasts for only several hours, as compared with 24 hr of suppression by controls. Dexamethasone suppression has been used as a test to distinguish between endogenous (major) and reactive depressions.

Schizophrenia

Schizophrenia occurs in .6% of the general population, 2% of families of schizophrenics, and about 6% of hospitalized psychiatric patients. It is the most overdiagnosed syndrome in American psychiatry. When modern diagnostic criteria are not used, it is the diagnosis made (usually incorrect) for 50% or more of psychiatric inpatients. According to the Taylor and Abrams criteria [8], schizophrenia is characterized by the presence of one or more of the following: Emotional blunting, first-rank signs of Schneider, and formal thinking disorder. Coarse brain disease, drug intoxication and affective disorder must be ruled out. Neuroleptics are the treatment of choice, and the prognosis for cure is poor. Most of the biochemical hyptheses of schizophrenia are oversimplifications.

The Dopamine Hypothesis of Schizophrenia

This theory holds that the crucial metabolic problem in schizophrenia is the hyperfunction of dopaminergic neurons in the brain. Data used to support this hypothesis includes the following: Neuroleptic drugs (which have therapeutic effect in schizophrenia) frequently produce a syndrome identical with Parkinson's disease, a condition associated with dopamine deficiency in the basal ganglia. Amphetamines, whose chronic toxicity produces a syndrome thought by some to resemble schizophrenia, may potentiate the effects of dopamine in the brain. The phenothiazine drugs (such as promethazine), which are ineffectual in the treatment of schizophrenia, do not decrease the levels of dopamine metabolites in the brain. In contrast, neuroleptics, which are effective in the treatment of schizophrenia, increase the quantity of dopamine metabolites.

The Transmethylation Hypothesis of Schizophrenia

Harley-Mason, Osmond and Symthies [13] speculated that since many hallucinogens were methylated substances with some resemblance to psychoactive brain monoamines, perhaps schizophrenia, which is sometimes associated with hallucinations, might be associated with the methylation of indoleamine and cathecolamine metabolites. In one study, patients thought to have schizophrenia were given methionine (a precursor of the methyl donor S-adenosyl methionine) and a monoamine oxidase inhibitor. This resulted in an exacerbation of symptoms. This also occurred when patients were given methionine alone.

Further support for the transmethylation hypothesis came when it was discovered that there was a dimethyltryptamine (DMT, a hallucinogen)-forming enzyme in human platelets, and that methylated indoleamine substances were found in the blood and urine of schizophrenics. Also, Wyatt, Potkin, and Murphy [14] found that people diagnosed as having chronic schizophrenia had low levels of platelet and white blood cell monoamine oxidase. This was thought to be significant because monoamine oxidase might be the enzyme which detoxifies methylated indoleamines, leaving larger quantities of these indoleamines acting in the brain.

Unfortunately for the hypothesis, DMT-producing enzymes and methylated indoleamine derivatives were found in normal subjects and in patients with psychiatric illnesses other than schizophrenia. Also, giving radiolabeled methionine [14] to humans and other animals does not increase the amount of radiolabeled S-adenosyl methionine in most body tissues, including the brain.

Autoimmunity Theory of Schizophrenia

Heath [15] postulated that the fundamental problem in schizophrenia is anhedonia, which is the result of an antigen-antibody reaction in the septum of the brain, where the antigen is the brain tissue itself, and the antibody is a γ-globulin called taraxein. He reported that serum γ-gobulins of schizophrenic patients, injected into the ventricular system of monkeys, caused the monkeys to act inappropriately. He also found that antibodies to the monkey septal region, injected into other monkeys, produced inappropriate behavior. Unfortunately for Heath's hypothesis, a number of investigators have been unable to replicate his findings.

Histamine in Schizophrenia

Several researchers have noted abnormal histamine levels, either elevated or reduced, in schizophrenic patients [16]. Others have found a diminished wheal-and-flare response to intradermally injected histamine. This suggests some problem of immune responsivity in schizophrenics. Unfortunately, many of these studies did not account for the fact that many of the patients were receiving neuroleptic drugs, which are known to affect histamine levels and responsivity to histamine [16].

Creatine Phosphokinase (CPK) and Psychosis

There are several isoenzymes of CPK in the body, one a muscle isoenzyme and another a brain insoenzyme. Meltzer and Crayton [17] found that the muscle isoenzyme was elevated in the serum of patients with severe acute psychiatric illnesses, including schizophrenia, and which could not be accounted for by intramuscular injections or exertion.

Curiously, brain CPK isoenzymes were not elevated in these illnesses. Meltzer and Crayton also found histological abnormalities, one of which is referred to as "Z-band spreading" in muscle biopsies from acute schizophrenic patients. The biopsy findings could be distinguished from the findings of biopsies from normal controls.

Endorphins and Schizophrenia

Wagemaker and Cade, quoted by Miller [4] and Snyder [18], reported preliminary studies of the successful treatment of schizophrenic patients with hemodialysis. They report that a β-endorphin molecule is found in the dialysate, and raise the possibility that this endorphin may play a role in the schizophrenic process. These results are from a small sample and the methodology is weak, but the possibilities are intriguing.

CONCLUSION

For many behavioral disorders, such as delirium secondary to hyproxia or hypoglycemia, the relationship between brain biochemistry and abnormal behavior is fairly clear. For affective disorders and schizophrenia, the relationships are far less clear, but because of the severity of these conditions it is crucial that brain biochemistry remain a major focus of study.

REFERENCES

1. Gilroy, J., and Meyer, J. *Medical Neurology.* Macmillan, New York (1969).
2. Kaplan, H., Sadock, B., and Freedman, A. Neurochemistry of behavior. Recent advances, in *Comprehensive Textbook of Psychiatry,* 2nd ed. A. Freedman, H. Kaplan, and B. Sadock, eds. Williams and Wilkins, Baltimore (1975), pp. 132-142.
3. Scriver, C., and Rosenberg, L. *Amino Acid Metabolism and Its Disorders.* Saunders, Philadelphia (1973).
4. Miller, R. The potential of endorphins. *Behav. Med.* 30-33.
5. Hughes, J. (ed.). *Centrally Acting Peptides.* Macmillan, New York (1978).
6. Hirschhorn, R., and Weissman, G. Genetic disorders of lysozymes, in *Progress in Medical Genetics.* A. Steinberg, A. Bearn, A. Motulsky, and B. Childs, eds. Saunders, Philadelphia (1976).
7. Sabelli, H., and Mosnaim, D. Phenylethylamine hypothesis of affective behavior. *Am. J. Psychiatry* 131:695-699 (1974).
8. Taylor, M., and Abrams, R. The prevalence of schizophrenia: A reassessment using modern diagnostic criteria. *Am. J. Psychiatry* 135:945-948 (1978).
9. Schildkraut, J. The biochemistry of affective disorders. A brief summary in *The Harvard Guide to Modern Psychiatry.* A Nicholi, ed. Belknap, Harvard, Cambridge, (1978), pp. 81-91.
10. Prange, A., Wilson, I., Lynn, C., Altop, L., and Stikeleather, R. L-Tryptophan in mania. Contributions to a permissive hypothesis of affective disorders. *Arch. Gen. Psychiatry* 30:56-62 (1974).
11. Coppen, A., and Noguera, R. L-Tryptophan in depression. *Lancet* 1:1111 (1970).
12. Sacher, E., Hellman, L., Roffwarg, H., Halpern, F., Fuhushima, D., and Gallagher, T. Disrupted 24 hour patterns of cortisol secretion in psychotic depression. *Arch. Gen. Psychiatry* 28:19-24 (1973).
13. Osmond, H., and Smythies, J.: Schizohrenia: A new approach. *J. Ment. Sci.* 98:309-315, 1952.

14. Wyatt, R., Potkin, S., and Murphy, D. Platelet monoamine oxidase activity in schizo-phrenia. A review of the data. *Am. J. Psychiatry* 136:377-385 (1979).

15. Heath, R. An antibrain globulin in schizophrenia, in *Biochemistry, Schizophrenias and Affective Illnesses*. H. Himwich, ed. Williams and Wilkins, Baltimore (1970), pp. 171-197.

16. Frazer, A., and Winokur, A. *Biological Bases of Psychiatric Disorders*. Spectrum, New York (1977).

17. Meltzer, H., and Crayton, J. Subterminal motor abnormalities in psychotic patients. *Nature (Lond.)* 249:373-375 (1974).

18. Snyder, S. The opiate receptor and morphine-like polypeptides in the brain. *Am. J. Psychiatry* 135:645-652 (1978).

6

Sleep

FREDERICK SIERLES and
CHARLES HILLENBRAND

INTRODUCTION

It is curious that sleep, an activity that occupies one-fourth to one-third of our lives, is accorded so little time in medical education. Knowledge about sleep is clinically helpful. Sleep problems are common, some are very disturbing, and one (sleep apnea) can even be fatal. In one study [1] of 1,006 randomly selected adults, the prevalence of current or previous sleep disorders was 52.1%

Sleep disturbance can be a symptom of an illness, aiding us in making a diagnosis; for example, early morning awakening is a symptom of endogenous depression. Normal sleep can be a time of exacerbation of certain medical conditions; for example, in peptic ulcer patients, there is an increase of unneutralized acid secretion during sleep [2].

HISTORY

Several milestones in the study of sleep are noteworthy. Berger, a psychiatrist, developed the electroencephalogram (EEG) in 1924. In 1935, Loomis, Harvey, and Hobart described five patterns of EEG activity during sleep. In 1953, Aserinsky and Kleitman described rapid eye movement (REM) sleep. Since then, there has been considerable sleep research resulting in the identification of some sleep disorders (such as sleep apnea) never before diagnosed. Sleep laboratories have assisted in the study of sleep. These labs, which often have a "homey" quality, have extensive recording machinery that includes electroencephalograms, electromyograms (EMGs), and electrooculograms (EOGs).

NEUROPHYSIOLOGY

Although the purposes of sleep are not known for sure, it is certain that sleep is much more than just a time of rest and relaxation. Considerable cerebral activity occurs. Hartmann [3-5], stating that sleep has a "restorative" function, speculates that sleep is a time of anabolism and establishment of new neuronal connections. Jouvet [6] and Broughton [7] have written about neuroanatomic pathways involved with sleep.

Sleep seems to be initiated by the median raphe nuclei of the pons, which inhibit the ascending reticular activating system (ARAS), the latter being responsible for the maintenance of consciousness. The median raphe nuclei have high concentrations of serotonin, which is apparently necessary for the initiation of sleep. The locus ceruleus in the pons inhibits the descending reticular activating systems (DRAS); this produces the muscle relaxation of REM sleep, for the DRAS helps to maintain muscle tone. The nucleus reticularis pontis caudalis seems to activate the ARAS and produce awakening.

As pictured in Figure 1, sleep is divided into six stages, which appear in succession. Stage 0 is the waking state, and momentary awakening occurs several times during the night. Stage 1 is light sleep, and it is easy to awaken the sleeper. The EEG (see Fig. 2) shows low-voltage fast activity. In stage 2, the sleeper also sleeps lightly. Sleep spindles and K-complexes are seen on the

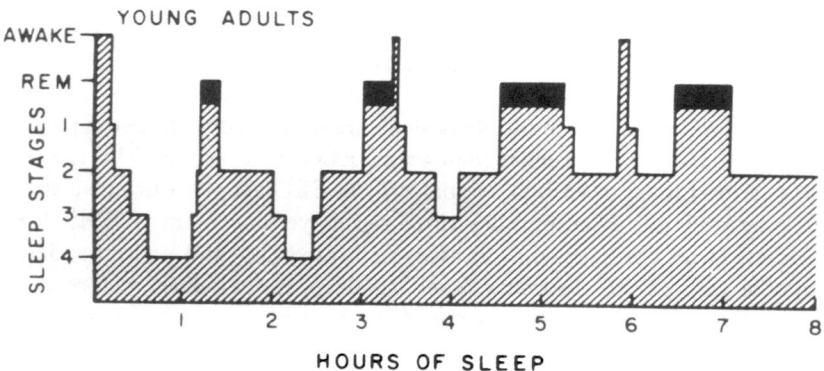

FIG. 1.   Stages of sleep. (From Berger, R: The sleep and dream cycle, in *Sleep: Pysiology and Pathology*, A. Kales, ed. Lippincott, Philadelphia (1969), with permission.)

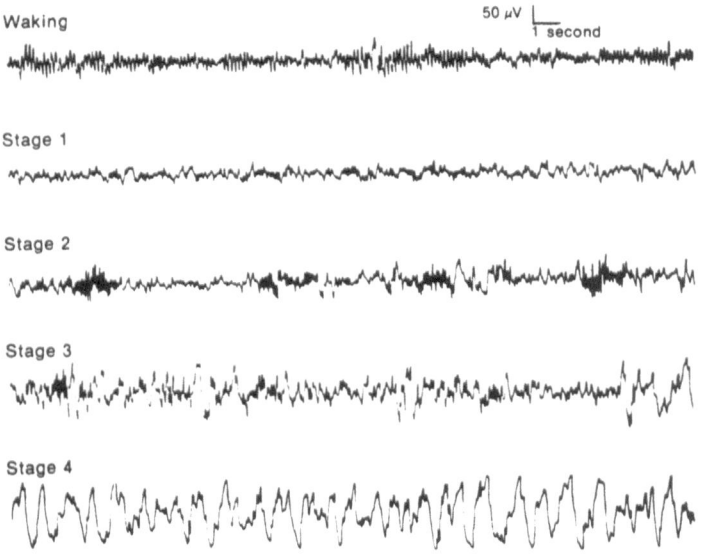

FIG. 2.   Electroencephalogram of five sleep stages. (From H. Hartmann. Sleep, in *Harvard Guide to Modern Psychiatry*. A. Nicholi, ed. Belknap, Harvard, Cambridge, 1978, with permission.)

EEG. In stage 3, there are moderate amounts of EEG delta (slow) wave activity. This is the first stage of deep sleep, from which it is hard to arouse the sleeper. In stage 4, delta wave activity predominates. As the night progesses, the proportion (compared with REM sleep) of stage 4 decreases. Stages 1-4 are called non-REM (NREM, synchronized, passive) sleep. Stages 3 and 4 are called deep or slow-wave sleep (SWS) [3-5]. Then REM (desynchronized, D-sleep, active, paradoxical) [3-5] sleep appears.

In REM sleep, the EEG is similar to the stage 1 EEG, and the sleeper is easily aroused. REM sleep is a time of increased autonomic activity, with increases in heart rate, systolic blood pressure, and voluntary muscle tone. Penile and clitoral engorgement with blood causes erections. Gross body movements decrease. If awakened, the sleeper will usually recall having just had a dream, since REM sleep is the time of dreaming. Dreams are in color, not black-and-white. REM sleep occurs every 90-110 min, and the first REM period begins 90-110 min after sleep onset. There are 3-5 REM periods per night. Normal sleep never begins with REM sleep. The duration of REM periods increases throughout the night, the first period lasting several minutes and the final period lasting 20-40 min.

If a person is deprived of REM sleep, such as by alcohol, anxiety, or medical illness, the following night he will start REM sleep sooner than 90-

110 min after sleep onset (shortened REM latency), and the length of each REM period will be lengthened. This phenomenon is called REM rebound. REM rebound may play a part in delirium tremens, for alcohol and prescription sedative-hypnotics are REM sleep suppressants.

AGE AND SLEEP

The average amounts of nightly sleep for each age group is fairly constant in all cultures. Williams and Karacan [8] cite data (Table 1) on mean values for sleep in 20 to 29-year-old men.

Table 1   Sleep in Young Men

Total time in bed:	442.23 min
Sleep period time:	424.64 min
Sleep efficiency index:	95%
Sleep latency:	14.55 min
Awakenings:	3.05 min
REM periods:	4.05 min
Percent Stage 0:	1.26%
Percent Stage 1:	4.44%
Percent Stage 2:	45.34%
Percent Stage 3:	6.21%
Percent Stage 4:	14.55%
Percent REM sleep:	28%

Source: From ref. 8, with permission.

Sleep period time is the time from lying down to sleep to the time of final awakening. Total sleep time is the sleep period time minus the time spent awake. The sleep efficiency index is

$$\frac{\text{Total sleep time}}{\text{Time in bed}} \text{ X } 100$$

Adult sleep patterns are stable on a night-to-night basis, unless the individual becomes ill, but there is considerable variation between individuals.

As age increases, the percentage of time in REM sleep decreases. REM sleep constitutes 50-80% of the sleep of premature infants. In normal-weight newborns, 40-60% of their sleep is REM sleep. The figures are 20-25% and 13-18% for young adults and older adults, respectively [5]. Beginning in a person's twenties, SWS declines, and may disappear after age 60.

People who sleep 6 or 7 hr nightly have the longest life expectancy, and people who sleep less than 4 hr or more than 10 hr have the lowest; however, there is no proof that this correlation represents a causal relationship.

QUALITY OF SLEEP

Quality of sleep is as important as quantity. The key is whether the individual sleeps sufficiently to be alert and refreshed the next day. People who regularly sleep 8 hr do not necessarily feel better than those who routinely sleep 6 hr. Therefore, the symptom of insomnia is a relative one.

DRUGS AND SLEEP

Barbiturates, alcohol, phenothiazines, meprobamate, benzodiazepenes, amphetamines, methylphenidate, monoamine oxidase (MAO) inhibitors, and tricyclic antidepressants all decrease REM sleep, regardless of whether they promote or impede total sleep time. Benzodiazepines are stage 4 sleep suppressants. Amphetamines and methylphenidate frequently cause initial insomnia; tricyclic antidepressants and MAO inhibitors, if taken just before bedtime, occasionally cause initial insomnia. Caffeine causes initial insomnia. Antihistamines, although they don't suppress REM sleep, do cause REM rebound when discontinued, and REM rebound can be experienced as vivid dreams or nightmares [9]. Barbiturates, other sedative-hypnotics, aliphatic and piperadine phenothiazines, antihistamines (including the over-the-counter hypnotic methapyriline), tryptophan, and benzodiazepines all have sleep-inducing effects, either as their primary use or as a side effect. On the other hand, continuous use of some sedative-hypnotics can cause insomnia. Tricyclic antidepressants may have sedation as a side effect. Drugs which improve the health of an individual (with trouble sleeping due to illness) promote sleep. Foods high in tryptophan content promote sleep, perhaps by increasing serotonin content in the median raphe nucleus [10].

SLEEP AND MEDICAL DISORDERS

Although sleep almost certainly serves important biological restorative functions, medically speaking, it is not necessarily the safest time for some patients. The arterial oxygen saturation falls during sleep and there is tachycardia in patients with chronic obstructive lung disease. The pulmonary arterial pressure increases during sleep in people with pulmonary hypertension. Some patients with angina pectoris are more likely to have angina attacks during REM sleep than while awake [2]. Premenstrually, the amount of REM sleep increases, and this may somehow be associated with premenstrual tension [5].

Although some illnesses are tiring and can induce sleep, it is more frequent for significant illness to impede sleep. Almost all illnesses that produce severe discomfort can decrease the quantity and quality of sleep. Just think of how difficult it is to sleep with pain, nausea, or even a common cold. The sudden onset of a serious psychiatric disorder is almost invariably associated with markedly reduced sleep time. When medical illness impedes sleep, treatment of the illness itself is the best treatment of the sleep problem, although use of sedative-hypnotics for a few days may be temporarily useful.

Of course, we must remember that because sleep has a restorative function, a good night's sleep is often therapeutic during the course of an acute illness. If sleep is impeded, as is frequently the case in intensive care units, general health may be affected (e.g., the development of delirium) as well [5].

THE SLEEP HISTORY

Every patient should be questioned about sleep. Questioning should include changes in sleep patterns, sleep period time, trouble falling asleep (initial insomnia), early morning awakening (terminal insomnia), medications, caffeine-containing drinks, daytime sleepiness, and snoring. More specific questions like "Do you ever fall to the ground when you laugh or get angry?" (cataplexy), should be asked when there is reason to suspect sleep pathology. Amounts of time spent awake are often exaggerated, and total sleeplessness is incredibly rare. However, the complaint of unsatisfactory or insufficient sleep (insomnia) should usually be taken at face value.

SPECIFIC SLEEP DISORDERS

Intense Moods

Intense moods such as anxiety, anger, and euphoria can impede sleep. These may be the product of illness, but usually they are not. If they are the product of illness (e.g., anxiety neurosis, depression, mania), the initiating cause should be diagnosed and treated. If they are the product of life circumstances (e.g., an argument, a disappointment, a success), banal, but sometimes effective, recommendations include reading, sex, housework, thinking of other things, resting (if this is not too frustrating), television, favorite foods, small doses of an anxiolytic agent (e.g., diazepam, 2-4 mg) or 250-1,500 mg L-tryptophan [22].

Narcolepsy

Guilleminault and Dement [12] studied a large group of patients with excessive daytime sleepiness and found that 62% had narcolepsy, 14% had upper airway sleep apnea, 4% had narcolepsy with sleep apnea, and 20% had other causes.

Narcolepsy is a syndrome consisting of excessive daytime sleepiness, daytime sleep attacks, cataplexy, and hypnagogic hallucinations. Sleep attacks are irresistible episodes of sleeping. Cataplexy is a sudden decrease in muscle tone, causing mild weakness or occasional falling to the ground, usually precipitated by a strong emotion (e.g., laughter, anger) or muscle exertion (e.g., swinging a baseball bat) [13]. Hypnagogic hallucinations are hallucinations upon falling asleep.

The excessive daytime sleepiness and sleep attacks are very disabling because the patient is drowsy, inattentive, or napping much of the day. Friends, associates, and relatives are disturbed by this, and sometimes take the sleeping personally, as an expression of boredom or rejection. The divorce rate for untreated narcoleptics approaches 100% [14].

The fundamental pathophysiology in sleep attacks and cataplexy is the onset of REM sleep during the day; the tendency of sleep attacks and cataplexy to occur every 90-110 min supports this explanation. The hypnagogic hallucinations are REM-period dreaming occurring in place of stage 1 at the onset of sleep. The diagnosis is confirmed by EEG and EOG; sleep onset begins with REM sleep.

Family members and close friends should be educated so they don't take the sleepiness personally. Methylphenidate (Ritalin), 5-10 mg 3 times daily, can be prescribed for the sleep attacks; imipramine, 25-50 mg 3 times daily, or protryptiline (Vivactil), 10 mg 3 times daily can be prescribed for cataplexy and hypnagogic hallucinations [15].

Sleep Apnea

During sleep of patients with sleep apnea, there is a cycle of 10-60 sec of apnea followed by snoring, gasping, rapid deep breathing, or awakening. Excessive daytime sleepiness is a common complaint. The pathophysiology lies in brain stem dysfunction (central sleep apnea) in some cases, and in upper airway obstruction (during sleep only) in others. The patient's bed partner or parent may give clues to the diagnosis by describing the pattern of breathing and snoring.

In adults, the condition is commoner in men than in women [14]. Obesity, hypertension, and morning headaches are quite common [14]. During sleep, the patient may experience cardiac arrhythmias and sudden death [14]. In pediatrics this syndrome explains some instances of sudden infant death syndrome (SIDS) [16].

The treatment of upper airway obstructive sleep apnea is tracheotomy, which is kept open by night and plugged by day. One treatment of central sleep apnea in children is theophylline. In infants who are at risk for sudden death, an electrical warning system, which awakens the mother when respirations decrease or cease, may be life-saving.

Sleep-Related Periodic Myoclonus

In this rare condition, the patient, often middle-aged, complains of insomnia and that "my legs jump at night." The reason is that he is having episodes of muscular jerking which waken him, sometimes as often as every 30 sec. The EEG reveals bursts of K-complex activity [17]. In some cases, the myoclonus is a side effect of tricyclic antidepressants or MAO inhibitors [17]. The patient should receive diazepam, 5-20 mg, at bedtime. If the patient has been taking tricyclic antidepressants or MAO inhibitors, the dose should be decreased or the drug discontinued.

Excessive Use of Sedative-Hypnotics

One of the commonest causes of insomnia is the chronic use of sedative-hypnotics. The treatment is to discontinue the sedative-hypnotic; the speed of discontinuation should depend on the quantity consumed daily.

Sleeptalking

This occurs during any non-REM sleep stage. The patient may talk fluently and can carry on a conversation, but what he says is meaningless and does not reveal personal secrets. The next morning he has no recollection of what he said. This phenomenon is quite common and completely benign, and requires no treatment.

Sleepwalking (Somnambulism)

In contrast to sleeptalking, sleepwalking is not benign. It is common among young children, most of whom "outgrow" it, but it can also occur in adulthood. During the "walk," which rarely lasts more than 2 min, the patient has a degree of visual agnosia [8] and his critical faculties and reactivity are impaired. Thus, he is at high risk for accidents; about half of all sleepwalks result in an accident, with or without injury. Complex activities, such as crimes, are not possible.

Because this occurs during stage 4 of sleep, it is difficult to arouse the patient during a walk. However, because of the risks, if anyone is awake in the house, the patient should be followed and awakened if necessary. Contrary to myth, awakened sleepwalkers do not act dangerously. If others are not immediately available, potentially dangerous objects should be removed and doors and windows locked. It may be necessary to tie a rope loosely from the patient's waist to a bedpost [10]. Benzodiazepines (stage 4 suppressants) can be employed, but success is limited.

Enuresis (Bedwetting)

This condition is also common, occurring in 22% of 500 unselected children between the ages of 4 and 14 [18], and has several causes, which include urologic disease, family stress such as the birth of a baby, and genetic transmission.

In this chapter, we will only discuss genetically related enuresis. Here, there is frequently a history of an enuretic family member whose condition disappeared during adolescence. The urination occurs primarily during stage 4 of sleep. In the sleep lab, distinct EEG changes are noted while the sleeping child is urinating. Bedtime imipramine is sometimes quite effective; for children, the starting dose should be about 25 mg, with increments up to 75 mg, if needed [9]. For adults, the starting dose should be 50 mg, with increments up to 150 mg, if needed. Behavior modification is another possibility [9].

Night Terrors (Pavor Nocturnus)

This condition, which runs in families, is commonest in children but it may also occur in adults. The affected child is often a sleepwalker. The child appears to awaken screaming and terrified, seems disoriented and does not recognize people, cannot be comforted, and is hard to awaken (if he is awakened, he cannot report a clear dream). The attack subsides after a few minutes, and the child falls back into a quiet sleep. When he awakens in the morning, he has no recollection of the night terror. These phenomena are understandable in light of the fact that this condition, like somnambulism and enuresis, occurs during stage 4 sleep. Bedtime benzodiazepines are the treatment of choice.

Night terrors must be distinguished from nightmares. The latter are anxiety-filled dreams which occur during REM sleep, and which can usually be remembered afterwards.

Sleep Deprivation

This is seen in patients in intensive care units, in people abusing amphetamines and cocaine, and in people who are compelled to stay awake under unusual circumstances. These include being on call in a medical service, participating in a sleep deprivation experiment, and being brainwashed in a prison camp. Signs and symptoms include fatigue, irritability, inability to concentrate, and consequent lapses of cognitive functioning [9].

Over 100 hr of sleeplessness may produce disorientation, illusions, and hallucinations; the hallucinations are typically visual or tactile. After 200 hr of sleeplessness, ptosis, nystagmus, and a find hand tremor have been noted [19]. The EEG is of low voltage, and production of 17-hydroxycorticosteroids is increased. Sleeping cures the condition [19].

REFERENCES

1. Bixler, E., Kales, A., Soldatos, C., Kales, J., and Healey, S. Prevalence of sleep disorders in the Los Angeles metopolitan area. *Am. J. Psychiatry* 136:1257-1262 (1979).
2. Kales, A., and Tan, T. Sleep alterations associated with medical illnesses, in *Sleep: Physiology and Pathology*. A.Kales, ed. Lippincott, Philadelphia (1969), pp. 148-157.
3. Hartmann, E. *The Sleeping Pill.* Yale, New Haven (1978).
4. Hartmann, E. Sleep, in *The Harvard Guide to Modern Psychiatry*. A. Nicholi, ed. Belknap, Harvard, Cambridge (1978).
5. Hartmann, E. *The Biology of Dreaming.* Thomas, Springfield, Ill. (1967).
6. Jouvet, M. The role of monoaminergic neurons in the regulation and function of sleep, in *Basic Sleep Mechanisms*. O. Petre-Quadens and J. Schlag, eds. Academic, New York (1974).
7. Broughton, R. Neurology and sleep research. *Can. Psychiatr. Assoc. J.* 16:283-293 (1971).
8. Williams, R., and Karacan, I. *Sleep Disorders: Diagnosis and treatment.* Wiley, New York (1978).
9. Kales, A., Malmstrom, E., Scharf, M., and Rubin, R. Psychophysiological and biochemical changes following use and withdrawal of hypnotics, in *Sleep: Physiology and pathology*. A. Kales ed.: Lippincott, Philadelphia (1969).
10. Hartmann, E., Cravens, J., and List, S. Hypnotic effects of L-tryptophan. *Arch. Gen. Psychiatry* 31:394-397 (1974).
11. Hartmann, E., and Spiniveber, C. Sleep induced by L-Tryptophan. Effects of dosages within the normal dietary intake. *J. Nerv. Ment. Dis.* 167:497-499 (1979).
12. Guilleminault, C., and Dement, W. 235 Cases of excessive daytime sleepiness. *J. Neurol. Sci.* 31:13 (1977).

13. Guilleminault, C. Cataplexy, in *Narcolepsy*. C. Guilleminault, W. Dement, and R. Passovant, eds. Spectrum, New York (1976).

14. Dement, W. Excessive daytime sleepiness. Paper presented at American Psychiatric Association Meeting, Toronto, May (1977).

15. Hauri, P. *The Sleep Disorders*. Upjohn, Kalamazoo (1977).

16. Guilleminault, C., Peraita, R., Souquet, M., and Dement, W. Apneas during sleep in infants. Possible relationship with SIDS. *Science* 190:677 (1965).

17. Dement, W., and Zarcone, V. Pharmacologic treatment of sleep disorders, in *Psychopharmacology: From theory to practice*. J. Barchas, P. Berger, R. Ciaranello, and G. Elliott, eds. Oxford, New York (1977).

18. Brathwaite, J. *Some problems connected with enuresis*. President's address. *Proc. R. Soc. Med.* 49:33 (1956).

19. Johnson, L. Psychological and physiologic changes following total sleep deprivation, in *Sleep: Physiology and pathology*. A. Kales ed. Lippincott, Philadelphia (1969).

7

Sex

FREDERICK SIERLES and EDWARD TYLER

INTRODUCTION

Human sexual behavior has many determinants, including the physiology of various organ systems, the physical and emotional health of the individuals, the relationship between the participants, and the social setting in which the sexual activity occurs. Inability to meet one's sexual expectations is a common source of discomfort. This may become disguised as a somatic illness for which the individual is inaccurately diagnosed and treated.

Some major contributions on the subject include Freud's theories of childhood sexuality [1], Kinsey's surveys of sexual behaviors in the general population [2], and Masters and Johnson's direct observations of the anatomy and physiology of people during sexual response [3-5]. The past three decades have witnessed the creation of sexual dysfunction clinics, the development of surgical procedures to treat certain sexual problems, the changing of attitudes about sexuality, the accumulation of a vast literature on human sexual performance, and the introduction of sex education for medical students and physicians.

SOCIAL ASPECTS

Since the late 1940s the "double standard," where men were encouraged to become sexually experienced and "proper" women were expected to be virgins until marriage, has been gradually replaced by a "convergence phenomenon." It is now more socially acceptable for women to masturbate, to "pet," to have intercourse outside of marriage, and to be the initiator of sexual activity. In a recent study of college women, a majority reported they had had intercourse by their senior year [6].

Of course longstanding, time-honored attitudes do not uniformly dissipate, and in traditional families among all socioeconomic, racial, and religious groups, more clear-cut sex role differentiations (i.e., what is expected of a woman as compared with a man) are more rigidly defined, with both partners accepting that the sexual needs of the man take priority over those of the woman. Also, the recognition of women as sexual beings, rather than as sexy objects, has precipitated significant conflicts in male-female relationships.

While women's rights activities have raised women's consciousness of their sexual as well as economic and political equality, sexual rights activities have not been limited to women's heterosexual freedoms. After years of hiding to avoid persecution, homosexuals took their fight for equality to the public, and the prestigious American Psychiatric Association removed homosexuality from its list of psychiatric diagnoses. Some public figures, including football player David Kopay [7], public health official Dr. Howard Brown [8], and playwright Tennessee Williams [9] announced their homosexuality. In 1977, Harvey Milk became the first publically acknowledged homosexual elected to public office (county supervisor in San Francisco). However, conflicts relating to homosexuality are still deep-rooted and may have accounted for Milk's assassination.

NEUROENDOCRINE ASPECTS

The neuroendocrine aspects of sexuality are complex and just beginning to be understood. The greatest vacuum is in causally relating overt sexual behavior with what is known endocrinologically. Although psychosocial influences on sexual behavior are vast, sexual function is also strongly influenced by neuroendocrine activity.

There is no "sex center" in the brain [10,11]. The diencephalon, limbic system, and cerebral cortex are all involved. Heath [12] wrote that electrical stimulation of the septum of the human brain could produce erotic sensations, and some of the subjects in his experiments voluntarily induced these erotic sensations when given the opportunity. Patients with temporal lobe epilepsy often manifest hyposexuality, although hypersexuality has been observed [13]. Frontal lobe dysfunction has been linked with inappropriate sexual behavior such as exhibitionism [14].

Understanding the role of the peripheral nervous system is complex and at times seems paradoxical. Penile and clitoral erection are functions of the parasympathetic nervous system, but ejaculation by the male is controlled by sympathetic nerves. Although penile and clitoral erection are usually initiated by cerebral function such as fantasy, many individuals with spinal cord transsections experience genital erectile function on a reflex basis as a result of local tactile stimulation. Those with prior-to-cord-injury sexual experience may even be able to experience orgasm.

The critical mechanism of neuroendocrine function is called feedback; the hypothalamus secretes hormones called releasing factors into the hypothalamic-pituitary portal vessel system. As a result, the anterior pituitary secretes gonadotropic hormones (e.g., follicle-stimulating hormone, FSH), which in turn stimulate target organs (e.g., the ovary), to produce hormones (e.g., estrogen). Feedback occurs when the circulating levels of the target organ's hormones affect the function of the hypothalamus and pituitary, resulting in alterations of levels of gonadotropic hormones; for example, an increase in circulating estrogen levels causes a decrease in the secretion of FSH.

Male and female patterns of gonadotropin and sex hormones secretion differ; the male pattern is tonic (continuous) and the female pattern is cyclic, the latter resulting in the biological rhythm of the menstrual cycle. The reasons for this difference are variable and multiple.

The brain plays an important role: In animal experiments, an ovary transplanted into a male animal continues to secrete estrogen, but does so in a tonic fashion. However, the brain is itself subject to hormonal influence: Administration of testosterone to female pig fetuses or to female rats several days after birth results in a tonic pattern of gonadotropin secretion [11].

Many behaviors of women appear to be related to phases of the menstrual cycle, although the causes of these variations are not understood. Forty-five percent of crimes committed by women, 46% of psychiatric admissions of women, 45% of instances of woman "calling in sick," 52% of all emergency room visits due to accidents, and 54% of all doctor visits by children brought in by their mothers, occur during the 4 premenstrual days and the first 4 days of menstruation [15]. Some women find it useful to let close family or intimate friends know their mood vulnerabilities during their menstrual cycles. Women report that their sexual functioning is frequently related to the cycle: Some report an increase in sexual enthusiasm during the first, or estrogen phase, of the menstrual cycle, often peaking at the time of ovulation; there is a slight tendency towards sexual withdrawal during the latter (luteal, progesterone) phase of the menstrual cycle [16]. However, the psychological meaning of sexual behavior may override the hormonal influences. To some women, premenstrual water retention may be associated with pelvic engorgement and be interpreted as sexual arousal. When a woman has been taught that sex is dirty but feels aroused, tension is a likely result of the conflict.

Testosterone stimulates sexual enthusiasm in both males and females, although it has no influence on sex object choice (who "turns one on"); For example, male homosexuals receiving testesterone for medical reasons experience increased sexual drive of a homosexual nature [10].

STAGES OF SEXUAL RESPONSE

For both sexes, there are four stages of sexual response: excitement, plateau, orgasm, and resolution [3,5].

Excitement

This is the initial stage, the stage of sexual arousal. Men have penile erection and elevation of the scrotal sac and testes. Women experience vaginal lubrication produced by transudation from the wall of the vagina. Their breasts show venous congestion, the nipples become erect, and the uterus ascends [3,5].

Plateau

There is intensification of sexual feeling and further physiological changes. Many (not all) males and females have a blotchy red, generalized, macular skin coloration, most prominently on the upper torso, which is called the sex flush, and which has been likened to a measles rash. Both sexes experience increased cardiovascular activity, with tachycardia sometimes as high as 175, systolic blood pressure increases of 10-40 mm, and an increased rate and intensity of respiration [17]. These visceral changes are usually more intense in the partner making the most thrusting actions, typically the one "on top." It is also more intensive when the partners have had limited experience with each other. Men continue to experience increased penile and testicular size. The woman's breasts increase slightly in size, the vaginal transudate becomes copious, the clitoral shaft withdraws within its prepuce, and the uterus contracts [3,5].

Orgasm

The intensity of sexual feeling reaches a climax. The sex flush remains. The pulse increases about 5 more beats per minute, the systolic rate increases. Perineal muscles contract rapidly, rhythmically, and involuntarily.

Males ejaculate, and there is a positive correlation between the quantity of ejaculate and the pleasure experienced. After ejaculation, there is a refractory period during which full erection, orgasm and ejaculation cannot occur. This varies in duration from a few minutes to hours. There is no refractory period in females, who are physiologically capable of multiple successive orgasms. In women, there are continued uterine contractions [3,5]. Is orgasm psychologically different for males and females? One study employing "blind" readings of volunteers' written descriptions of their emotions during orgasm failed to distinguish between descriptions by male and female volunteers.

Resolution

In this phase, which usually takes between 5 and 30 min, there is a return of all parameters to a baseline level [3,5].

MASTURBATION

Children begin playing with their genitals as early as the first year of life, but this is not usually considered masturbation until the child is over 3 years old. Masturbation can be a source of pleasure as any age, and a source of relief from anxiety as well as a sexual outlet. It may be a substitute for intercourse when a partner is unavailable, and/or a regular behavior among adults who are married or have an available sex partner. Because many people feel guilty about masturbation, and are fearful of its consequences, physicians' advice and council is frequently sought. Without hesitation the physician should assure the patient that there are no physically damaging consequences. Masturbation is used as a technique in the treatment of certain sexual dysfunctions [4,5,18,19]. To obtain sperm samples for infertility studies or artificial impregnation, the subject must masturbate. Of course, the physician must be curious when masturbation is the only source of sexual pleasure, used in preference to sharing pleasures with partners, or when it is performed compulsively. These latter situations require a psychosocial evaluation.

AGE AND SEX

It is commonly reported that the intensity of the physiological experience of sex is greatest for men in their late teens and for women in their thirties. Intercourse can and does occur among couples in geriatric age groups, including into the eighties and nineties, although there is a tendency for a decline in frequency of coitus after 60 [2]. In general, the greater the frequency and enjoyment of sex in early and midlife, the greater the frequency and enjoyment after 60 [2]. A major problem for many individuals over 65 is lack of a partner, particularly for women over 65, since they outnumber men over 65 by 138:100 [20]. When the individual has grown accustomed to sex only in a primary relationship, this adds yet another resistance to finding partners. On the other hand, boredom with sameness can decrease desire when couples remain in a very long monogamous relationship.

MENSTRUATION AND SEX

Intercourse can occur safely and pleasantly during the time of menstrual flow. This is also a time when conception is least likely. Many men and women feel less enthusiastic about sex during the time of menstruation. There is considerable ignorance about menstruation, regardless of class, cultural, or educational factors. Thoughtful preparation by a parent or older sibling about menstruation can alleviate anxiety about, and increase the acceptance of, menstruation and the menstrual cycle by adolescents of both sexes.

HOMOSEXUALITY

The frequency of exclusive homosexuality (Kinsey Scale 5 or 6 — see below) in the general population is probably about 4% [2,21]. It was formerly labeled an illness, which may psychiatrists felt originated in disturbed parent-child relationships.

Bieber [22] wrote that the majority of homosexuals hadn't had loving relationships with their fathers. He reported that some homosexuals sought treatment in hope of becoming heterosexual, claimed that psychoanalysis was the treatment of choice, and that 27% became exclusively heterosexual [22]. One problem with Bieber's research was that he saw a skewed sample which didn't represent the general homosexual population. The vast majority of homosexuals do not believe homosexuality is an illness and do not seek to become heterosexual.

Freud wrote that all humans were born with bisexual potential [1]. Both Kinsey [2] and Masters and Johnson [5] describe a spectrum of sexual object choice preference, using a scale of 0 (absolutely no homosexual experiences) to 3 (about an equal frequency of homosexual and heterosexual experiences) to 6 (exclusively homosexual). Recently, Masters and Johnson described a group they called ambisexual [5]. These are people in Kinsey category 3 who have sex with men and women with equal frequency, have no sex object preference, and prefer not to maintain committed sexual relationships with anyone.

In *Homosexuality in Perspective* [5], Masters and Johnson discuss sexual response in homosexuals. They found that (1) the anatomy and physiology of sexual response was the same for homosexuals as for heterosexuals; (2) committed homosexual couples were more verbally expressive about their needs during lovemaking than committed heterosexual couples; (3) committed homosexual couples were more apt to engage in preorgasmic teasing than committed heterosexual couples, the latter being more concerned with getting right to coitus; (4) homosexuals experienced heterosexual sex fantasies and heterosexuals had homosexual fantasies; and (5) some homosexuals experienced sexual dysfunctions. Masters and Johnson do point out that their sample of volunteers was skewed, having been selected on the basis of prior effective sexual functioning, and being volunteers.

Homosexuals have been discriminated against in some cultures for centuries, while other cultures accepted homosexuality and bisexuality during certain phases of development.

Physicians must recognize that "gay" individuals are as sensitive about their life style choices as anyone else. Gays also suffer from the same illnesses and seek the same quality of care as "straight" people.

Table 1 is a list compiled by Masters and Johnson [5] of the fantasies most frequently experienced by both homosexual and heterosexual individuals.

Table 2 is useful for considering the differences between heterosexuality, homosexuality, transsexuality, and transvestitism (i.e., cross-dressing).

Table 1   Comparative Content of Fantasy Material:
Frequency of Occurrence

Homosexual male (N = 30)	*Heterosexual male (N = 30)*
1. Imagery of sexual anatomy	1. Replacement of established partner
2. Forced sexual encounters	2. Forced sexual encounter
3. Cross-preference encounters	3. Observation of sexual activity
4. Idyllic encounters with unknown men	4. Cross-preference encounters
5. Group sex experiences	5. Group sex experiences
Homosexual female (N = 30)	*Heterosexual female (N = 30)*
1. Forced sexual encounters	1. Replacement of established partner
2. Idyllic encounter with established partner	2. Forced sexual encounter
3. Cross-preference encounters	3. Observation of sexual activity
4. Recall of past sexual experiences	4. Idyllic encounters with unknown men
5. Sadistic imagery	5. Cross-preference encounters

Source: From W. Masters and V. Johnson. *Homosexuality in Perspective.* Little, Brown, Boston, 1979, with permission (Ref. 5).

Table 2   Sexual Variations

	Anatomy	Identification	Dress	Love object
Heterosexual	Same	Same	Same	Opposite
Homosexual	Same	Same	Same	Same
Transsexual	Same	Opposite	Opposite	Same
Transvestite	Same	Same	Opposite	Opposite

For example, a male homosexual has the anatomy of a male, identifies himself as a male, dresses as a male, and prefers a male sexual partner.

SEXUAL PROBLEMS

In the course of the average primary care physician's practice, he will be confronted with a number of persons complaining of sexual problems. Ninety percent of these will be unrelated to medical illness or side effects of medication.

Problems Due to Drugs [8]

Chlorpromazine (Thorazine), throridazine (Mellaril) and mesoridazine (Serentil) can produce impotence or failure to ejaculate ("dry orgasm"). α-Methyldopa (Aldomet), guanethidine (Ismelin), phenoxybenzamine (Dibenzyline), mecamylamine (Inolesine), pentolinium (Ansolysen), and rauwolfia (Reserpine) can all produce impotence or disinterest [18]. Chronic opioid abuse can diminish sex drive, and intoxication with large amounts of alcohol can produce temporary impotence; however, one drink may alleviate inhibitions, allowing better sexual functioning. Disulfiram (Antabuse) can be associated with impotence [23]. None of these substances produces permanent sexual dysfunction, so the treatment of the dysfunction is to withhold the medication.

Disease That May Cause Sexual Dysfunction

Impotence is common in diabetics. Sometimes it is due to pathology of peripheral nerves which initiate erection. It can also result from occlusion of the aortic bifurcation (Leriche syndrome), and from psychological causes such as predicting poor performance.

It helps to ask the patient if he has morning erections, or can masturbate. If he does, his perineal nerves and vascular function are probably intact. Leriche syndrome requires surgery. Impotence from performance anxiety is treated by sex therapy (to be described later).

Disease of the cauda equina can produce sexual dysfunction. There is a high frequency of sexual disinterest in endogenous depressions, where the treatment of choice is electroconvulsive therapy. Mania is often associated with hypersexuality, which can overtax and distress the manic patient's partner. Painful intercourse can be caused by a number of conditions, many of which are listed in Table 3 [19].

Disinterest in Sex Due to Acute Medical Illness [24]

People who have acute medical illnesses may not be interested in sex because they are preoccupied with, or disabled by, their medical condition. The physician's task is to treat the medical illness; sexual enthusiasm should return as the medical condition resolves.

Physical Incapacity with Desire to Have Sex [25]

In many chronic medical conditions, usual sexual behaviors (e.g., the "missionary" position) are awkward, painful, or embarrassing. Examples include bone fractures, colostomies and paraplegia. The physician must do more than treat the primary medical illness; he must also give the patient and his partner "permission" to experiment with different sexual techniques and positions.

Although patients with anatomic or functional spinal cord transsections (e.g., paraplegics and quadriplegics) have genital cutaneous anesthesia and may be unable to initiate genital physiological changes by mental imagery, many can have genital physiological responses by way of reflexes initiated by touching the area. Patients with catheters may remove and replace them with sterile technique, or position the catheter to minimize its blockage of the sex act [25]: Women can bend it upwards, and men can fold it within a lubricated condom [25]. Here, the intercourse should be gentle to avoid trauma.

There is no evidence that marriages of paraplegics or quadriplegics to able-bodied spouses are less stable or less sexually gratifying than other marriages [24]. There are several good educational films available to patients and physicians that deal with the sexuality of paraplegics and quadriplegics.

Fear of the Consequences of Sex on General Health [24]

Many patients with serious medical illnesses, or their sexual partners,

Table 3   Pelvic Causes of Painful Intercourse for Women and Men

WOMEN

Trauma
Torn hymen
Vaginal or perineal damage from rape
Vaginal or cervical lacerations
Torn broad ligaments

Infection or Inflammation
Enlargement of Bartholin glands
Vaginal or cervical infection
Pelvic and inflammatory disease
Endometriosis

Surgery
Postepisiotomy
Postvaginal repair
Postsurgical complications from tumors,
    cyst, or cancer

Other factors
Clitoral irritation from adhesions or smegma
    under the foreskin
Postmenopausal sensitivity
Rash from contraceptive cream, jellies,
    suppositories, foam, foam tablets,
    douche powders, condoms, or diaphragms,
    poison ivy, herpes

Treatment
Postradiation atrophy
Postmenopausal atrophy

MEN

Sensitivity of the glans following
    ejaculation
Irritation of the foreskin from infection
Phimosis
Skin sensitivity—dermatitis

Prostatitis, urethritis, epidedymitis
Trauma to the penis with posttraumatic
    angulation of the penis
Prolonged foreplay
Peyronie's disease
Hydrocele
Poison ivy, herpes

Source: From D. Kentsmith and M. Eaton. *Treating Sexual Problems in Medical Practice.* Arco, New York, 1979, with permission (Ref. 18).

perceive intercourse as very risky, and may fear that having intercourse is tantamount to committing suicide (e.g., the patient may "die in the saddle"). Some cardiac patients experience impotence as a result of this kind of thinking. It is important for the physician to know the risks and to initiate discussion about activity guidelines. Wagner [17], citing Hellerstein and Friedman [26], writes:

> . . . for the middle-class long-married man, the physiologic cost of sexual activity is modest, especially when compared to the physiologic impact of sexuality upon young volunteers in laboratory settings. Heart rate response with the older patients was minimal, with peak heart rate averaging 117.4 per min (range 90-140) . . . Responses are similar to those observed in the same individuals during regular daily activity such as driving a car, discussing business matters, or climbing one or two flights of stairs.

Ueno [27] writes that in deaths in the saddle the victim is usually a middle-aged or older man having an affair with a much younger woman in a clandestine setting. Various criteria have been used to decide when a patient can resume intercourse after myocardial infarction; Wagner [17] states that sexual intercourse can resume when the patient is cleared to climb a flight of stairs or resume work. Eliot and Miles [28] write, "If a heart patient can walk on a treadmill at 3 or 4 M.P.H., or climb stairs, or do a single Masters' test asymptomatically and without EKG charges, his exercise capacity exceeds demands required for sexual intercourse." Masturbation can be a useful first reassuring sexual activity, and in fact is often engaged in spontaneously while the patient is still hospitalized [17].

Pregnancy, while certainly not an illness, sometimes evokes similar fears. Butler and Wagner [29], reviewing sexuality during pregnancy and postpartum, state:

1. Although one study revealed a relationship between premature labor and multiple orgasms during pregnancy, there is no evidence that coitus to single orgasm in the first two trimesters, or coitus without orgasm until the 34th week, presents a risk to the mother or fetus in an uncomplicated pregnancy.

2. Between the 13th and 34th weeks the side-by-side or rear entry positions are generally more comfortable and popular.

3. When the fetal head becomes engaged between the 34th and 38th weeks, coitus may produce considerable discomfort, so other forms of sexual activity should be considered.

4. Cunnilingus is a good substitute. An infrequently used form of cunnilingus, where the man blows air into the vagina, has been linked to several maternal deaths due to embolism, and should therefore be avoided.

5. The risk of maternal infection associated with intercourse is increased late in gestation in women with an incompetent cervical os, ruptured membranes, or an effaced or dilated cervix.

6. Sex should be avoided if there is vaginal bleeding; the bleeding should be reported immediately to the doctor.

7. Once the episiotomy is healed (2-4 weeks postpartum), the couple can resume sex.

Nonsexual Interpersonal Problems

Sex can be pleasurable for a couple not in love, but the pleasure of intimate involvement is missing. Sex as an expression of love rather than as an athletic event is a distinctly different experience for a majority of humans.

Many couples refuse to have sex after an argument, while others use sex as a means of "patching things up." Refusal of sex may be a means of punishing a partner, or a way of controlling the relationship. Medical illness can be used as an excuse to avoid sex. In the latter three situations, marital counseling may help.

Mild Sexual Problems

The majority of sex problems have little to do with systemic medical illness; other causes have been postulated. Fear of pregnancy is one, and education about reproductive physiology and and contraception may be helpful. However, individuals who are knowledgeable about reproductive physiology and contraception may also become unnecessarily worried. Many individuals view coitus as a means of proving masculinity, femininity, attractiveness, or desirability, rather than as an activity whose primary goal is one's sensual pleasure. Sex acquires the quality of a performance, which when the *partner* is not satisfied, tends to be viewed as a personal failure. Thus, there can be anxiety during initial "performances," or anxiety following a previous performance viewed as a failure. In cases of one-or-two episode impotence, lack of lubrication, or lack of orgasm due to performance anxiety, the physician should (1) reassure the patient that this is a common experience and that there is no evidence that this will become a longstanding problem requiring sex therapy, and (2) tell the person he should give himself permission to "hang loose" and enjoy giving and receiving sensual pleasure rather than "performing on the sexual athletic field."

Partners should be encouraged to communicate their needs and preferences. Thus, "selfish" needs of each partner can be met in the mutual experience, but only if they are known.

More Complex Sexual Dysfunctions

Certain sexual dysfunctions should be referred to a trained sex therapist. A number of cities have sexual dysfunction clinics and programs for training sex therapists, and will accept nonpsychiatric physicians and other professionals as trainees. Some of the complex sex dysfunctions treated in these clinics include premature ejaculation, vaginismus, orgasmic dysfunctions, and impotence.

In the treatment of these dysfunctions, the couple contract ("doctor's orders") not to engage in coitus during the initial phases of treatment. This removes the demand for performance, and enables the couple to concentrate on enjoyment, on expression of needs, and on specific therapeutic exercises.

Premature Ejaculation

In *premature ejaculation,* the man "comes" almost immediately after penetration, much too soon for full enjoyment by both partners. This is treated by teaching the couple either a *squeeze technique* [4,18,19] or a stop-start [19] method. The old method of encouraging the man to concentrate on nonsexual matters, such as multiplication tables, is no longer used. In both the squeeze technique and the stop-start method, the couple first learns "ejaculatory control" as the woman masturbates the man. As the man enters the late plateau phase, and senses orgasm approaching, he tells his partner. At this point, in the squeeze technique, the woman grasps the penis at the frenulum between her thumb and forefinger; this stops the progression to orgasm. At this time, in the stop-start method, the couple simply stops the masturbation. Then the masturbation, and its cessation, is repeated several times. This increases tolerance of sexual stimulation and arousal. At the end of the session, the man is masturbated to orgasm and the woman, if she chooses, is stimulated or brought to orgasm noncoitally. After the therapist and the couple feel that the couple has reached ejaculatory control in masturbation, a similar process is repeated, whereby repeated coital penetration is followed by plateau-phase squeeze or stop-start termination. At the end of the session, the man may ejaculate intravaginally. By the end of this phase of the treatment, ejaculatory control is sufficient for sex to be resumed as desired. If the premature ejaculation recurs, the couple returns to the earlier exercises.

Vaginismus

This condition is characterized by involuntary contraction of the woman's paravaginal muscles whenever penile penetration is attempted. The woman and her partner should be reassured that the vaginismus is not voluntary—that it doesn't represent rejection of the man. The treatment is to desensitize the woman to having something inserted in her vagina [4,18,19]. She is instructed to insert one of her fingers into her vagina; when she can do this comfortably, she proceeds to two fingers, and so on until she can insert five fingers. After she can do this comfortably, her partner inserts one finger, and progresses from one to five digits. After this, he can then insert his penis. If the woman is squeamish about using her fingers, the physician may use Hegar dilators [4,18,19] of increasing size.

Orgasmic Dysfunction

For women, dysfunctions in experiencing sexual pleasure range from lack of pleasure in any sex play, to lack of orgasm under any circumstances, to having orgasm by masturbation or oral sex but not by coitus, to frequency of orgasm not frequent enough for her satisfaction. All of these can be categorized as orgasmic dysfunction. Of course, considerable pleasure can and does occur without orgasm, and treatment for the woman is indicated only if her expectations are not being met. The meaning of orgasm for the woman must be investigated; some women may be anxious about "losing control"; some see orgasm as a "success" and may feel trepidation about being successful; others may feel guilt about having sexual pleasure, having been warned as teenagers about "going too far." It is essential that she learns to accept her own orgasms as natural biological process over which she has the right of control.

For women who experience almost no pleasure in sex play of any type, and wish to experience this pleasure, treatment consists of recommending the following progression of sessions [19]:

1. As she lies prone in bed, she instructs her partner to stroke and caress her body in whatever manner she chooses, while learning at what locations the stroking is most enjoyable. It is a rare person who derives no pleasure from stroking and caressing by a partner.

2. In later sessions, she lies supine and again requests stroking in nongenital areas at her pleasure.

3. Then she asks for stroking of her genitals in a manner of her choosing, while penile penetration still not permitted.

4. Next, the couple is to have "nondemand coitus": When the woman feels stimulated and lubricated by her partner's stroking, she takes the female superior (woman-on-top) position, places his penis inside her vagina, and thrusts in whatever manner she chooses, her own pleasure being the only objective. There may be several rest periods in which the penis is removed. Each session ends when the woman has an orgasm (an infrequent occurrence at this point) or has had enough for that encounter.

5. In the concluding sessions, once the woman has been erotically responsive from nondemand coitus, the couple's goal is coitus with orgasm for both partners. As before, the woman must have the right to take the lead by expressing her wishes and by controlling the pace and method of the pelvic thrusting.

For the woman who experiences erotic responsiveness in the excitement and plateau phases, but no orgasm, the procedure is somewhat different [18,19]. In early sessions, she is encouraged to masturbate alone for pleasure. The therapist should make sure that she is aware of her genital anatomy, and that she includes clitoral stimulation as part of the process. In this phase, her partner is to be absent and there is no coitus. Once she can masturbate to orgasm alone, her partner masturbates her to orgasm in the next sessions. This should include clitoral stimulation, and other genital and nongenital teasing, which she is to direct at her pleasure, but no intercourse. Several techniques are applied at this point [19]. First, after the sessions when the woman masturbates to orgasm, the couple has sessions in which they have coitus, and then the woman masturbates to orgasm in her partner's presence, followed by sessions in which he masturbates her to orgasm. In the final sessions, nondemand coitus, using the female-superior position with the woman directing the activity, should lead to orgasm. If not, a "bridge maneuver" is used, where the couple has coitus while the woman simultaneously masturbates herself by clitoral stimulation, or has her partner simultaneously masturbate her by clitoral stimulation. Some women will never experience coital orgasm but will be very satisfied with pre- or postintercourse masturbatory orgasms given to herself or by her partner.

Impotence

This male sexual dysfunction has no identifiable physical cause about 85% of the time [19]. The treatment is similar to that of lack of sexual enjoyment for a woman. The first sessions involve nongenital "pleasuring" (stroking and caressing) by the woman with the man in the prone position. Here, and in future exercises, the man determines what is pleasurable for *him*. The next sessions emphasize nongenital pleasuring with the man in the supine position. In the exercises that follow, the woman strokes the man's genitals until he experiences erections, but penile penetration and coitus are forbidden. In the next exercises, the woman sits upright, and places his penis in her vagina to let him experience vaginal containment, but makes no demand for her satisfaction. Subsequently, he will thrust for his own pleasure, but not to ejaculation. In the final exercises, he will engage in penile thrusting, at a pace which he chooses for his own pleasure, until he ejaculates. Next he attempts to engage in mutual orgasmic satisfaction. If impotence occurs during any of the later sessions, the couple returns to earlier sequences.

REFERENCES

1. Freud, S. *Three Contributions to the Theory of Sex.* Dutton, New York (1962).
2. Kinsey, A., Pomeroy, W., and Martin, C. *Sexual Behavior in the Human Male.* Saunders, Philadelphia (1948).
3. Masters, W., and Johnson, V. *Human Sexual Response.* Little, Brown, Boston (1966).
4. Masters, W.. and Johnson, V. *Human Sexual Inadequacy.* Little, Brown, Boston (1970).
5. Masters, W., and Johnson, V. *Homosexuality in Perspective.* Little, Brown, Boston (1979).
6. Oswalt, R. Sexual contraceptive behavior of college females. *J. Am. Coll. Health Assoc.* 22:329 (1974).

7. Kopay, D., and Young, P. *The David Kopay Story*. Arbor, New York (1977).

8. Brown, H. *Familiar Faces, Hidden Lives*. Harcourt, Brace, Jovanovich, New York (1976).

9. Williams, T. *Memoirs*. Bantam (1976).

10. Morris, N. *The Neuroendocrinology of Sexuality*. Unpublished manuscript (1978).

11. Money, J., and Ehrhardt, A. *Man and Woman, Boy and Girl*. Johns Hopkins, Baltimore (1972).

12. Heath, R. Pleasure response of human subjects to direct stimulation of the brain. Physiologic and psychodynamic considerations, in *The Role of Pleasure in Behavior*. R. Health, ed. Hoeber, New York (1964).

13. Bear, D., and Fedio, P. Quantitative analysis of interictal behavior in temporal lobe epilepsy. *Arch. Gen. Neurol.* 34:454-467 (1977).

14. Sherwin, I., and Geschwind, N. Neural substrates of behavior, in *The Harvard Guide to Modern Psychiatry*. A. Nicholi, ed. Harvard, Cambridge (1978).

15. Sherman, J. *On the Psychology of Women: A survey of empirical studies*. Thomas, Springfield, Ill. (1971).

16. Benedek, T. *Psychoanalytic Investigations*. Quadrangle, New York (1973).

17. Wagner, N. Sexuality and the cardiac patient, in *Human Sexuality: A health practicioner's text*. R. Green, ed. Williams and Wilkins, Baltimore (1975).

18. Kentsmith, D., and Eaton, M. *Treating Sexual Problems in Medical Practice*. Arco, New York (1979).

19. Kaplan, H. *The Illustrated Manual of Sex Therapy*. Quadrangle, New York (1975).

20. Brotman, H. Who are the aging? In *Mental Illness in Later Life*. E. Busse and E. Pfeiffer, eds. Am. Psychiatr. Assoc., Washington, D.C. (1973).

21. Marmor, J. Homosexuality and sexual orientation disturbances, in *Comprehensive Textbook of Psychiatry*, Vol. II. A. Friedman, H. Kaplan, and B. Sadock, eds. Williams and Wilkins, Baltimore (1975).

22. Bieber, I. (ed.). *Homosexuality in Perspective*. Random, New York (1962).

23. *Physician's Desk Reference*. Medical Economics, Oradell, N.J. (1979).

24. Tyler, E. Sex and medical illness, in *Comprehensive Textbook of Psychiatry*, Vol. II. A. Freedman, H. Kaplan, and B. Saddock, eds. Williams and Wilkins, Baltimore (1975).

25. Cole, T. Sexuality and the spinal cord injured, in *Human Sexuality: A health practitioner's text*. R. Green, ed. Williams and Wilkins, Baltimore (1975).

26. Hellerstein, H., and Friedman, E. Sexual activity and the post coronary patient. *Arch. Intern. Med.* 125:987-999 (1970).

27. Ueno, M. The so-called coition death. *Jap. J. Legal Med.* 17:333 (1967).

28. Eliot, R., and Miles, R. Advising the cardiac patient about sexual intercourse. *Med. Aspects Hum. Sexual.* 9:49-50 (1975).

29. Butler, J., and Wagner, N. Sexuality during pregnancy and postpartum, in *Human Sexuality: A health practitioner's text*. R. Green, ed. Williams and Wilkins, Baltimore (1975).

8

Psychopathology

FREDERICK SIERLES

INTRODUCTION

A disease is a tissue and organ malfunction with the potential for producing discomfort, disability, or death. What society considers a disease also plays a part. For example, the dermatosis dyschromic spirochetosis (pinta) is not considered a disease in certain South American tribes; in these tribes, having the skin discolorations of pinta increases marriageability [1].

A disease is identified, classified, and distinguished from other diseases when it shows characteristic patterns in the following areas [2-4]:

1. Causes
2. Demographic and family patterns
3. Signs and symptoms
4. Lab findings
5. Response to treatment
6. Prognosis

A syndrome is a group of symptoms, signs, and lab findings which tend to occur together. Examples include hypertension, chronic renal failure, delirium, major depression, nephrotic syndrome, mental retardation, and carpal tunnel syndrome. The difference between a syndrome and a disease is that a syndrome does not have a known predominant cause; for example, the syndrome of mental retardation (impaired performance of tasks of daily living due to intellectual impairment originating during child development) is associated with many diseases (e.g., phenylketonuria, Down's syndrome) with definite causes (e.g., autosomal recessive inheritance, trisomy 21). Sometimes, a syndrome is composed both of diseases and more-precisely-defined syndromes; for example, the syndrome hypertension is associated with (among other abnormalities) the disease pheochromocytoma and the syndrome essential hypertension.

RELIABILITY AND VALIDITY OF DIAGNOSIS

By requiring proof of cause if we are to call a condition a disease, we see that many medical conditions are syndromes. Applying this standard to psychiatry, we see that, with the exception of many of the coarse brain diseases, the major psychiatric conditions are syndromes.

A genetic causal component has been demonstrated by adoption studies in major affective illnesses [5], schizophrenia [6,7], sociopathy [8], and alcoholism (in men) [9]. Based on twin studies, a genetic causal component appears possible in the neuroses [10]. However, additional nongenetic causes of these syndromes can be inferred from the data as well; the primacy of genetic causation has not been established as it has for phenylketonuria, Down's syndrome, Huntington's chorea, and hemophilia.

Critics of psychiatric diagnosis [2,11], with varying objectivity and vehemence, have questioned the validity of identifying some or all of the conditions "assigned" to psychiatry as biologically discrete syndromes. Some of this criticism has been fair for, prior to the 1960s, systems of diagnostic classification were based upon clinical "impression," not scientific studies. Of course, it is important to start with clinical impressions in developing diagnostic classifications. But unless impressions undergo scientific scrutiny, anybody can claim anything for his or her diagnoses and treatments.

Reliability

For a diagnosis to be valid, the diagnostic system must be reliable. This means that different observers using the sasme system on the same patients will usually make the same diagnosis. If reliability is demonstrated for a set of criteria, and the criteria are applied conscientiously, then medical communications and conclusions have more meaning. For example, if a physician reports that a group of patients with primary affective disorder, depression, according to Washington-St. Louis criteria [3,12], responds a certian way to electroconvulsive therapy, then the reader can easily comprehend the effectiveness of electroconvulsive therapy (ECT) in that series of patients. Before research criteria, diagnosis was less meaningful. Journal readers read articles with statements like "A diagnosis of schizophrenia was made for these patients by two board-certified psychiatrists and one board-eligible psychiatrist," as if the psychiatrists' credentials were all that was required.

Table 1   Agreement Between Two Raters Using Research Diagnostic Criteria for the Diagnosis of Schizophrenia

Diagnostic system	Kappa	Percentage of sample diagnosed schizophrenic by both raters
New Haven Schizophrenic Index	0.83	42
(Carpenter and Strauss)		
4 items	0.69	29
5 items	0.53	11
6 items	0.64	6
7 items	0.47	3
Washington University (Feighner)	0.87	11
Taylor-Abrams (Modification of Feighner)	1.00	6
Research Diagnostic Criteria		
Schizophrenia and schizoaffective disorders	0.83	44
Schizophrenia only	0.72	14
Schizoaffective only	0.61	22

Source: From R. Spitzer, J. Fleiss, and J. Endicott. Problems of classification in *Psychopharmacology: A Generation of Progress.* M. Lipton, A. DiMascio, and K. Kellain, eds. Raven, 1978, with permission (Ref. 14).

A number of groups, listed in Table 1 [13], created research criteria and subjected them to interrater reliability studies. Tests for interrater reliability include (1) percentage of agreement, (2) "specific agreement," and (3) "weighted kappa," the latter being the best because it takes chance agreement into account [13]. The formula for weighted kappa is $K = (P_0/1 - P_c)$, where P_0 is the percentage of interrater agreement and $P_c =$ the probability of chance agreement. A K of 1.0 means perfect agreement: Satisfactory Ks range from .7 to 1.0. Kappas for the diagnosis of schizophrenia by five systems are listed in Table 1 [14]. These results are on a par with those of a number of studies in other branches of medicine, and are better than some [15-19].

Validity

Evidence for validity of some syndromes has come from twin and adoption studies, family and sex distributions, signs and symptoms, lab tests, response to treatment, and prognosis.

A tendency in families has been established for major affective disorders, schizophrenia, sociopathy, Briquet's syndrome, alcoholism, drug dependence, and the neuroses. Major affective disorders, Briquet's syndrome, and the neuroses are more common in women, and schizophrenia, sociopathy, alcoholism, and drug dependence are more common in men.

There are laboratory tests for some psychiatric syndromes which reportedly can help distinguish between disorders. These include infusion of sodium lactate for diagnosing anxiety neurosis (lactate infusion precipitates anxiety attacks in anxiety neurotics) [20]; administration of oral lithium, with measurement of subsequent 36-hr urine lithium excretion, for diagnosing mania (manics retain lithium more than others) [21]; the sedation threshold test for distinguishing reactive from endogenous depression (reactively depressed people are less readily sedated by amobarbital than are endogenously depressed patients) [22]; the penetration into, and efflux from, red blood cells by lithium as a test for major affective disorders (patients with major affective disorders have a higher RBC lithium index) [23]; and the dexamethasone suppression test for identifying endogenous depression (endogenously depressed patients respond minimally to attempted suppression of the pituitary gland by dexamethasone) [24].

Most of these tests are not used routinely for a number of reasons, which include lack of familiarity of physicians with the existence of these tests; lack of absolute diagnostic specificity; and conflicting results obtained in studies attempting to replicate results of the amytal sedation threshold test, lactate infusion test, and RBC lithium index. Because of its recently-documented [24] specificity and ease of administration, the dexamethasone suppression test will likely become popular.

Response to treatment helps establish diagnostic validity. Eighty percent of manic patients respond well to lithium, but few schizophrenics do. Patients with major affective disorders respond well to electroconvulsive therapy, and 85% of patients with major depression become asymptomatic with ECT, but reactively depressed people and schizophrenics do not [25]. Patients with major depression respond well to tricyclic antidepressants 50-70% of the time [25], but patients with reactive depression rarely benefit [26]. Patients with either sociopathy [2] or Briquet's syndrome do not respond well to any known treatment [2].

Prognosis is important. For a syndrome to be considered a separate biological entity, followup should reveal that patients either have improved or manifest the syndrome first diagnosed. Continuity over time has been demonstrated for schizophrenia [2,27,28], sociopathy [28], Briquet's syndrome [29], alcoholism [29], drug dependence [29], major affective disorders [30], obsessive-compulsive neurosis [31], and phobic neurosis [32].

The case of so-called "good-prognosis schizophrenia" and "bad-prognosis schizophrenia" is a classic example of the use of prognosis and other criteria for establishing validity. Several groups observed that some patients with schizophrenia improved over time (good prognosis) and some failed to improve (poor prognosis) [4,8,27]. They found that the two groups could be differentiated by other characteristics as well: Those with good prognosis were more likely to have a family history of affective disorder, good pre-morbid adjustment, acute onset, a broad affect, and confusion; those with poor prognosis had family histories of schizophrenia, schizoid premorbid adjustment, insidious onset, a blunted affect, and clear consciousness. This strongly suggested that the good prognosis and poor prognosis conditions were separate syndromes. Later, other researchers, applying the above-mentioned standards for validity, found that patients with good prognosis schizophrenia were indistinguishable from patients with major affective disorders; thus, good-prognosis schizophrenia was not a separate biological entity [33].

SPECIFIC SYNDROMES

In discussing syndromes, I will use the criteria I use in my own practice, applying Taylor and Abrams [34] criteria to some syndromes, and Washington-St. Louis criteria to others [3,12]. I must add that *at least* 20% (the figure quoted by the Washington-St. Louis group) of patients do not meet research criteria. In such cases, the patient should be treated from the perspectives that (1) life-threatening situations (e.g., acute coarse brain disease, suicidal intent) must be ruled out and, if present, treated immediately; and (2) when symptoms and signs of two major disorders coexist in the same patient (the commonest dilemma is between schizophrenia and major affective illness), treat for the syndrome with the better prognosis (e.g. the major affective illness) and the more benign treatment (e.g., lithium is more benign than neuroleptics in terms of long-range side effects). Interrater reliability of Washington-St. Louis criteria for 12 syndromes are listed in Table 2 [15].

MAJOR AFFECTIVE SYNDROMES

Mania (Manic Episode)

Mania occurs in about .1% of the population [35]. It is commoner in women than in men, and runs in families. Inclusion criteria (criteria which must be met for the diagnosis to be certain) are motor hyperactivity, rapid or pressured speech, a euphoric, expansive or irritable mood, and a broad (not blunted) affect [34]. Exclusion criteria (conditions which must be ruled out) are coarse brain disease, psychostimulant drug abuse in the past month, and systemic illnesses known to produce manic symptoms [34]. Other symptoms seen in mania are in Table 3 [36]. Untreated manic episodes have a mean duration of about 6 months. Many patients with initial manic episodes

Table 2   Interrater Diagnostic Agreement (With and Without Undiagnosed
Patients) of Washington-St. Louis Criteria

	Kappa	
Diagnosis	All patients	Excluding undiagnosed
Depression	.55	.70
Mania	.82	.93
Anxiety neurosis	.76	.84
Schizophrenia	.58	.66
Antisocial personality	.81	.85
Alcoholism	.74	.73
Drug dependence	.84	.85
Hysteria (female subjects only)	.72	.72
Obsessional illness	.78	.79
Homosexuality	.85	.79
Organic brain syndrome	.29	.36
Average concordance	.66	.75

Source: From J. Helzer, R. Clayton, R. Pambikian, T. Reich, R. Woodruff and M. Reveley. Reliability of psychiatric diagnosis. *Arch. Gen. Psychiatry* 34:136-141, 1977, with permission (Ref. 15).

develop major depression some time later. The significance of this will be discussed later.

Lithium carbonate, in a starting dose of 1,200-1,800 mg/day, is the treatment of choice, although haloperidol or ECT may have be used for severe irritability or combativeness, or if the patient refuses to take lithium. Lithium carbonate should be prescribed prophylactically after the acute episode resolves.

Major (Endogenous) Depression (Major Depressive Episode)

This syndrome occurs in about 1-2% of the population [35,37] and is commoner in women than in man [35]. Inclusion of criteria are (1) a sustained sad, dysphoric, or anxious mood, and (2) three of the following six: early morning awakening; diurnal mood swing, anorexia with a weight loss of at least 5 lb in the 3 previous weeks; motor retardation or agitation; suicidal thoughts or behavior; and feelings of guilt, self-reproach, hopelessness or worthlessness. Exclusion criteria are (1) coarse brain disease, (2) use of reserpine or steroids within the past month, and (3) medical illnesses known to cause depressive symptoms. Untreated, the mean duration of major depression is 9 months. The treatment of choice is ECT, with six to eight treat-

Table 3   Frequency of Various Symptoms in 52 Manic Patients

Symptoms	% Patients affected
Mood disorder	100
Irritable	80.8
Expansive	65.5
Euphoric	30.8
Labile, with depression	28.8
Hyperactivity	100
Rapid/pressured speech	100
Flight-of-ideas	76.9
Grandiose delusions	59.6
Assaultive/threatening behavior	48.1
Incomplete auditory hallucinations	48.1
Persecutory delusions	42.3
Confusion	32.7
Singing/dancing	32.7
Head decoration	32.7
Autochthonous ideas	26.9
Visual hallucinations	26.9
Nudity/sexual exposure	23.1
Fecal incontinence/smearing	19.2
Olfactory hallucinations	15.4
Catatonia (posturing, catalepsy, mannerisms, sterotypes, automatic cooperation)	13.5
First-rank symptoms of Schneider	11.5

Source: From M. Taylor and R. Abrams. The phenomenology of mania. *Arch. Gen. Psychiatry* 29:520–522, 1973, with permission (Ref. 36).

ments usually sufficing. If the patient refuses ECT, tricyclic antidepressants or lithium may be effective.

Many people with initial depressive episodes have manic episodes some time later, and vice versa. There is a sizeable literature dividing the major affective syndromes into "bipolar" disorder (one or more episodes of mania, with or without episodes of major depressoin), and "unipolar" affective illness (major depressions only, no episodes of mania). The problem with this dichotomy is twofold: (1) there are many relatives with bipolar illness in the families of patients with unipolar illness, and vice versa, and (2) lithium carbonate produces similar clinical responsivity to both acute and maintenance treatment for people with unipolar affective illness as well as for bipolar affective illness [35].

Schizophrenia

This is the most overdiagnosed condition in American psychiatry; I was taught as a resident that 50% of hospitalized psychiatric patients had it. This error results from applying criteria that are too broad, allowing good-prognosis schizophrenia (see pages 96 and 97) to be included with poor-prognosis schizophrenia. Using narrower (and more valid) criteria, a number of researchers have established that schizophrenia occurs in about .6% of the population, 2-3% of relatives of schizophrenics, and 5-6% of hospitalized psychiatric patients [34]. It is commoner in men than in women.

Inclusion criteria are: (1) clear consciousness with intact memory and orientation; and (2) at least one of the following: emotional blunting, a formal thinking disorder, or one or more first-rank signs of Schneider. Exclusion criteria are: (1) diagnosable major affective disorder, (2) coarse brain disease, (3) use of hallucinogens or stimulant drugs, and (4) systemic illness known to cause psychiatric symptoms [34]. Electroencephalographic, computerized tomographic, and aphasia screening test abnormalities are common [38,39].

The treatment of choice is a neuroleptic. The prognosis is poor, and there is a high risk of irreversible extrapyramidal side effects due to continuous neuroleptic use.

Coarse Brain Disease (Organic Mental Disorder)

Another for coarse brain disease is "organic brain disease," which is misleading because it implies that there are manifestations of brain dysfunction that are inorganic. The brain consists largely of organic compounds. A coarse brain disease is one with identifiable structural damage in the brain (e.g., infarction) or pathognomonic measurable biochemical abnormalities (e.g., hypoglycemia) known to produce brain dysfunction. By way of contrast, a "fine" brain dysfunction (e.g., anxiety neurosis, sociopathy) is one where no such abnormalities can be demonstrated.

A full discussion of the coarse brain diseases is beyond the scope of this book. The headings under which coarse disease fall are the same as those found in pathology textbooks. These include:

1. Trauma (e.g., subdural hematoma)
2. Infection (e.g., meningitis)
3. Neoplasm (e.g., metastatic lung cancer)
4. Hematologic (e.g., thrombotic thrombocytopenic purpura)
5. Vascular (e.g., ruptured berry aneurysm)

6. Metabolic (e.g., "myxedema madness")
7. Autoimmune (e.g., lupus erythematosus)
8. Degenerative (e.g., Alzheimer-senile brain disease)

Some of the degenerative diseases are "assigned" to the field of psychiatry; these include Alzheimer-senile brain disease and Pick's disease.

Coarse brain disease as a cause of abnormal behavior is probable when the patient has noncognitive (e.g., spastic paralysis) signs of brain disease; laboratory findings (e.g., lesion seen on computerized tomographic scan) documenting a brain lesion, or signs (e.g., pallor) or laboratory findings (e.g., anemia) of systemic illness (e.g., megaloblastic anemia) known to affect the brain. Coarse brain disease must be ruled out in any patient with abnormalities on the behavioral neurological examination (Chap. 3), Aphasia Screening Test [4], or Minimental State Examination.

It must also be considered in *any* patient with *any* significant behavioral abnormality; this is because the brain, like any other organ, has a limited repertoire of responses to injury, a repertoire which includes delirium (Chap. 13), dementia (Chaps. 4, 23), signs of focal brain dysfunction (Chaps. 3, 4) and signs (e.g., euphoria, formal thinking disorder, anxiety attacks) mimicking those seen in any of the fine (e.g., mania, schizophrenia, anxiety neurosis) brain dysfunctions. Thus, a thorough history and physical, including a behavioral neurological examination (or at least an Aphasia Screening Test and Minimental State Examination) must be done on all patients with significant behavioral abnormalities.

A clinically crucial question is to what extent can a patient's behavior help us to localize dynsfunction and identify the cause. The answer is that behavioral abnormalities can be highly specific for *identifying* diffuse brain dysfunction (delirium, dementia) and localizing focal brain dysfunction, but our ability to *identify precise pathological diagnoses* based upon behavior alone is very limited. True, certain diseases have a predilection for specific regions in the brain. These include (1) Korsakoff's encephalopathy and the mammillary bodies and thalamus; (2) Marchiafava-Bignami syndrome and the corpus callosum; (3) Pick's disease and the frontal and temporal lobes, insula, and corpus callosum; (4) cerebrovascular accidents and the convexities of the frontal and temporal lobes; and (5) temporal lobe epilepsy and, naturally, the temporal lobes. A few illnesses are associated with specific behavioral abnormalities (e.g., reserpine toxicity and depression; thyrotoxicosis or pheochromocytoma and anxiety). However, for the most part, medical illnesses do not have strong proclivities for specific regions of the brain.

The treatment for coarse brain disease is first try to diagnose and treat the cause.

Sociopathy (Antisocial Personality Disorder, Psychopathy)

This syndrome occurs in 2.3% of adoptees [8]; its frequency in the general population is unknown [3]. It is much more common in men than in women. Family history reveals an increased frequency of sociopathy, Briquet's syndrome, alcoholism, drug abuse, and criminality [29]. The onset is in childhood or adolescence; a history of childhood or adolescent onset is required for a definite diagnosis. The patient must meet four of the following for a probable diagnosis, and five for a definite diagnosis [3,12]:

    1. Major school problems (e.g., suspension, expulsion or frequent fighting)

    2. Running away from parents' home overnight

    3. Frequent or serious trouble with the police

    4. Poor work history (e.g., frequent job changes, firings, or unemployment)

    5. Marital difficulties (e.g., deserting family, two or more divorces, cruelty to spouse, or recurring infidelity)

    6. Repeated outbursts of rage or fighting, or one episode of use of a weapon

    7. Sexual problems (e.g., prostitution, pimping, more than one episode of veneral disease, or flagrant promiscuity)

    8. Vagrancy or wanderlust

    9. Using an alias or repeated lying

Associated findings include drug abuse, alcoholism, and conversion reactions. The syndrome is incurable, but some authors note slight improvement in some cases after the age of 30. Despite the prognosis, we can be of help to a sociopath by treating him for superimposed problems (e.g., childhood hyperactivity persisting into adulthood, drug withdrawal, complications of "mainlining"), and by *not* building up your hopes, his hopes, or the hopes of his family for a complete cure.

Briquet's Syndrome (Somatization Disorder, Hysteria)

This syndrome occurs in 1-2% of females, and is much commoner in women [3,40]. The family history reveals an increased frequency of sociopathy, alcoholism, drug abuse, and criminality. For diagnosis, the onset must be before age 30, and the patient must report 20-24 medically unexplained symptoms for a probable diagnosis, and 25 or over medically unexplained symptoms for a definite diagnosis, from 9 of the 10 groups listed in Table 4 [3,12]. This long list needs to be used only if the review of systems reveals large numbers of medically unexplained symptoms.

Table 4   Symptoms of Briquet's Syndrome by Group

Group 1

Headaches
Sickly majority of life

Group 2

Blindness
Paralysis
Anesthesia
Aphonia
Fits or convulsions
Unconsciousness
Amnesia
Deafness
Hallucinations
Urinary retention
Trouble walking
Other unexplained "neurological"
  symptoms

Group 3

Fatigue
Lump in throat
Fainting spells
Visual blurring
Weakness
Dysuria

Group 4

Breathing difficulty
Palpitation
Anxiety attacks
Chest pain
Dizziness

Group 5

Anorexia
Weight loss
Marked fluctuations in weight
Nausea
Abdominal bloating
Food intolerances
Diarrhea
Constipation

Group 6

Abdominal pain
Vomiting

Group 7

Dysmenorrhea
Menstrual irregularity
Amenorrhea
Excessive bleeding

Group 8

Sexual indifference
Frigidity
Dyspareunia
Other sexual difficulties
Vomiting all nine months of pregnancy at
  least once, or hospitalization for
  hypermesis gravidarum

Group 9

Back pain
Joint pain
Extremity pain
Burning pains of the sexual organs, mouth,
  or rectum

Group 10

Nervousness
Fears
Depressed feelings
Need to quit working, or inability to carry
  on regular duties because of feeling sick
Crying easily
Feeling life hopeless
Thinking a good deal about dying
Wanting to die
Thinking about suicide
Suicide attempts

Source: From J. Feighner, E. Robins, S. Guze, R. Woodruff, G. Winokur, and R. Munoz. Diagnostic criteria for use in psychiatric research. *Arch. Gen. Psychiatry* 26:56-63, 1972.

There is a high frequency of unnecessary surgery; if Briquet's syndrome is diagnosed, surgery should be avoided when the need is not well documented. Conversion ractions are common [2]. A conversion reaction is a symptom or sign which mimics neurological disease (e.g., blindness, anesthesia), but where the findings do not conform to standard neuroanatomic pathways (e.g., hemianesthesia exactly to the midline, "stocking" or "glove" anesthesia) or neurophysiological functioning (e.g., presence of optokinetic nystagmus), and no tissue diagnosis can be made. Some conversion reactions remit spontaneously, some respond to behavior modification, and some transform into significant medical disease at the same site [41].

There is no successful treatment for Briquet's syndrome [3], but some patients may benefit from an explanation and a tentative statement of prognosis.

Anxiety Neurosis (Panic Disorder)

This common condition occurs in about 5% of the population [42] and is twice as common in women as in men [2]. For definite diagnosis, the onset must be prior to age 40 [3,12]. The patient experiences chronic nervousness and anxiety attacks. Pheochromocytoma, temporal lobe epilepsy, mitral valve prolapse, thyrotoxicosis, and caffeinism specifically, and coarse brain disease in general, must be ruled out [43]. Treatments that have had some success include behavior modification, monoamine oxidase (MAO inhibitors, and imipramine. Benzodiazepenes can be given during acute anxiety attacks. Psychoanalysts claim satisfactory results.

Phobic Neurosis (Phobic Disorder)

Phobias are a major complaint in 2-3% of psychiatic patients, and 7.7% of the general population [44]. For a definite diagnosis, the onset must be before age 40 [3,12]. It is more common in women than in men.

Phobias are intense fears of certain objects or situations, which include the following: Insects, animals, heights (acrophobia), closed spaces (claustrophobia), and open spaces (agoraphobia). Patients experience panic when exposed to the feared situation, so they will go to great lengths to avoid these situations. Phobias can be mild or incapacitating; for example, an acrophobic patient may refuse to stand on a chair to fix a light bulb, and an agoraphobic patient may become housebound. The treatment of choice for most monosymptomatic phobias (one phobia only) is behavior modification (usually systematic desensitization). For agoraphobia or multiple phobias, MAO inhibitors or imipramine may be helpful. Benzodiazepenes may be used for situations when patients have to face a phobic situation, such as when a acrophobic patient has to make a plane flight. Psychoanalysts claim satisfactory results in the treatment of phobias.

Obsessive-Compulsive Neurosis (Obsessive-Compulsive Disorder)

The frequency of this syndrome in the general population is unknown. It occurs in slightly less than 5% of psychiatric inpatients [45]. It occurs about as frequently in men as in women. Patients with this syndrome are more likely to be from higher social classes, to be better educated, and to have higher IQs than the psychiatric patient population in general [3,46].

To make a definite diagnosis [3], the age of onset must be under 40; the patient must have recurrent intrusive thoughts (obsessions) which are "foreign" and unacceptable to the patient, and/or repetitive urges or behaviors (compulsions) also perceived as foreign, and usually a response to the obsessions. The treatment is the same as for anxiety neurosis.

Transsexualism

This syndrome, the prevalence of which is one in 40,000-100,000 men and one in 100,000-400,000 women, is manifested by a lifelong feeling that one is a member of the wrong sex, and by a desire to be a member of the opposite sex [3]. This often leads to a dressing as a member of the opposite sex and seeking sex-change surgery. The patient should be evaluated for other disorders; if these are ruled out, he should be referred to a clinic specializing in evaluating and treating such problems. In some centers, those considered candidates for sex-change surgery are given hormones of the opposite sex, instructed to dress as a member of the opposite sex, and regularly reevaluated during an observation period of 1-2 years. If all goes well, a sex-change operation is performed. Long-term follow-up after such surgery, however, raises questions about its status as a treatment of choice [47].

Anorexia Nervosa

This rare condition is more common in women than in men by a ratio of 9:1. Its onset is usually in adolescence. Usually following a period of perceiving herself as obese, the patient goes on a diet, or eats and regurgitates, and eventually loses over 25% of her body weight [3]. This predisposes her to developing inanition and to dying. Amenorrhea, lanugo hairs, bradycardia, periods of bulimia, periods of overactivity, and denial of illness are all very common. The patient should be hospitalized, told she is very ill (too ill to leave the hospital until her health is restored), given sustagen or intravenous hyperalimentation as treatment for her illness, and given behavior modifica-

Table 5   Other Psychiatric Syndromes

Diagnosis	Clinical characteristics	Source
Hysterical psychosis (brief reactive psychosis)	Follows stressful event; signs of psychosis (loss of touch with reality); broad dramatic effect; duration several weeks or less; amnesia for period of psychosis	Hollander and Hirsch [49]
Paranoid disorders	Core signs are called "paranoid syndrome"; characterized by suspiciousness, mistrust, hostility, hyperalertness, grandiosity, and litigiousness. Other signs may include delusions or hallucinations	Swanson, Bohnert, and Smith [50]
Borderline personality disorder	Depression due to emptiness, not guilt; frequent anger; intense dependent relationships; impulsivity; absence of psychosis or transient psychosis.	Gunderson and Kolb [51]
Narcissistic personality disorder	Faulty self-esteem regulation; impaired self-esteem; feelings of emptiness; work difficulties; perverse sexuality	Kohut [52]
Transient situational disturbance (adjustment disorder)	Following major stressful life events, symptoms resembling neuroses or psychoses; full recovery over time	Looney and Gunderson [53]
Hysterical personality disorder	Histrionic, vain, dependent; prone to conversion reactions	Horowitz [54]
Masochistic personality disorder	Chronic guilt and suffering	Panken [55]
Cyclothymic personality disorder	Long history of mood swings	Brody and Sata [56]
Dependent personality disorder	Excessive dependence upon others	Brody and Sata [56]
Schizoid personality disorder	Loner, isolate	Brody and Sata [56]
Compulsive personality disorder	Meticulous, controlling, ambivalent; inexpressive of feelings	Salzman [57]

tion or psychotherapy. A recent paper shows a family association with affective disorder [48].

Other Syndromes

Temporal lobe epilepsy, alcoholism, drug abuse, minimal brain dysfunction (MBD)/hyperactivity and homosexuality have been discussed in other chapters. In addition, there are a number of diagnoses for which more research will be needed to establish validity. These are summarize^d briefly in Table 5.

REFERENCES

1. Mumford, E. Culture: Life perspectives and the social meanings of illness, in *Understanding Human Behavior in Health and Illness*. R. Simons and H. Pardes, eds. Williams and Wilkins, Baltimore (1977).
2. Guze, S. The diagnosis of hysteria. What are we trying to do? *Am. J. Psychiatry* 124:4 491-498 (1967).
3. Woodruff, R., Goodwin, D., and Guze, S. *Psychiatric Diagnosis*. Oxford, New York (1974).
4. Robins, E., and Guze, S. Establishment of diagnostic validity in psychiatric illness. Its application to schizophrenia. *Am. J. Psychiatry* 126:983-987 (1970).
5. Mendlewicz, J., and Rainer, J. Adoption study supporting genetic transmission in manic depressive illness. *Nature (Lond.)* 268:327-329 (1977).
6. Rosenthal, D., Wender, P., Kety, S., et al. Schizophrenic's offspring reared in adoptive homes, in *The Transmission of Schizophrenia*. D. Rosenthal and S. Kety, eds. Pergamon, New York (1968).
7. Heston, L. Psychiatric disorders in foster-home reared children of schizophrenic mothers. *Br. J. Psychiatry* 112:819-825 (1966).
8. Crowe, R. An adoptive study of antisocial personality. *Arch. Gen. Psychiatry* 31:785-791 (1974).
9. Goodwin, D., Shulsinger, F., and Hermansen, L. Alcohol problems in adoptees raised apart from alcoholic biologic parents. *Arch. Gen. Psychiatry* 28:238-243 (1973).
10. Shields, J. Genetic factors in neurosis, in *Research in Neurosis*. H. Van Praag, ed. Spectrum, New York (1978).
11. Szasz, T. *The Second Sin*. Doubleday, New York (1973).
12. Feighner, J., Robins, E., Guze, S., Woodruff, R., Winokur, G., and Munoz, R. Diagnostic criteria for use in psychiatric research. *Arch. Gen. Psychiatry* 26:56-63 (1972).
13. Helzer, J., Robins, L., Taibleson, M., Woodruff, R., and Reich, T. Reliability of psychiatric diagnosis, I. *Arch. Gen. Psychiatry* 34:129-133 (1977).
14. Spitzer, R., Fleiss, J., and Endicott, J. Problems of classification, in *Psychopharmacology: A Generation of Progress*. M. Lipton, A. DiMascio, and K. Kellam, eds. Raven, New York (1978).
15. Helzer, J., Clayton, P., Pambakian, R., Reich, T., Woodruff, R., and Reveley, M. Reliability of psychiatric diagnosis, II. *Arch. Gen. Psychiatry* 34:136-141 (1977).
16. Koran, L. The reliability of clinical methods, data and judgments, part 1. *N. Engl. J. Med.* 293:642-646 (1975).

17. Koran, L. The reliability of clinical methods, data and judgments, part 2. *N. Engl. J. Med.* 293:695-701 (1975).

18. Norden, C., Philipps, E., Levy, P., and Kass, E. Variation in interpretation of intravenous pyelograms. *Am. J. Epidemiol.* 91:155-160 (1970).

19. Felson, B., Morgan, W., Bristol, L., Pendergass, E., Dessen, E., Linton, O., and Reger, R. Observations on the results of multiple readings of chest films in coal miners pneumoconious. *Radiology* 109:19-23 (1973).

20. Pitts, F., and McClure, J. Lactate metabolism in anxiety neurosis. *N. Engl. J. Med.* 277:1329-1336 (1967).

21. Almy, G., and Taylor, M. Lithium retention in mania. *Arch. Gen. Psychiatry* 29:232-234 (1973).

22. Shagass, C., Naiman, J., and Mihalik, J. An objective test which differentiates neurotic from psychotic depression. *Arch. Neurol. Psychiatry* 75:461-471 (1955).

23. Rybakowski, J. Pharmacogenetic aspects of red blood cell lithium index in manic depressive psychosis. *Biol. Psychiatry* 12:425-429 (1977).

24. Feinberg, M., Greden, J., Tarika, J., Albala, A., Haskett, R., James, N., Kronfol, Z., Lohr, N., Steiner, M., De Vigne, J., and Young, E. A specific laboratory test for the diagnosis of melancholia. *Arch. Gen. Psychiatry* 38:15-23 (1981).

25. Abrams, R. The ECT controversy. *Psychiatr. Opinion* 11:15 (1979).

26. Kiloh, L., and Garside, R. The independence of neurotic depression and endogenous depression. *Br. J. Psychiatry* 109:451-463 (1963).

27. Fowler, R., McCabe, M., Cadoret, R., and Winokur, G. The validity of good prognosis schizophrenia. *Arch. Gen. Psychiatry* 26:182-185 (1972).

28. Stephens, J. Long-term prognosis and follow-up in schizophrenia. *Schizophrenia Bull.* 4:25-47 (1978).

29. Guze, S. *Criminality and Psychiatric Disorders.* Oxford, New York (1975).

30. Murphy, G., Woodruff, R., Herjanic, M., and Fischer, J. Validity of the diagnosis of primary affective disorder. A prospective study with a five-year followup. *Arch. Gen. Psychiatry* 30:751-756 (1974).

31. Goodwin, D., Guze, S., and Robins, E. Followup studies in obsessive neurosis. *Arch. Gen. Psychiatry* 20:182-187 (1969).

32. Agras, W., Chapin, H., and Olivean, D. The natural history of phobia. *Arch. Gen. Psychiatry* 26:315-321 (1972).

33. Taylor, M., and Abrams, R. Manic depressive illness and good-prognosis schizophrenia. *Am. J. Psychiatry* 132:741-742 (1975).

34. Taylor, M., and Abrams, R. The prevalence of schizophrenia: A reassessment using modern diagnostic criteria. *Am. J. Psychiatry* 135:945-948 (1978).

35. Abrams, R., and Taylor, M. A comparison of unipolar and bipolar depressive illness. *Am. J. Psychiatry* 137:1084-1087 (1980).

36. Taylor, M., and Abrams, R. The phenomenology of mania. *Arch. Gen. Psychiatry* 29:520-522 (1973).

37. Helgason, T. Epidemiology of mental disorders in Iceland. *Acta Psychiatr. Scand. (Suppl.)* 29:520-522 (1973).

38. Taylor, M., Greenspan, B., and Abrams, R. Lateralized neuropsychological dysfunction in affective disorder and schizophrenia. *A. J. Psychiatry* 136:1031-1034 (1979).

39. Abrams, R., and Taylor, M. Differential EEG patterns in affective disorder and schizophrenia. *Arch. Gen. Psychiatry* 36:1355-1358 (1979).

40. Woodruff, R., Clayton, P., and Guze, S. Hysteria: Studies of diagnosis, outcome and prevalence. *JAMA* 215:425-428 (1971).

41. Lazare, A. Hysteria, in *Handbook of General Hospital Psychiatry*. T. Hackett and N. Cassem, eds. Mosby, St. Louis (1978).

42. Cohen, M., and White, P. Life situations, emotions and neurocirculatory asthenia. *Assoc. Res. Nerv. Dis. Proc.* 29:832-869 (1950).

43. Taylor, M. *The Neuropsychiatric Mental Status: Examination*. Spectrum, New York (1981).

44. Agras, S., Sylvester, D., and Oliveau, D. The epidemiology of common fears and phobia. *Compr. Psychiatry* 10:151-156 (1969).

45. Goodwin, D., Guze, S., and Robins, E. Followup studies in obsessional neurosis. *Arch. Gen. Psychiatry* 20:182-187 (1969).

46. Ingram, I. Obsessional illness in mental hospital patients. *J. Ment. Sci.* 107:382-402 (1961).

47. Meyer, J., and Reter, D. Sex reassignment. Followup. *Arch. Gen. Psychiatry* 36:1010-1015 (1979).

48. Cantwell, D., Sturzenberger, S., Burroughs, J., Salkin, B., and Green, J. Anorexia nervosa. An affective disorder? *Arch. Gen. Psychiatry* 34:1087-1093 (1977).

49. Hollander, M., and Hirsch, S. Hysterical psychosis. *Am. J. Psychiatry* 120:1066-1074 (1964).

50. Swanson, D., Bohnert, P., and Smith, J. *The Paranoid*. Little, Brown, Boston (1970).

51. Gunderson, J., and Kolb, J. Discriminating features of borderline patients. *Am. J. Psychiatry* 135:792-796 (1978).

52. Kohut, H. *Psychology of the Self*. Int. Univ., New York (1971).

53. Looney, J., and Gunderson, E. Transient situational disturbances. Course and outcome. *Am. J. Psychiatry* 135:660-663 (1978).

54. Horowitz, M. *The Hysterical Personality*. Aronson, New York (1977).

55. Panken, S. *The Joy of Suffering*. Aronson, New York (1973).

56. Brody, E., and Sata, L. Personality disorders 1. Trait and pattern disturbances, in *Comprehensive Textbook of Psychiatry*, A. Freedman and H. Kaplan, eds. Williams and Wilkins, Baltimore (1967).

57. Salzman, L. *The Obsessive Personality*. Aronson, New York (1973).

9

Psychopharmacology

RICHARD ABRAMS

INTRODUCTION

The bioavailability of psychoactive agents is intimately related to their therapeutic efficacy, and is affected by several variables, each of which requires careful consideration.

Dose

There is a linear relation between the dose of a drug and its blood level, and therapeutic failures often result from inadequate dosage. Manufacturers' recommended doses are only rough guidelines and frequently must be exceeded in order to attain maximum therapeutic benefit.

Preparation and Route of Administration

The highest blood levels are achieved through parenteral administration, with the intramuscular route preferred to the intravenous except in the case of the benzodiazepines chlordiazepoxide and diazepam. Oral preparations are less well absorbed than parenteral, and are also subject to a "first-pass" effect through the hepatic portal circulation, undergoing a degree of metabolism befor entering the general circulation. Of the oral preparations, liquid concentrates provide the highest blood levels and are virtually impossible to secrete in the cheek or under the tongue; this is a decided advantage when treating uncooperative patients. When prescribing certain classes of drugs, such as neuroleptics or antidepressants, care should be taken not to administer them with food or on a full stomach, as their absorption would thereby be severely impaired.

Drug Interactions

As most psychoactive drugs, except lithium, undergo extensive hepatic biotransformation, the enzyme-inducing or inhibiting effects of coadministering other compounds must be carefully considered. For example, barbiturates are enzyme-inducing and may lower blood levels of antidepressants and related drugs. The substitution of a nonbarbiturate sedative such as chlordiazepoxide will yield the desired hypnotic effect with very little enzyme induction. Conversely, enzyme-inhibiting drugs such as the stimulant methylphenidate have been administered with tricyclic antidepressants in order to *raise* blood levels of these agents and augment their therapeutic effect.

Pharmacodynamics

Certain psychoactive agents, specifically the antidepressants and neuroleptics, share some physical and pharmacokinetic properties which affect their bioavailability. As noted above, these drugs are primarily metabolized in the liver, with only insignificant amounts excreted unchanged in the urine. They are highly lipid-soluble, pass rapidly into the central nervous system, and are stored in fat cells. They are extensively bound to plasma protein, with clinical activity limited to the unbound portion (generally 10-20% of the total). All of these factors result in these drugs having a long half-life, so that once-a-day administration is usually satisfactory, and drug-free holidays can be given without risk of immediate relapse.

Effective use of psychoactive agents requires additional important considerations.

Choice of Drugs

There is almost no data to suggest that, within classes of psychoactive drugs (e.g., neuroleptics), one drug is superior to another in the treatment of any symptom or group of symptoms; frequent change of prescriptions rarely results in dramatic improvement, and is discouraging to both the patient and his physician. Drug "failures" in psychiatry often result from inadequate dosage, and it is generally wiser to increase the dose of a compound than to replace it with another of the same class.

Side Effects

Although severe side effects may prevent a patient from taking a drug, mild or moderate side effects serve notice to the physician that a pharmacologically active dose has been achieved, and that patient cooperation and drug bioavailability are satisfactory.

Drug Combinations

True synergism among psychopharmacological drugs remains to be demonstrated, and combining these agents often serves only to accentuate their side effects. Fixed-drug combinations of a tricyclic antidepressant with a neuroleptic have no scientific basis and should not be prescribed.

THE DRUGS

There are four classes of psychopharmacologic agents in general use: neuroleptics, antidepressants, anxiolytics, and lithium.

Neuroleptics

These compounds were introduced in the early 1950s for the treatment of psychotic patients, and had the distinct advantage over the barbiturates in that they induced sedation, emotional quieting, and affective indifference without sleep. Furthermore, their duration of action was markedly prolonged, in comparison with the barbiturates, and they exhibited specific activity against hallucinations and delusions, the first time such antipsychotic properties had been obtainable with any drug.

Pharmacologically, the neuroleptics are potent blockers of α-adrenergic receptors, and exert powerful antiemetic effects through inhibition of the chemoreceptor trigger zone in the hypothalamus. Of greatest theoretical interest, however, is the fact that all neuroleptics block dopamine receptors, an observation which has been incorporated into a dopamine hypothesis of psychosis. Blockade of dopamine receptors in the nigrostriatal systems is responsible for one of the most common side effects of neuroleptic therapy, the induction of a pseudoparkinsonian syndrome.

In normal humans, modest doses of neuroleptics may have very little effect, but higher doses impair speed on performance tasks and increase reaction time.

The several classes of neuroleptic drugs presently available in this country include the tricyclic neuroleptics of the phenothiazine and thioxanthene types, the butyrophenones, the dibenzoxazepenes, and the dihydroindolones. Table 1 shows the classes of neuroleptic drugs, with only prototypical examples given. The most experience to date has been garnered with the phenothiazines, thioxanthenes, and haloperidol; no specific therapeutic advance

Table 1   The Classes of Neuroleptic Drugs, with Some Prototypical
Examples

Class	Prototype
Tricyclics	
Phenothiazines	
Aliphatic	Chlorpromazine
Piperazine	Fluphenazine
Piperidine	Thioridazine
Thioxanthenes	
Aliphatic	Chlorprothixene
Piperazine	Thiothixene*
Dibenzoxazepines	Loxapine*
Butyrophenones	Haloperidol*
Dihydroindolones	Molindone*
Rauwolfia alkaloids†	Reserpine

*The only representative presently available for prescription in the United States.
†No longer used in psychiatry.

can yet be attributed to the addition of the dibenzoxazepenes or dihydro-indolones.

In general, most commonly prescribed neuroleptics can be divided into those with low potency (the aliphatic and piperidine tricyclics) and high potency (the piperazine tricyclics and haloperidol) per milligram. Low-potency neuroleptics require higher dosages, are more sedating, and exhibit more cardiovascular effects (electrocardiogram [EKG] changes, hypotension). High potency neuroleptics induce extrapyramidal side effects (e.g., pseudoparkinsonism, dystonia, akathisia) more frequently.

There is scant data to demonstrate the clinical superiority of any individual neuroleptic drug or group of drugs, and the choice of which to prescribe will often depend upon the availability of specific preparations and the profile of side effects. For example, if a colorless, odorless, and tasteless concentrate is required, haloperidol will be the choice; if a long-acting intramuscular injection is needed, fluphenazine will be used; and if a compound with the lowest incidence of pseudoparkinsonism is desired, thioridazine will fill the bill.

Clinical Indications

The neuroleptics are demonstrably effective only in patients suffering from psychoses secondary to one of three major diagnostic groups—schizophrenia, mania, and organic brain disease. In general, a "target symptom" approach has been successful, with certain syndromes or symptom-clusters responsive to treatment regardless of the primary diagnoses.

Psychotic excitement states These states of increased and heightened psychomotor activity are characterized by overactivity, intense affect, and a "driven" quality which is unresponsive to external controls. They are often characterized by threatening behavior and actual assaults upon property and person, and if left unchecked, they may progress to states of unremitting excitement, leading to exhaustion, dehydration, fever, and even death. Neuroleptic drugs are usually rapidly effective in such states, and treatment must be initiated parenterally and with high dosages. A very effective regimen is the prescription of an initial intramuscular injection of 20 mg haloperidol, to be continued twice daily for 48-72 hr, after which time an oral preparation may be substituted at a 20% increase in dose. The initial treatment of such patients with oral medication is rarely effective, regardless of dose, and a prescription written "as needed" (PRN) is merely an invitation to repeated crescendoes of overactivity as each individual injection wears off. Other injectable neuroleptics of the high potency variety may also be used (e.g., thiothixene), but low-potency compounds such as chlorpromazine may produce dangerous hypotension if given parenterally in dosages large enough to block psychotic excitement states.

If 4-5 days of high-dose, parenteral, neuroleptic therapy fails to inhibit an excitement state, neuroleptics should be discontinued and electroconvulsive therapy (ECT) given in order to avoid the risk of a psychotic exhaustion death.

Paranoid-hallucinatory syndrome Delusional mood, persecutory delusions, and auditory and visual hallucinations all may accompany psychotic excitement, but may also exist in the absence of such excitement, often in patients with schizophrenia or organic psychosyndromes. In the absence of menacing or assultive behavior, treatment can be initiated with an oral preparation and the dosage increased daily until the desired effect is achieved or troublesome side effects supervene. For example, an initial prescription of chlorpromazine concentrate 200 mg BID might well be increased to a total daily dosage of 800-1,000 mg by the end of the first week of treatment, at which time it would usually be well tolerated as a single, bedtime dose. Hallucinations and delusions are less rapidly responsive to neuroleptics than is psychomotor excitement, and 1 or 2 weeks may pass before definitive improvement occurs. In general, hallucinations are first to respond, followed by the emotional response to the delusional content, and finally by the delusions themselves.

Formal thought disorder   Even less rapidly responsive are the manifestations of formal thought disorder, defined here as specific abnormalities of language, akin to aphasic disorders rather than disorders of logical thinking. Nonetheless, significant improvement is often seen, reaching maximum benefit in certain instances only after weeks of continued neuroleptic therapy.

Other symptoms asssociated with the major psychoses, such as catatonia and emotional blunting, are generally unresponsive to neuroleptics and may even be aggravated by them. Occasionally, however, an unexpected positive response occurs, and these drugs are worth a trial in patients with these symptoms if other measures (e.g., ECT) fail.

Side Effects, Precautions, and Contraindication

Central nervous system (CNS)   The most frequent side effects are in the central nervous system and derive from blockade of dopaminergic transmission in the nigrostriatal system. These extrapyramidal syndromes occur most often with the high-potency neuroleptics and consist of parkinsonism, dystonia, and akathisia. The parkinsonian triad of tremor, rigidity, and bradykinesia generally occurs after the first week or two, and may be accompanied by other classic symptoms such as unblinking gaze, hypersalivation, and festinating gait. Treatment with antiparkinson agents such as benztropine or amantidine is usually effective, and these compounds may often be discontinued after several weeks without a return of symptoms.

Acute dystonia is manifested by a spastic contraction of head, neck, and orofacial musculature, and may be accompanied by oculogyrus. It occurs most frequently after initiation of parenteral therapy in younger patients, usually males, and is readily relieved by 25-50 mg diphenhydramine intravenously. The syndrome may be painful and distressing, but is not life-threatening. Akathisia, a syndrome of motor restlessness and inability to sit still, may mimic an agitated state, resulting in the erroneous administration of an increased dose of the neuroleptic drug. While antiparkinson agents are occasionally useful in treating this symptom, dose-reduction is often the only effective remedy.

The most serious central nervous system side effect of neuroleptics is tardive dyskinesia, a syndrome of involuntary choreiform movements (analagous to Huntington's disease) which is accentuated by withdrawing the drug, and which is usually permanent. Oral dyskinesias are most frequent, with tongue protrusion, lip-smacking, and puffing movements of the cheeks, but athetoid hyperextension of the wrist and fingers also occurs, as well pelvic torsion and peculiar gaits. There is no effective treatment for tardive dyskinesia. The observation that reinstitution of neuroleptic therapy inhibits the symptoms has led to the hypothesis of dopamine receptor hypersensitivity as its underlying pathophysiology.

Cardiovascular Orthostatic hypotension is a frequent side effect of the low-potency neuroleptics, particularly after parenteral administration. EKG changes are also common, especially with thioridazine, and are generally limited to repolarization abnormalities (T-wave inversion, notching, splitting) believed to be benign.

Hematopoetic Agranulocytosis and pancytopenia are rare complications, due to an idiosyncratic allergic response to neuroleptics. Agranulocytosis often presents with painful oropharyngeal infections and, for this reason, any complaint of sore throat in a patient on neuroleptics must be taken very seriously.

Skin and eye These ectodermal derivatives may suffer both acute (photosensitivity) and chronic (pigmentation, corneal opocities) changes with neuroleptics, especially with the low-potency compounds. And one drug, thioridazine, is capable of inducing retinitis pigmentosa leading to blindness in doses exceeding 1,200/day.

Hepatic A benign, intrahepatic, cholestatic jaundice was occasionally reported in the earlier days of neuroleptic therapy, most frequently with chlorpromazine. For reasons which are unclear this complication is now less frequent.

Hormonal A pseudopregnancy syndrome occurs, secondary to the serum prolactin increase which results from dopamine blockade in the tuberoinfundibular system. Impaired glucose tolerance, especially in women, is also reported, and is benign.

Fatalities Rare instances of unexplained sudden death in patients receiving neuroleptics have been atributed to hyperpyrexia, asphyxiation by food bolus, circulatory collapse, and cardiac arrhythmias.

Precautions

In the event of circulatory collapse secondary to neuroleptics, epinephrine should not be used, as the resulting α-adrenergic blockade of its blood pressure raising effects will leave its blood pressure lowering activity unopposed. Although specific evidence for birth defects with neuroleptics does not exist, these and other drugs should be avoided in the first trimester of pregnancy. These drugs are excreted in mothers' milk and should not be given to nursing mothers.

Contraindications

Prostatic hypertrophy and narrow-angle glaucoma may be severely aggravated by the anticholinergic properties of the neuroleptics, especially thioridazine.

Antidepressants

There are two groups of antidepressant drugs available in the United States, the tricyclics and the monoamine oxidase inhibitors:

1. Tricyclics

These compounds are closely related structurally to the tricyclic phenothiazines, although their pharmacology differs in several essential ways. They do not posses dopamine-blocking activity, and therefore do not cause either the acute or the chronic extrapyramidal syndromes seen with the neuroleptics. Instead, they possess the ability to block the reuptake of biogenic amines (serotonin, norepinephrine) into the presynaptic neuron, a fact which formed the basis for an amine hypothesis of the etiology of affective disorders.

Pharmocokinetics

Plasma level studies have revealed two types of relationships between steady-state drug levels and therapeutic response. The first is the classic linear (or sigmoid) dose-response curve, as observed with imipramine, in which higher plasma levels are associated with a better outcome. The second is curvilinear, resembling an inverted "U." It is characterized by increasing improvement with increasing plasma levels during the initial dosage increment, and a fall-off of therapeutic effect at the higher doses and blood levels, producing a "therapeutic window," a dosage range whose boundaries should not be crossed if the drug is to be effective. Nortriptyline displays such a curve.

Choice of Drug

Imipramine and amitriptyline are the two original compounds from which most of the others have been derived through demethylation or slight alterations of the central ring (desipramine, nortriptyline, protriptyline, doxepin). There is no hard evidence that any of these derivatives is clinically more effective than the parent compounds, which are still the most widely prescribed tricyclic antidepressants. There is little to choose between imipramine and amitriptyline, although a summary of all their comparisons would yield perhaps a slight advantage for the latter drug. One study found imipramine more useful for the younger, retarded depressive, and amitriptyline superior for the older agitated depressive.

Preparation and Dosage

Although parenteral formulations exist for both imipramine and amitriptyline, treatment is invariably by the oral route. Adequate dosage is the key to successful treatment with these drugs, and there is good data to suggest that their therapuetic range lies between 200 and 300 mg/day. Several studies have demonstrated single daily doses of the tricyclics to be both safe and effective. A typical treatment regimen might begin with 50 mg of either compound at bedtime, with nightly increases of 50 mg until a dose of 200-300 mg is reached or undesirable side effects supervene.

Indications and Treatment Results

The primary indication for treatment with tricyclic antidepressants is the syndrome of endogenous depression, characterized by early morning waking, significant weight loss, retardation or agitation, diurnal mood swing (worse in the morning), suicidal ruminations, and feelings of guilt, hopelessness, and worthlessness. Approximately 60-70% of such patients will respond favorably to tricyclics, but there is usually a 2-week delay before the first signs of clinical improvement are seen. When such improvement occurs, it generally reaches its maximum at 3-5 weeks after treatment is begun, at which point the dose can be reduced to a maintenance level of 150 mg/day and continued for an additional 2-3 months to prevent relapse. There is no evidence that prolonged tricyclic treatment (e.g., more than 6 months) will prevent future recurrence of illness; if this is desired, lithium should then be prescribed.

When a rapid clinical effect is needed, or where suicidal risk, poor physical condition, severe agitation, or psychotic symptoms of hallucinations or delusions dominate the clinical picture, ECT is the initial treatment of choice. Compared with tricyclics, ECT has a significantly better overall response rate, as well as a better quality of improvement (a greater proportion of fully recovered patients).

Tricyclics, especially imipramine, are also used in the management of nocturnal enuresis.

Side Effects, Precautions, and Contraindications

The tricyclics, amitriptyline in particular, have significant anticholinergic properties, and frequently induce dry mouth, stuffed nose, blurred vision, constipation, and urinary problems. Their most important side effects are on the cardiovascular system, through effects on cardiac conduction and blood pressure.

EKG changes The tricyclics inhibit atrioventricular conduction, yielding prolongation of the PR, QRS, and QT intervals at therapeutic blood levels. Caution should be observed when prescribing these drugs for patients with bundle-branch disease, as heart block has been reported under such circumstances. Toxic blood levels of tricyclics are associated with a variety of arrhythmias, including ventricular tachycardia and, in lethal cases, ventricular fibrillation.

Hypotension Therapeutic doses of tricyclics frequently induce orthostatic hypotension, which is more severe in patients with preexisting cardiovascular disease. Orthostatic blood pressure drops have been associated with death due to acute myocardial infarction, as well as syncopal episodes with resultant skull or hip fractures.

2. Monoamine Oxidase Inhibitors (MAOIs)

These drugs are chemically unrelated to the tricyclics and have a different spectrum of clinical indications as well. Their characteristic pharmacological property is the inhibition of intracellular monoamine oxidase, with a resultant increase in brain biogenic amine concentration. No specific evidence has yet been adduced, however, for any relation between this property and the therapeutic effects of these compounds in psychiatric patients.

Choice of Drug There are two presently available MAOIs of demonstrated effectiveness in psychiatry, phenelzine and tranylcypromine. Of the two, phenelzine is more widely used because of its lower incidence of toxicity, and tranylcypromine is often reserved for the more severely ill or treatment-resistant patient. An advantage of tranylcypromine is an initial stimulating effect which derives from an amphetamine-like structure.

Preparation and Dosage The MAOIs are available in oral form only. Phenelzine has been more carefully studied with regard to dose-response relationships than has tranylcypromine. The optimal dosage is in the range of 1.0 mg/kg body weight, or about 60-75 mg/day. Unlike the tricyclics, the MAOIs should not be given in a single bedtime dose, as their stimulant properties may cause insomnia. As a general rule they are given twice a day, with the second dose administered no later than 6:00 p.m. The usual dose range with tranylcypromine is 30-40 mg/day, but in light of recent studies showing the inadequacy of the previously accepted standard phenelzine dose of 45 mg/day, this too may be suboptimal.

There is a delay in the onset of the therapeutic effects with the MAOIs which may be even longer than that seen with the tricyclic antidepressants, and at least 3 weeks of treatment should be given before discontinuing the medications as a failure.

Clinical Indications and Treatment Response   Large-scale studies comparing tricyclics with MAOIs in the treatment of endogenous depression have not shown significant improvement induced by the latter group of drugs. Rather, it is the patients with atypical, reactive, neurotic, or anxious depression who seem to respond favorably to MAOIs, and who present with symptoms of anxiety (somatic and psychic), initial insomnia, self-pity, lability, fluctuation in the depressed mood, and hysterical personality traits.

In addition to this group, other neurotic patients are reported to benefit from MAOIs, especially those with phobic anxiety states characterized by agoraphobia and depersonalization.

Improvement rates with MAOIs (phenelzine in particular) in neurotic depression are in the 50-60% range which, although not as high as that seen with tricyclics in endogenous depression, still compares very favorably with placebo response rates of 25-35%, as usually reported.

Side Effects, Precautions, and Contraindications   The preeminent risk with MAOI therapy derives from their interaction with pressor amines. Before this was known, in the early days of treatment with these drugs, a number of episodes of severe paroxysmal hypertension were reported which, in a few instances, led to subarachnoid hemmorrhage and death. A careful investigation of these occurrences revealed that each episode followed the ingestion of foodstuffs that had high concentrations of tyramine, a pressor amine which is normally a substrate for monoamine oxidase. All patients receiving MAOIs must therefore strictly adhere to a low-tyramine diet, and eschew such foods as cheese, liver, pickled herring, wine or beer, raw yeast, and commercial meat extracts such as Marmite and Bovril. Italian broad (Fava) beans are also prohibited, due to their high L-dopa content, as are all diet pills, decongestants, nose drops, and other over-the-counter nostrums containing pressor amines.

Although it has traditionally been asserted that MAOIs should never be combined with tricyclic antidepressants, no specific data exists demonstrating a dangerous interaction between these drugs and there have been a few recent reports of such combined therapy without significant side effects.

MAOIs also cause orthostatic hypotension, as well as lowering of recumbent blood pressure; this side effect has been made use of by medical practitioners who prescribe the MAOI pargyline for the treatment of hypertension.

Anxiolytic Sedatives

These are perhaps the most widely prescribed ethical pharmaceuticals in the United States and have replaced the barbiturates for the temporary palliation of anxiety and tension in patients with a variety of nonpsychotic diagnoses. Benzodiazepines such as chlordiazepoxide and diazepam constitute the overwhelming majority of these drugs prescribed, although the substituted diols meprobamate and tybamate are also used.

Pharmacology

The anxiolytics share many properties of the barbiturates, including the development of habituation, tolerance, and addiction; the suppression of epileptic seizure activity; the production of muscle relaxation through inhibition of the spinal interneuronal pool; and the occurrence of delirium and seizures when the drugs are abruptly discontinued after prolonged high dosage. Specific advantages of the benzodiazepines over the barbiturates derive from a lesser degree of respiratory depression, reduced induction of hepatic enzyme systems, and diminished suppression of rapid eye movement sleep with the former compounds.

Preparations and Dosage

As the benzodiazepines are the most widely used anxiolytics, and as the compounds chlordiazepoxide and diazepam have not yet been significantly improved upon, these drugs will serve as prototypes for the class. Oral and parenteral preparations are available; however, absorption after intramuscular injection is poor, and intravenous administration is generally used where a very rapid effect is required (e.g., in the treatment of status epilepticus). Although both drugs are available in low-dose units (e.g., 5-mg capsules of chlordiazepoxide), higher dosages are invariably required for clinical effectiveness. There is no delay in onset of activity with these compounds; their effect is immediate when given intravenously, and within 30 min when given orally. Their duration of action is short, and doses must generally be given every 4-6 hr to maintain the desired effect.

Clinical Indications and Treatment Results

The primary psychiatric indication for anxiolytic drugs is the actue anxiety attack, manifested by the sudden onset of unexplained fear, dread, or dysphoria, and the physical symptoms of tremor, sweating, tachycardia, "butterflies in the stomach," rapid respiration, and faintness or dizziness. Hyperventilation may also lead to feelings of numbness or tingling in the hands and feet, and extreme degrees of depersonalization. Oral doses of 25 mg chlordizepoxide or 15 mg diazepam are generally required in such patients, and may be repeated as needed, up to 4 times daily. As the acute state is inhibited, the dose should be rapidly reduced and the drug discontinued as soon as possible (preferably within 3-4 days). The long-term management of chronic anxiety states is not satisfactory with anxiolytics, as increasing doses must be administered in order to maintain the same clinical effect. MAOIs are the pharmacological agents most useful in these patients.

Delirium Tremens Benzodiazepines are the treatment of choice for patients with early or frank delirium tremens, and alcohol-withdrawal syndrome manifested by tremor, apprehension, clouding of consciousness, disorientation, amnesia, and typical visual illusions and hallucinations. Such patients may be unable to keep anything in their stomach due to alcoholic gastritis, and treatment is often initiated with a parenteral benzodiazepine such as chlordiazepoxide, 100 mg intravenously every 4-6 hr. Such a regimen is rapidly effective in delirium tremens, and a change to the oral route can usually be accomplished after 24-48 hr.

Other Uses While anxiolytics are frequently useful as nighttime hypnotics or for medical or surgical patients requiring sedation, their use in the treatment of day-to-day "nervous tension" or to ameliorate the stresses and strains of adult life is deplorable, and such prescription is responsible for the high rates of habituation to these compounds in the United States today. Unfortunately the manufacturers of these drugs have done nothing to discourage their inappropriate prescription, and have instead covertly supported such use through misleading advertisements.

Side Effects, Precautions, and Contraindications

The principal side effects of the anxiolytics is the production of excessive drowsiness, interfering with daily activities. As with the other cortical depressant effects, patients "adapt" to this over time through the development of tolerance, which of necessity also leads to adaptation to the anxiolytic properties as well. With increasing doses, patients may develop ataxia, nystagmus, and slurred speech, exactly as with the barbiturates. Patients who have been taking high doses of these drugs for a long period of time (e.g., 60 mg diazepam daily for over a month) should not be abruptly terminated from therapy for fear of withdrawal seizures or delirium. A gradual step-wise "tapering-off" of dosage should instead be instituted to prevent such phenomena. Patients should be warned of the synergism between these compounds and alcohol; there is little doubt that the thoughtless combination of these two central nervous system depressants has led to many vehicular fatalities as well as unplanned "suicides." A so-called paradoxical agitation has been reported with the benzodiazepines. This is nothing other than the familiar agitated response to barbiturates when given in inadequate dosage to patients with pain or to the very old or young.

Lithium Carbonate

Lithium is unique among psychopharmacological agents in this country as it alone was incontrovertibly demonstrated to be effective prior to its introduction for general clinical use. Its therapeutic effect in manic-depressive illness has rendered psychodynamic explorations of this disorder moot, and stimulated myriad investigations of its biological underpinnings. Even the most dyed-in-the-wool analyst now finds it impolitic to maintain that mania is a "flight into health," when a simple univalent cation without substantial sedative properties resolves the syndrome in 1-3 weeks in 80% of cases.

Physiology and Pharmacology

Lithium is well absorbed from the gut (better than 95% of an orally administered dose can be recovered from the urine), and exists in an ionized, unbound form in the blood, where it diffuses freely into the glomerular filtrate. About 80% of this is reabsorbed (mostly in the proximal tubule) by the same active transport mechanism which handles sodium and, in the blood, red blood cell (RBC)/plasma lithium ratio is maintained at equilibrium through active extrusion of lithium from inside the cell, using the same mechanism for sodium (the "sodium pump").

Lithium is excreted in the urine totally unchanged and has a half-life in normal subjects of about 18 hr. Its half-life in manic patients is almost twice as long, suggesting lithium retention in this diagnostic group, which also shows greater RBC/plasma lithium ratios than normals.

Preparations and Dosage

Lithium is presently available as the carbonate salt, in 300-mg oral doses only. It is absorbed when given with food, but should not be given with antacids, as insoluble precipitates will form. Due to the fairly short half-life, lithium can not usually be administered in a single daily dose and is given in three or four divided doses. The usual range is 900-1,800 mg/day, and serum lithium determinations are readily available as a guide to patient compliance and adequacy of drug dosage.

Clinical Indications and Treatment Results

Lithium is indicated in the treatment and prevention of mania and major (endogenous) depression.

Mania   Lithium is the initial treatment of choice in acute mania, as manifested by hyperactivity, rapid and pressured speech, elevated or irritable mood, flight of ideas, and grandiosity.

After determining that normal kidney function is present, treatment is initiated with 1,200-1,800 mg/day lithium carbonate in three to four divided doses. Serum lithium levels are obtained twice weekly during the induction phase, and levels around 1.5 mEq/liter are sought. A clinical response is usually observed 4-7 days after starting treatment, and reaches its maximum in about 2 weeks. Approximately 80% of manics will show marked improvement or complete recovery on this regimen. For the patient unable or unwilling to cooperate with oral drug therapy, treatment may be initiated with a parenteral neuroleptic (e.g., haloperidol, 20 mg IM, BID), and lithium added a few days later when the patient has shown some improvement. In such cases the aim will be to reduce and discontinue the neuroleptic drug once stable lithium levels have been achieved in the therapeutic range.

Following stable improvement or recovery, the dose of lithium is reduced to a level which will yield a serum level in the range of 0.5-1.0 mEq/liter (generally 900-1,200 mg/day), a usual maintenance dose. Continuation of treatment in this way has been shown to prevent relapse or recurrence in 80% of patients followed over the years. Once a stable serum lithium level has been achieved, blood tests need only to be taken once a month.

Endogenous depression There is not much data on the efficacy of lithium during the acute phase of a depressive illness, although a number of uncontrolled trials have shown direct antidepressant properties of this ion. However, there is no doubt about the effects of long-term maintenance lithium in the prevention of future recurrences of depression, and this is true for unipolar as well as bipolar patients (see p. 99 for definitions).

Side Effects, Precautions, and Contraindications

As the kidney is the main route for lithium excretion, normal renal function is virtually a prerequisite for lithium therapy. A normal serum creatinine provides satisfactory evidence of this, and it is only under exceptional circumstances and with great circumspection that lithium will be prescribed in the face of an elevated creatinine. Patients on low-salt diets should never receive lithium, as an adequate sodium load must be presented to the kidney if lithium is not to be excessively retained. Brief use of diuretics (e.g., furosemide "push") does not have profound effects on lithium excretion, but long-term diuretic therapy, especially with thiazides, is incompatible with lithium administration.

Lithium is an inhibitor of the adenyl cyclase/cyclic adenosine monophosphate (AMP) membrane system, and interferes with hormones whose effect is mediated thereby. Lithium can block the action of antidiuretic hormone (ADH) at the renal level, inducing a diabetes insipidus-like syndrome characterized by polydipsia and the output of a large volume of dilute urine. In a very small percentage of patients, especially with a history of lithium toxicity, this syndrome may be permanent, but no cases of chronic renal disease ("end-stage kidney") have been reported to date. Inhibition of the release of thyroid hormone may also occur, producing goiter, elevated thyroid-stimulating hormone (TSH) levels, and clinical signs of hypothyroidism in about 1% of patients on lithium.

Lithium should not be prescribed concomitantly with indomethacin, as large (50%) increases in serum lithium levels may occur. If patients on lithium require ECT, the drug must be discontinued during the course of treatment, as lithium prolongs the neuromuscular block with succinylcholine, the drug used to achieve muscle relaxation during ECT.

The most frequent side effects of lithium, usually occurring at blood levels of 2.0 mEq/liter and greater, are on the central nervous system and gastrointestinal tract. Tremor, slurring of speech, ataxia, and drowsiness are frequently-observed symptoms of mild-to-moderate toxicity, often in association with nausea and loose stools. If not caught in time, this may progress to coarse muscle twitching, myoclonic jerks, nystagmus, seizures, stupor, coma, and death. Persistent vomiting and profuse diarrhea may be harbingers of this state. Treatment involves stopping lithium and encouraging adequate food and fluid intake. If detected early, mild-to-moderate toxicity generally requires only a day or so off lithium, with resumption at a lower dose. For severe lithium toxicity, as with overdoses, renal dialysis is advisable.

SELECTED BIBLIOGRAPHY

AMA Department of Drugs. *AMA Drug Evaluations,* PSG Pub. Co., Acton, Mass. (1977).

Baldessarini, R. J. *Chemotherapy in Psychiatry.* Harvard, Cambridge (1977).

Barchas, J. D., Berger, P. A., Ciaranello, R. D., and Elliott, G. R. *Psychopharmacology from Theory to Practice.* Oxford, New York (1977).

Jefferson, J. W., and Greist, J. H. *Primer of Lithium Therapy.* Williams and Wilkins, Baltimore (1977).

Johnson, F. N. (ed.). *Lithium Research and Therapy.* Academic, New York (1975).

Kornetzky, C. *Pharmacology: Drugs Affecting Behavior.* Wiley, New York (1976).

Lipton, M. A., DiMascio, A., and Killam, K. F. (eds.). *Psychopharmacology: A Generation of Progress.* Raven, New York (1978).

Sellers, E. M. *Clinical Pharmacology of Psychoactive Drugs.* Addiction Res. Found., Ontario (1975).

Shader, R. I. (ed). *Manual of Psychiatric Therapeutics.* Little, Brown, Boston (1975).

Van Praag, H. M. *Psychotropic Drugs: A Guide for the Practitioner.* Brunner/Mazel, New York (1978).

10

Alcoholism

FREDERICK SIERLES

INTRODUCTION

In order to practice medicine properly, a physician must have a working knowledge of alcoholism. Five to nine million Americans are alcoholics [1] and alcoholism costs the American economy about $15 billion per year in job absenteeism, inefficiency, and medical treatment [2]. Alcoholism causes a huge number of medical and social complications, many of which can be fatal or can have a profound disruptive effect on the lives of alcoholics and their families.

DEFINITION

The definition of alcoholism is simple for advanced cases. Such people demonstrate the following:

Impairment of work and social function due to alcohol
Preoccupation with alcohol
Large daily intake of alcohol
Signs of withdrawal in the absence of alcohol
Medical complications of alcohol

Early cases meet only some of the criteria, and this may lead to a missed diagnosis. Several research teams have set out specific criteria for a diagnosis of alcoholism. The Washington-St. Louis criteria [1,3] are listed in the Appendix.

ETIOLOGY AND CORRELATES

A full comprehension of the etiology of alcoholism still eludes us, even though much is known:

1. *Genetics:* Compared to the general population, many more alcoholics have a father or a sibling who is alcoholic [4]. The prevalence of alcoholism is higher in monozygotic twins than in dizygotic twins [5]. None of the above prove genetic etiology, but the fact that adopted-away sons of alcoholic biological parents have a higher prevalence of alcoholism than a control group of adoptees does demonstrate a genetic causal component in at least some cases [4].

2. *Ethnic Group:* Alcoholism is more prevalent among Irish-Americans, American Indians [6], and poor black Americans [7] than it is in the general population. Alcoholism is very prevalent in France and in Russia [8].

3. *Parental Loss:* A significant number of alcoholics are the product of marriages that ended in divorce or separation [9].

4. *Other Substance Abuse:* Over 95% of alcoholics are cigarette smokers [10], and many alcoholics abuse other drugs in addition to alcohol.

5. *Socioeconomic Status:* There is considerable alcoholism in all social classes, and only about 5% of alcoholics inhabit skid row [2].

6. *Sex:* Alcoholism is more common in men than in women, by a ratio of about 2:1 [1], but the gap is narrowing.

7. *Animal Experimentation:* Animals can be bred or conditioned to develop alcohol-seeking behavior.

COMPLICATIONS

The complications of alcoholism are numerous and often fatal. They will be divided into general medical complications of excessive intake, neuropsychiatric complications of excessive intake and withdrawal, and social complications.

General Medical Complications

Skin

Rhinophyma: The patient has a large, bulbous nose, like W. C. Fields'.

Rosacea: The skin of the cheeks and nose shows a macular blotchy reddening.

Alcoholic Facies: The skin turgor of the face is diminished and the face may have a "leonine" or "leathery" quality.

Petechiae or Ecchymoses: These spotty or patchy discolorations of the skin proceed, in a stepwise fashion, from red to blue to yellow, and represent bleeding into the skin due to hematologic abnormalities or trauma.

Spider Angiomata: These are red macules several millimeters in diameter which blanch (turn white) when pressed, and then turn red again when the pressing finger is released. These are areas of increased vascularity associated with Laennec's cirrhosis.

Susceptibility to the Effect of Cold: Alcohol intoxication is associated with peripheral vasodilation, and this impedes the normal retention of heat associated with vasoconstriction in response to cold.

Lungs

Aspiration Pneumonia: This is an infection of one or more lobes of the lungs due to accidentally inhaling (aspirating) alcohol or food while intoxicated. Organisms other than diplococcus (e.g., *Klebsiella*) are frequently found. Alcoholics have an increased incidence of pulmonary tuberculosis.

Gastrointestinal Tract

Gastritis: The stomach mucosa is inflamed and the patient may experience nausea, retching, vomiting, hematemesis, melena, and abdominal pain.

Duodenal Peptic Ulcer: This may be exacerbated by drinking alcohol.

Hemorrhoids: These are swollen veins protruding from the mucosa of the rectum or from the skin of the anus, and frequently cause hematochezia (blood in the stools). They may be secondary to portal hypertension associated with alcoholic (Laennec's) cirrhosis.

Esophageal Varices: These are dilated esophageal veins which may bleed, producing hematemesis or melena; the condition is often fatal. Like hemorrhoids, esophageal varices may be secondary to portal vein hypertension.

The Liver

Laennec Cirrhosis: The liver becomes enlarged, fibrotic, and palpable below the right costal margin. Often there is blood dyscrasia, hypoproteinemia, or portal hypertension. Hepatic coma may ensue.

Alcoholic Hepatitis (Acute Fatty Liver): The liver shows areas of necrosis and fatty degeneration. It is initially enlarged, tender, and palpable, and the patient often has fever.

Pancreas

Pancreatitis: The patient usually has abdominal pain and tenderness, and often shows dehydration and electrolyte imbalance. Serum amylase is elevated.

Cardiovascular System

Cardiomyopathy: The heart is enlarged and very susceptible to heart failure.

Neuromuscular System

Peripheral Neuropathy: The ankle jerk reflexes are diminished or absent, and calf muscles are atrophic. The patient may experience weakness and parasthesias, and may be unable to walk.

Myopathy: The patient's extremities show proximal muscle weakening and atrophy.

Brain Injuries Due to Accidents: Alcoholics are accident-prone while drinking, and accidents often result in fractures. Sometimes the brain is injured due to subdural hematoma, epidural hematoma, contusion, or laceration.

Cerebellar Degeneration: This is far more common (11:1) in men than in women [11]. The cerebellum, especially the vermis, shows degeneration, and the patient demonstrates cerebellar signs like ataxia and intention tremor.

Marchiafava-Bignami Syndrome: There is discoloration and degeneration of the center of the corpus callosum [11]. Frontal lobe signs, seizures, dementia, and dyspraxias (perhaps due to interhemispheric dysconnection) may occur [11]. The syndrome was first described in Italian red wine drinkers [12], but is certainly not confined to that group.

Central Pontine Myelinolysis: This can occur in advanced chronic alcoholism, or in other diseases which produce cachexia, like cancer [11]. There are patches of demyelination in the pons. If these patches are small, there are no clinical signs. If large, the patient may show decreased consciousness or long-tract (e.g., pyramidal or spinothalamic tract) signs [11].

Hematopoeitic System

Blood Dyscrasias: The patient may develop *anemia* (associated with weakness, shortness of breath, functional heart murmurs, overtaxing of the heart) or *thrombocytopenia*, characterized by a bleeding tendency and petechial hemorrhages in the skin.

Vitamin Deficiency Disease: The patient may develop *scurvy, beri-beri, Wernicke's encephalopathy,* and *pellagra* as a result of excessive drinking with insufficient vitamin intake.

Neuropsychiatric Complications

Withdrawal States

These are conditions which occur when the alcoholic patient discontinues drinking or greatly diminishes his intake.

Alcohol withdrawal "shakes" The patient experiences a coarse tremor (in resting and intention) of the extremities; if severe, there is tremor of the trunk and tongue as well. The patient is quite anxious and has tachycardia. Anorexia, nausea, retching, vomiting, and abdominal cramps occasionally occur. Intellectual functioning is intact and there are no hallucinations or delusions. If the condition goes untreated, the patient will develop delirium tremens. The treatment of "the shakes" is chlordiazepoxide (Librium) 100 mg every 4 hr orally (if the patient has no gastritis or vomiting), by deep intramuscular injection, or intravenously (which is most effective in urgent situations). Diazepam (Valium) 10-15 mg may be substituted for 100 mg chlordiazepoxide.

Delirium tremens ("The DTs") In order to make a definite diagnosis of the DTs, the patient must have a coarse tremor, diffuse intellectual impairment (which may be due to a concentration deficit), and hallucinations (often visual or tactile, but they can be in any sensory modality). In addition, the patient often shows tachycardia, fever, irritability, muttering, suggestibility, dehydration, electrolyte imbalances, and albuminuria. The patient may develop seizures, Korsakoff's psychosis, and may die (depending on the study, mortality rates vary from 1-37%, most commonly 10-15%) due to injury, status epilepticus, hyperthermia, secondary infections, or cardiac arrhythmias. Incomplete variations of the DTs may also occur during alcohol withdrawal. For example, the patient might show only irritability and intellectual impairment. The treatment of the DTs or variants of the DTs is to give 100 mg chlordiazepoxide intravenously every 2-4 hr until the patient falls asleep or the condition is cured.

Diazepam (10-20 mg) could be used in place of chlordiazepoxide. If the patient is dehydrated, he should be given fluids to drink or an IV should be started. If he is not dehydrated, fluids should not be rushed. Electrolyte abnormalities (e.g., hypokalemia, hypomagnesemia) should be corrected. The room should be dimly lit to minimize overstimulation or understimulation. Histopathologically, the brain is usually normal-looking, but edema has been reported. Neuroleptics and barbiturates are contraindicated, the former because they lower the seizure threshold, the latter because they may increase the risk of arrhythmias. Paraldehyde (10-12 cc orally every 4 hr) is also an excellent treatment, but the paraldehyde must be fresh, and the patient's breath will be unpleasant while he is taking it.

Withdrawal seizures Within several days after markedly reducing or discontinuing alcohol a patient may have a grand mal seizure. This occasionally leads to status epilepticus (a continuous seizure treated with diazepam approximately 10 mg slowly IV) or DTs. If not, the doctor should draw blood for a magnesium level, give 100 mg thiamine HCl IM, and 25-50 mg chlordiazepoxide deep IM or slowly IV. If the patient has epilpsy unrelated to alcoholism, his antiepileptic medication should be given. Other causes of seizures should be considered. Some authors suggest diphenylhydantoin, with or without a loading dose, in addition to thiamine and chlordiazepoxide.

Complications of Chronic Use

Korsakoff's Psychosis

There is degeneration in the diencephalon, hippocampus, and other portions of the limbic system, such as the fornix, degenerate as well. The patient usually has a severe disturbance of short-term and recent memory, and sometime confabulates (makes up answers) to fill in memory gaps. This memory deficit is part of a diffuse deficit of intellectual functioning (dementia). Sometimes there is an associated peripheral neuropathy, with paresthesias, muscle atrophy, and diminished ankle jerks. The treatment of Korsakoff's psychosis is for the patient to "go on the wagon" (become abstinent) and to be given a well-balanced diet, 100 mg thiamine hydrochloride daily, and a multivitamin daily. Complete recovery occurs only 20% of the time [11]; when Korsakoff's psychosis occurs simultaneously with Wernicke's encephalopathy; it is called the Wernicke-Korsakoff syndrome.

Wernicke's Encephalopathy

The brain shows necrotic lesions in the gray matter surrounding the aqueduct of Sylvius, pathology in the thalamus, hypothalmus, and mamillary bodies, and some diffuse brain involvement as well [11]. The patient shows diffuse intellectual impairment and "eye signs," consisting of nystagmus (horizontal and vertical) or extraocular muscle movement palsies (typically abducens palsy) or both. Ataxia is common. There may be a modest elevation in cerebrospinal fluid protein, diffuse electroencephalogram slowing, elevated blood pyruvate [11], or decreased blood transketolase [11]. Wernicke's encephalopathy is a medical emergency and, in severe cases, the patient may die. If a diagnosis of Wernicke's encephalopathy is made, the patient should receive 200 mg thiamine hydrochloride IM and then receive 100 mg thiamine orally each day. Wernicke's encephalopathy is occasionally seen in non-alcoholics, and there is a genetic predisposition to it.

Alcoholic Delusional-Hallucinatory State

This is the result of damage to the brain due to chronic use of alcohol, and is commonest in middle-aged males, many of whom have not had other disabling sequelae of alcoholism. The predominant, and sometimes the only, symptoms are vivid hallucinations and/or delusions. The patient does not usually have extensive intellectual impairment, and may have none at all. He does not show coarse tremor, muttering, or suggestibility, as in the case with withdrawal states. The hallucinations may be so vivid and frightening that the patient may take drastic action in response. I know a patient who jumped off a bridge onto an expressway (and sustained numerous fractures) while fleeing hallucinated police cars. Because of the possible presence of complete auditory hallucinations with a clear consciousness, the condition may be confused with schizophrenia, but there is no demonstrated connection between this illness and schizophrenia. The treatment of this condition is to use neuroleptics such as chlorpromazine (Thorazine) or haloperidol (Haldol). The dosages depends on the acuteness and severity of the presenting symptoms and signs. A similar clinical picture is sometimes seen in alcohol withdrawal states, but in the acute withdrawal states, there is a history of recent withdrawal or diminished intake, and the patient usually has some motoric, cognitive, or systemic signs of delirium tremens. When the cause of the delusional-hallucinatory state is uncertain, it is probably better to begin by treating with chlordiazepoxide or diazepam as if the patient has delirium tremens.

Alcoholic "Blackouts"

This occurs early in an alcoholic's drinking career (as opposed to DTs, seizures, and Wernicke's and Korsakoff's syndromes, which are usually seen after several years of drinking), and continues as long as he continues to drink. Here, while drinking, the patient has periods of time, from hours to weeks, about which he will have no recollection in the future. His behaviors during the blacked-out period are his characteristic behaviors when he is intoxicated, ranging from friendly sociability to irritable combativeness. The blacked-out period is sometimes referred to as the "lost weekend." Often, months later, the alcoholic and his family find empty whiskey or beer bottles, and have no recollection of how they got there. The only treatment for this complication is to stop drinking. The term alcoholic blackouts should be distinguished from other types of blackouts, the latter being a lay term for fainting or unconsciousness of any cause.

Pathological Intoxication

This phenomenon, whose existence is challenged by some, is seen in nonalcoholics as well as alcoholics, and follows ingestion of small amounts of alcohol, as well as considerable amounts. After taking a drink, the patient becomes belligerent, combative, irritable and mistrustful, and shows intellectual impairment. The episode usually terminates with the patient falling asleep [13], after which he is amnesic for the period when he was pathologically intoxicated. Other causes of intellectual impairment or irritability should be ruled out. Since pathological intoxication subsides soon after the effect of the alcohol wears off, the key in treatment is to keep the patient in a seclusion room or in restraints until he is no longer intoxicated. Giving 10 ms diazepam or 50 mg chlordiazepoxide might be helpful, but not curative. The patient should receive an extensive neurological workup when the episode is over.

Regular Intoxication (Drunkenness)

The intoxicated person may be euphoric, angry, anxious, or sad, or have any other emotions. When is common is that the drinker is usually less inhibited than when sober. Simple drunkenness is one of the commonest causes of combativeness or irritability in hospital emergency rooms, and alcohol intoxication may be confused with acute mania and other severe psychiatric conditions. Nystagmus may be noted and the speech may be slurred and rambling, and the gait is often ataxic. The breath usually smells of digesting alcohol. Blood alcohol levels are occasionally drawn for legal purposes, and the point of intoxication is usually 100-150 mg/100 ml, depending on the locality, which corresponds to taking two or more strong drinks. The treatment of simple drunkenness is to treat the patient firmly but respectfully, offer him something to eat, and wait until the effect of the alcohol wears off. If he is combative, and cannot be "talked down" or left alone, he should be treated as if he were pathologically intoxicated.

Social Complications

Alcoholics have a high rate of impaired work functioning and divorce. Plant supervisors frequently comment that many of the workers spend part of their day intoxicated, and this greatly affects the efficiency of the plant. Some farsighted employers have programs for referring and monitoring alcoholic employees. Organizations like Alanon and Alateen provide support for spouses and children of alcoholic patients.

THE TREATMENT OF ALCOHOLISM IN GENERAL

Data-Gathering Phase

A careful history and physical should be done, with emphasis on common complications of alcoholism. Routine lab tests done on hospitalized medical patients should detect common complications of alcoholism. In taking the history, the doctor should not be judgmental about alcoholism. If the doctor is critical and judgmental, the patient will sense this and be less compliant with treatment regimens.

One noncritical way of inquiring about alcohol intake is to ask "Are you a drinking man (or drinking person)?" with a tone of voice that can be construed as tolerant of drinking. In assessing the amount of intake, it is often useful for the doctor to exaggerate the amount in his questioning. For example, when the patient describes himself as a drinker, the doctor might as "What do you drink, two quarts a day?" and the patient, rarely surprised by the question, will often say something like "Oh no, I only drink a pint."

Withdrawal Phase

If the patient has been drinking heavily until the time of admission, he should be hospitalized. If the patient has one of the complications described earlier in this chapter, this should be treated. If the patient has no apparent complications he should be given a balanced diet, 100 mg thiamine per day, and a multivitamin; he should also receive 100 mg chlordiazepoxide per day (or diazepam 20-40 mg/day) orally in divided doses, as prophylactic against withdrawal phenomena. During the withdrawal phase, regardless of complications, almost all alcoholics should receive daily thiamine. The anxiolytic agent can be discontinued in about a week.

One of the hallmarks of this phase of the treatment is that the alcoholic often sees that he can function well physically and emotionally while abstinent. During this phase he should be approached to discuss long-term treatment.

Long-Term Treatment

No one has done a controlled study demonstrating long-term treatment of alcoholism to be better than no treatment at all [14]. However, since no one has ever proven the opposite and it is common practice to attempt some form of treatment and since the alcoholic patient is asking for help in "getting on the wagon," the physician should attempt one of the conventional forms of long-term treatment, or refer the patient to someone who regularly treats alcoholics. The treatment methods are as follows, and can be used alone or in any combination acceptable to the doctor and the patient.

Disulfiram (Antabuse)

Twelve hours or longer after the patient has had his last drink, he is given 500 mg Antabuse orally once daily for a week, and then 250 mg orally per day, (or 500 mg orally every other day) indefinitely. He is instructed that if he drinks alcohol in any form, applies alcohol-containing shaving lotions, or takes wine sauce on meat or fish, he is likely to have excruciating physical distress for several hours. The signs and symptoms of the Antabuse-alcohol reaction are nausea and vomiting, cough and shortness of breath, malaise and weakness, flushing, and headache. This is the result of the buildup of acetaldehyde in the patient's bloodstream. In rare cases, if the patient has a severe medical illness, the Antabuse-alcohol reaction can be fatal. If the patient has significant medical illness of any cause, a family physician or specialist should be consulted before using Antabuse. The treatment of the Antabuse-alcohol reaction is to give diphenhydramine (Benadryl) 50 mg intramuscularly and have the patient inhale oxygen by nasal cannula. Patients should not drink for 2 weeks after Antabuse has been discontinued lest they experience the alcohol-Antabuse reaction.

Psychotherapies

This category encompasses many forms of treatment by talking, including Alcoholics Anonymous, behavior therapy, individual psychotherapy, group psychotherapy, and family therapy, alone, in combination with each other, or with Antabuse. It may be initiated in the hospital during the withdrawal phase, and continued after the patient is discharged. Many claims are made for good results, with various criteria used for measuring improvement, but as stated before, no one has been able to prove that any form of treatment for alcoholism is better than no treatment at all. Chafetz' *Frontiers of Alcoholism* [14] tabulates alcohol tratment studies prior to 1970.

Alcoholics Anonymous (AA) is a national organization with chapters in most cities, and has long experience in treating alcoholics. It was founded, and is run, by alcoholics, who must be abstinent to work as counselors. They hold weekly (or more frequent) meetings. Members are offered support during difficult periods, and are encouraged to call other members if the urge to resume drinking is strong. Abstinent members have made the organization and abstinence a major element, a raison d'etre, in their lives and this may help them to achieve and maintain abstinence. They believe that alcoholism is a disease like diabetes, and that alcoholics must be abstinent just as diabetics must take insulin. Members are told that they must take each day at a time, instead of having to contemplate continuous suffering to remain abstinent. This organization used to function outside the medical community, and the use of Antabuse was frowned upon as a "crutch" by AA. More recently, both AA and many of the alcohologists in the medical profession have come to accept the other's position and to work together.

PROGNOSIS

Alcoholism is a tough disease to treat successfully. Many alcoholics (the percentages vary with the study) never attempt to achieve abstinence, and many never even believe they are alcoholics. Some have periods of several months or years of abstinence, and then return to drinking for various intervals. But even if there is a recurrence after abstinence, the patient's diseased organs will have had a chance to heal, the patient has had a chance to see that abstinence is possible, and the patient may have contributed productively to his family and society. A small, but very real percentage of patients become continuously abstinent, and serve as a model for others to follow.

REFERENCES

1. Woodruff, R., Goodwin, D., and Guze, S. *Psychiatric Diagnosis*. Oxford, New York (1974).
2. Chafetz, M. Alcoholism and alcoholic psychosis in *Comprehensive Textbook of Psychiatry II*. A. Freedman, H. Kaplan, and B. Sadock, eds. Williams and Wilkins, Baltimore (1975).
3. Feighner, J., Robins, E., Guze, S., Woodruff, R., Winokur, G., and Munoz, R. Diagnostic criteria for use in psychiatric research. *Arch. Gen. Psychiatry* 26:56-63 (1972).
4. Goodwin, D. Family and adoption studies of alcoholism, in *Biosocial Bases of Criminal Behavior*. S. Mednick and K. Christiansen, eds. Gardner, New York (1977).
5. Kaij, L. *Studies on the Etiology and Sequels of Use of Alcohol*. Lund: Department of Psychiatry, University of Lund (1960).
6. Dozier, E. Problem drinking among American Indians: The role of sociocultural deprivation. *Quart. J. Studies of Alcohol* 27:72-87 (1966).
7. Robins, L., Murphy, G., and Breckinridge, M. Drinking behavior of young Negro men. *Quart. J. Studies of Alcohol* 29:657-684 (1968).
8. Sadoun, R., Lolli, G., and Silverman, M. *Drinking in French Culture*. Monographs of the Rutgers Center of Alcoholic Studies No. 5. College and University Press, New Haven (1965).

9. Westermeyer, J. *Primer on Chemical Dependency*. Williams and Wilkins, Baltimore (1976).
10. Walton, R. Smoking and alcoholism: A brief report. *Am. J. Psychiatry* 128:139-140 (1972).
11. Adams, R., and Victor, M. *Principles of Neurology*. McGraw-Hill, New York (1977).
12. Marchiafava, E., and Bignami, A. Sopra un alterazione del corpo calloso osservata in soggetti alcoolisti. *Riv. Patol. Nerv* 8:544 (1903).
13. Kosbab, F., and Kuhnley, E. Pathologic intoxication. *Psychiatric Opinion* 15:35-38 (1978).
14. Chafetz, M., Blane, H., and Hill, M. *Frontiers of Alcoholism*. Science House, New York (1970).

APPENDIX: WASHINGTON-ST. LOUIS CRITERIA FOR ALCOHOLISM*

ALCOHOLISM: A "definite" diagnosis is made when symptoms occur in at least three of the four groups. A "probable" diagnosis is made when symptoms occur in only two groups.

Group One: (1) Any manifestations of alcohol withdrawal such as tremulousness, convulsions, hallucinations, or delirium. (2) History of medical complications, e.g., cirrhosis, gastritis, pancreatitis, myopathy, polyneuropathy, Wernicke-Korsakoff's syndrome. (3) Alcoholic blackouts, e.g., amnesic episodes during drinking not accounted for by head trauma. (4) Alcoholic binges or benders (48 hr or more of drinking associated with default of usual obligations: Must have occurred more than once to be scored as positive).

Group Two: (1) Patient has not been able to stop drinking when he wanted to do so. (2) Patient has tried to control drinking by allowing himself to drink only under certain circumstances, such as only after 5:00 p.m., only on weekends, or only with other people. (3) Drinking before breakfast. (4) Drinking nonbeverage forms of alcohol, e.g., hair tonic, mouthwash, Sterno, etc.

Group Three: (1) Arrested for drinking. (2) Traffic difficulties associated with drinking. (3) Trouble at work because of drinking. (4) Fighting associated with drinking.

Group Four: (1) Patient thinks he drinks too much. (2) Family objects to his drinking. (3) Loss of friends because of drinking. (4) Other people object to his drinking. (5) Feels guilty about drinking.

Source: From J. Feighner, E. Robins, S. Guze, R. Woodruff, G. Winokur, and R.Munoz. Diagnostic criteria for use in psychiatric research. *Arch. Gen. Psychiatry* 26:56-63, 1972.

11

Drug Abuse

FREDERICK SIERLES

INTRODUCTION

I will define drug abuse as the excessive or physiologically unnecessary use, for psychological effects, of a substance for which the ingestion, continued use, or withdrawal may be dangerous. This definition, while imprecise, bypasses the problems presented by defining it based on whether the drug is prescribed or whether it is approved of by society.

CATEGORIES OF DRUGS

The following drugs will be discussed in this chapter:
Barbiturates and other sedative-hypnotics
Anxiolytics
Opiates and opioids
Amphetamines
Cocaine
Anticholinergic substances
Glue and other volatile substances
Hallucinogens
Volatile nitrites
All psychoactive substances can be abused, but we will not cover them here. Alcoholism is discussed in Chapter 10.

EXTENT OF THE PROBLEM

The abuse of drugs is widespread, although no drug on our list is abused as much as alcohol. In 1973, the Federal Bureau of Narcotics and Dangerous Drugs estimated that opioid addicts numbered about 560,000, which is about .3% of the American population. Diazepam (Valium) is the most commonly prescribed drug in America, and it is both abused and overprescribed, but addiction to it is rare. In 1973, Callan and Patterson studied all midwestern military inductees (N = 19,948) for a 6-month period, and provided the results listed in Table 1 [1]. A sample of midwestern military inductees is certainly not demographically similar to the general population, but the study may provide some idea of the *relative* frequency which the drugs listed are used by young Americans in general.

Table 1   Drug Abuse by Military Inductees

Name of drug	Percentage of Inductees using the drug
Marijuana	24
Hashish	16
Amphetamines	12
LSD	9
Mescaline	9
Barbiturates	9
Glue	4
Opium	4
Cocaine	4
Psilocybin	3
Heroin	3
DMT	2
STP	2
Morphine	2

Source: Modified form J. Callan and C. Patterson. Drug abuse among military inductees. *Am. J. Psychiatry* 130:260-264, 1973.

In the late 1960s and early 1970s the frequency of drug abuse was steadily increasing, and has probably been close to a plateau for the past several years. Rapid changes occur, often on a regional basis. For example, the abuse of a combination of pentazocine (Talwin) and pyribenzamine (the combination is sometimes called "Ts and blues"), reached epidemic proportions in Chicago in 1978. Wars are frequently associated with changes in drug abuse patterns. Woodruff, Goodwin, and Guze [2] estimate that "perhaps half of the American soldiers in Vietnam during 1971 experimented with opium, although only 20% used it frequently and many were able to discontinue the drug upon returning to the states." Japanese (and possibly American and British) pilots in World War II were given amphetamines by their superiors.

ADDICTION

Addiction is the combination of psychological dependence, tolerance (where a progressively increasing dose is required to obtain the original effect), and withdrawal (where physical signs occur during abstinence). The etiology of addiction is not known. Barbiturates and other sedative-hypnotics, alcohol, anxiolytics, and opioids are addicting. The hallucinogens, neuroleptics, monoamine oxidase (MAO) inhibitors, tricyclic antidepressants, and volatile nitrites are not addicting. Withdrawal from barbiturates, other sedative-hypnotics, anxiolytics, and alcohol may be fatal.

EXTENT OF USE

Fortunately, the majority of people who abuse drugs do so only occasionally, and not everyone using addicting drugs becomes addicted. For example, Zinberg and Jacobson [3] describe "chipping," the occasional use of opioids by nonaddicted individuals. On the other hand, many individuals abuse several drugs simultaneously ("polydrug abusers"). There are many addicts.

CORRELATES OF DRUG ABUSE

Sex

The abuse of "street" drugs is commoner in men than in women; the abuse of prescribed drugs, especially the anxiolytics and sedative-hypnotics, is commoner in women than in men.

Age

The majority of street drug abusers are adolescents and young adults. Glue-sniffing is commonest in early adolescence. Although abuse of street sedative-hypnotics is commoner in adolescents and young adults, the abuse of prescribed sedative-hypnotics is associated with middle age.

Occupation

Drug abuse is very common in physicians, nurses, and criminals.

Ethnic and Religious Groups

Callan and Patterson's previously mentioned study of midwestern military inductees [1] showed the following: Whites and blacks have an approximately equal total drug abuse rate; among religious groups, Jews and "unaffiliated" people have the highest total drug abuse rates. The rates for Catholics and Protestants are approximately equal.

Within the total drug abuse picture, there are differing patterns, with young adult Jews abusing hallucinogens more frequently, middle-aged Jews abusing prescription sedative-hypnotics more frequently [4], and young adult blacks abusing opioids more frequently [5].

Associated Psychiatric Illnesses

This is a controversial area, with conflicting data and no certainty that correlations correspond to a causal relationship. Grant and Judd [6] demonstrated that of a sample of polydrug abusers, 37% had deficits in neuropsychological functioning (as measured by the Halstead-Reitan battery), compared with 26% for psychiatric patients and 8% for controls. Whether the drugs caused the dysfunction is hard to assess, since polydrug users also had higher rates of head trauma and were school dropouts prior to the onset of drug abuse. Acord and Barker [7] found an increased prevalence of deficits in neuropsychological functioning in hallucinogenic drug users.

Stefanis et al. [8] found a rate of personality disorder and neurosis significantly higher in chronic hashish users than in controls, with sociopathy being the commonest personality disorder. Guze [9] found an association between drug abuse, sociopathy, and Briquet's syndrome in convicted felons.

On the other hand, Beaubrun and Knight [10] found no increase in psychopathology in chronic cannabis users as compared with controls. Weissman et al. [11] found that 30% of addicts in a methadone program had clinically significant depression. The incidence of suicide is increased among drug abusers.

INDIVIDUAL VARIATIONS

Hofmann and Hofmann [12] write: "The nature of individual drug experiences, which can vary greatly, is probably largely determined by the drug (including dose and route of administration), the user's response to the drug's effects, and the environment in which the drug is taken."

DIAGNOSIS AND MANAGEMENT OF INTOXICATIONS AND WITHDRAWAL

Barbiturates and Other Sedative-Hypnotics

Names

The barbiturates include amobarbital (Amytal), secobarbital (Seconal), pentobarbital (Nembutal), Amobarbital-pentobarbital combination (Tuinal), and phenobarbital (Luminal). The other sedative-hypnotics include methaqualone (Quaalude), ethchlorvinyl (Placidyl), chloral hydrate (Noctec), chloral etaine, paralydehyde (Paral), glutethamide (Doriden), methyprylon (Noludar), and ethinamate (Valmid).

Intoxication

Intoxication with these substances is virtually identical with alcohol intoxication, but unless the patient has also been drinking, there is no odor of digesting alcohol on the breath. The behavior is often uninhibited; irritability and combaitveness are common. Drowsiness and euphoria are also common. Ataxia, slurred speech, and nystagmus are characteristic. Treatment of barbiturate intoxication is the same for alcohol intoxication; wait the episode out and try to prevent (by talk, restraints, or seclusion) violence if the patient is irritable or combative. There is no specific antidote. These substances can be detected in the blood and urine by hospital toxicology labs.

Addiction

These substances are highly addicting, with significant withdrawal signs occurring after more than a few weeks' use of addicting doses (Table 2) [13]:

Table 2   Addicting Doses of Sedative-Hypnotics

Drug	Addicting dose (mg/day)
Phenobarbital	300
Pentobarbital	400-600
Amobarbital	600
Secobarbital	600
Methaqualone	600
Ethchlorvinyl	2,000
Methyprylon	2,400
Gluthethamide	2,500
Ethinamate	1,300

Source: From R. Shader, E. Caine, and R. Meyer. Treatment of dependence on Barbiturates and sedative-hypnotics, in *Manual of Psychiatric Therapeutics.* R. Shader, ed. Little, Brown, Boston, 1975, with permission (Ref. 13).

After 6-8 weeks' use of these or greater doses of these drugs, over 80% of patients have definite withdrawal signs. From 4-6 weeks, over 50% of patients experience significant withdrawal signs.

Withdrawal

Signs of withdrawal from these substances include anxiety with tachycardia and sweating, coarse tremor, fever, muscle twitching, cramping, nausea and vomiting, dysphoria, delirium tremens (see Chap. 10) and grand mal seizures. The seizures may occur alone, and may be the first sign of withdrawal. Treatment of the sedative-hypnotic withdrawal syndrome is best accomplished in the hospital and is based on the following: (1) the patient may die in "DTs" or with seizures, so treatment must be aggressive, and (2) all of these sedative-hypnotics have cross-tolerance, so each could be substituted for the other. Withdrawal is usually carried out by using the original addicting substance or by substituting an equivalent amount of phenobarbital. Phenobarbital is preferred because of its long duration of action, providing for stability of blood level.

Here are the mechanics of the treatment process:

1. Ask the patient for his approximate daily amount of the addicting drug.

2. Give one-fourth the daily amount of the addicting drug (or its equivalent in phenobarbital) orally or intramuscularly as a test dose. If you are totally unsure of his daily intake, 200 mg pentobarbital or 60 mg phenobarbital could be used as a test dose.

3. If the patient achieves a "safe drunk" or a "mild high" ½-1 hr after the test dose, prescribe the test dose every 6 hr for a day or two. A mild high is reached when the patient feels comfortable, has nystagmus and mild ataxia, and has no withdrawal signs.

4. After a day of relative comfort for the patient, begin decreasing the drug by 5-10% (of the original baseline daily dose required to produce the mild high) per day over 10-20 days.

If the patient still has withdrawal signs ½-1 hr after the test dose, add a supplemental amount to the test dose. If the patient manifests life-threatening withdrawal signs, he should be given intramuscular amobarbital or pentobarbital, which are faster-acting than phenobarbital. Then the original abused substances or phenobarbital can be substituted. If the patient falls asleep ½-1 hr after the test dose, and has been abstinent for the 2 or 3 hr prior to the test dose, he should receive a second but smaller test dose 6 hr after the original test dose. Table 3 is a list of equivalent doses of sedative-hypnotics [13].

Table 3 Substitution Doses of Sedative-Hypnotics

Drug	Equivalent dose (mg)
Phenobarbital	30
Secobarbital	100
Pentobarbital	100
Chloral hydrate	250
Gluthethamide	250

Source: From R. Shader, E. Caine, and R. Meyer. Treatment of dependence on barbiturates and sedative-hypnotics, in *Manual of Psychiatric Therapeutics.* R. Shader, ed. Little, Brown, Boston, 1975, with permission (Ref. 13).

Anxiolytic Agents: Benzodiazepines and Prophylendeiols

Names

The benzodiazepines include diazepam (Valium), chlordiazepoxide (Librium), oxazepam (Serax), and chlorazepate (Tranxene). The propylenediols include meprobamate (Miltown, Equanil) and tybamate.

Intoxication

Clinically noticeable intoxication with these substances is uncommon, although I have seen severe chlordiazepoxide intoxication due to advanced liver cirrhosis. When it occurs, the intoxication mimics barbiturate or alcohol intoxication, and the treatment is the same as for sedative-hypnotic intoxication.

Addiction

Addiction to benzodiazepines does occur, although it is uncommon. The addicting doses of chlordiazepoxide and diazepam are 300 mg/day and 120 mg/day, respectively. The propylenediols are more highly addicting, with significant withdrawal symptoms occuring at 2,400 mg/day for meprobamate. The equivalent doses are listed in Table 4 [13].

Withdrawal

Withdrawal signs and symptoms, when they do occur, are identical to those of sedative-hypnotic withdrawal, and should be treated the same way,

Table 4   Substitution Doses of Anxiolytic Agents and Sedative-Hypnotics

Drug	Equivalent dose (mg)
Diazepam	5
Chlordiazepoxide	25
Meprobamate	200
Phenobarbital	30

Source: From R. Shader, E. Caine, and R. Meyer. Treatment of dependence on barbiturates and sedative-hypnotics, in *Manual of Psychiatric Therapeutics*. R. Shader, ed. Little, Brown, Boston, 1975, with permission (Ref. 13).

bearing in mind that these substances also have cross-tolerance with the barbiturates and other sedative-hypnotics.

Withdrawal in Neonates

The symptoms resemble those of opioid withdrawal in the newborn, and are treated with very small doses of a barbiturate with a daily decrement over 7-10 days.

Opiates and Opioids

Names

These include codeine, dolophine (Methadone), heroin, hyodrmorphone (Dilavdid), meperidine (Demerol), morphine, opium, pentazocine (Talwin), and propoxyphene (Darvon). Opiates are naturally occurring substances; opioids are synthetic.

Intoxication

In the early stages euphoria is common, often associated with drowsiness and falling asleep while sitting ("nodding"). The first contact with opiates may also be disagreeable, for nausea and vomiting may occur. The pupils are pinpoint in size, for reasons not yet known. People intoxicated with opioids rarely request treatment for the intoxication, but patients may be brought to the hospital in a coma due to a deliberate or accidental overdose. Patients comatose from opioid intoxication should be given .4 mg naloxone (Narcan, an opiate antagonist) slowly intravenously. If the first dose of naloxone doesn't work, this dose can be repeated twice more at 3-min intervals. If the third dose does not work, the diagnosis was probably wrong. Opiates can be detected in blood or urine samples by a toxicology lab.

Addiction

Because street drugs are mixed with powders and diluents such as quinine, procaine, baking soda, talc, starch, and mannite (an Italian laxative), actual metric doses are not usually mentioned. Instead intake is reported as "dollars per day" habits, with addicts usually taking between $50-200 per day of opiates, or as "bags per day," with each bag containing 4-15 mg pure heroin. Government-supported methadone maintenance programs, designed to reduce crime by providing free dolophine, usually give addicts between 40 and 100 mg dolophine per day.

Medical complications of intravenous drug use include the following:

1. Bacterial endocarditis—this is often due to antibiotic resistant bacteria or fungi.

2. Pulmonary edema—the cause of this is uncertain. It may be related to the powders or diluents.

3. Tetanus—this is most likely to occur in addicts who "skin pop" (inject subcutaneously).

4. Quartan malaria—this is rare nowadays.

5. Thrombophlebitis and cellulitis.

6. Bacterial pneumonia.

7. Viral hepatitis—this is typically serum hepatitis, which is usually Australia-antigen-positive early in the illness.

8. Delayed or absent ejaculation and diminished sexual interest.

9. Generalized glomerular sclerosis.

10. Fibrotic scars—most opioid addicts have fibrotic scars on the skin of their hands, forearms, and antecubital fossa veins. These can be treated by a plastic surgeon.

11. Cigarette burns—these are on the anterior chest and result from "nodding."

Withdrawal

Signs of withdrawal include yawning, anxiety, tachycardia, rise in blood pressure, rhinorrhea, lacrimation, piloerection, nausea, vomiting, muscle twitching or kicking, abdominal, back or joint pains, pains in almost any location, and leukocytosis. Spontaneous orgasm may occur [12]. Opioid withdrawal is not fatal, unless it is superimposed upon an illness which could itself produce sudden death. Thus, addicts can be treated "cold turkey" (no substitute drugs), as is done in some drug treatment programs or jails. One can obtain more comfortable withdrawal by giving 10-20 mg dolophine, orally or intramuscularly, twice daily for 1 day, and reducing the dose by 10-20% per day over 5-10 days. If milligram dosage of heroin is known to the addict, 1 mg methadone = 1 mg heroin, up to 40 mg. On alternate days, when the morning and evening doses are not equal, the nighttime dose should be the higher dose. If the patient is in a methadone program, the withdrawal process should begin with a higher starting dose and a longer withdrawal period. Mild physiological disturbances may occur up to 6 months following withdrawal.

Withdrawal in Neonates

An infant born to an opioid-addicted mother may be born lethargic and, within 24 hr after birth, become irritable, raise his legs to the abdomen as though having abdominal cramps, have fever, yawning, sneezing, lacrimation, nasal congestion, loose stools, or erratic breathing. Rarely, seizures, depressed respirations, and cyanosis can occur. There is a high morbidity and low mortality. The treatment, if the withdrawal syndrome is mild, is to observe. If severe, small amounts of tincture of opium, paregoric, dolophine, barbiturates, or diazepam may be used. A definite treatment of choice has not been established.

Amphetamines

Names

This group includes amphetamine, dextroamphetamine, methamphetamine.

Intoxication

Amphetamines have adrenergic properties, and amphetamine intoxication may be associated with mild hypertension and tachycardia, dilated pupils with occasional blurred vision, and dry mouth with occasional trouble swallowing. Anxiety, increased alertness, and anorexia are quite common. The respiratory rate may be increased and hyperthermia may occur. Occasionally, the patient will go into an adrenergic crisis with hypertension and hyperpyrexia.

Intoxication may produce euphoria and alertness, although depression may be seen. Heightened sexuality may occur. Continuing high-dosage usage often produces emotional blunting, suspiciousness, delusions of persecution, sterotyped behavior, and visual or auditory hallucinations. The latter five symptoms, which may become permanent, have caused chronic amphetamine intoxication to be confused with schizophrenia. Bruxism (uncontrollable gnashing of the teeth) may also occur.

A patient with amphetamine intoxication should be "talked down," and if unremitting anxiety is the only sign, could get a benzodiazepine. If the patient is psychotic and not improving, he should get haloperidol intramuscularly as often as every half hour. Haloperidol has a specific antiamphetamine effect. For an adrenergic crisis with tachycardia, hypertension, and hyperpyrexia, 1-2 mg propranolol (Inderal) intravenously or 20-40 mg orally has a specific antidote effect. The presence of amphetamines can be detected in urine and blood samples by toxicology labs.

Addiction

Tolerance develops rapidly, and patients may take as much as 3000 mg amphetamine per day orally, and up to 13,000 mg per day intravenously [12]. The extent of this tolerance is best comprehended by knowing that the standard therapeutic dose of amphetamines is 15-45 mg/day. Seizures, delirium tremens, muscle twitching, pains, and fever do not occur in amphetamine withdrawal, even if the withdrawal is abrupt.

Withdrawal

Patients withdrawing after high-dosage daily use of amphetamines may experience depression, sleepiness, and increased appetite. However, the amphetamine can and should be withdrawn totally and abruptly. Treatment for the depression depends on the type of depressive syndrome which presents.

Cocaine

Names

This is a single drug, not a category of drugs. It is an adrenergic drug which is similar to the amphetamines, and has recently become popular.

Intoxication

Like the amphetamines, cocaine intoxication may produce mild hypertension, tachycardia, anxiety, and increased alertness. Small doses of cocaine produce euphoria, moderate doses produce depression, and continuing high dosages produce persecurory delusions. The progression from euphoria to depression to psychosis has been called a "kindling effect" analogous to small burning sticks of kindling wood finally resulting in a large fire of bigger logs [14]. In addition, interesting perceptual disturbances may occur. These include polyopia (seeing numerous "carbon copies" of a single image), dysmegalopsia (objects become smaller or larger), tactile hallucinations (called formication, "cocaine bugs," or Magnan's sign), and geometrical hallucinations similar to those occurring with migraine headaches. [15]. Like amphetamine psychosis, cocaine psychosis has occasionally been confused with schizophrenia, and the treatment for intoxication is the same as for amphetamine toxicity.

Addiction

The drug can be abruptly discontinued without a risk of death. Chronic cocaine inhalers develop ulcerations of the nasal septum.

Withdrawal

In withdrawal from cocaine, the patient may experience drowsiness or depression. The depression is treated based upon whether it is endogenous or reactive.

Anticholinergic Drugs

Names

The toxic effects of anticholinergic (atropinic) substances often occur with legal (prescribed or over-the-counter) anticholinergic drugs such as atropine, scopolamine (used in many over-the-counter medications), benztropine (Cogentin), diphenhydramine (Benadryl), tricyclic antidepressants, and neuroleptics. "Cold tablets" often contain atropinic substances. Occasionally, large doses of anticholinergics are used for a hallucinogenic effect.

Intoxication

The syndrome of anticholinergic toxicity is summarized as "dry as a bone (decreased sweating and salivation with lip-licking), red as a beet (flushing), and mad as a hatter (delirium)." The patient often has fever, and sometimes has hyperpyrexia. Temperatures up to 109°F have been observed in anticholinergic toxicity in children.

Occasionally, the patient may hallucinate in the absence of a full-blown delirium. Delirium and hallucinations may occur with low doses of anticholinergics, but usually require high doses. The patient may develop cardiac arrhythmias. The treatment of anticholinergic toxicity is to give 1-2 mg physostigmine (a specific antidote) subcutaneously as often as every 15 min to a total of four doses. Neuroleptics are contraindicated because they have anticholinergic properties. The anticholinergics can be discontinued abruptly without complications.

Glue and Other Volatile Solvents

Names

These substances are hydrocarbons. The group includes glue, plastic cement, nail polish remover, lacquer thinner, lighter fluid, spot remover, gasoline, antifreeze, marking pencils, aerosols, and solvents.

Intoxication

These substances are commonly inhaled from a plastic bag held tightly over the mouth and nose. When any of these substances is inhaled, the patient may experience drowsiness, euphoria, analgesia, slurred speech, diplopia, photophobia, tinnitus, rhinitis, nausea, vomiting, chest pain, diarrhea, dizziness, ataxia, disinhibition, combativeness, hallucinations, and illusions. Cases have been reported where a patient inhaled a solvent and then experienced a "flashback" of a past hallucinogenic drug "trip." Intoxicated patients should be "talked down", and a benzodiazepine can be given if the only sign is unremitting anxiety. For psychosis that does not resolve, a neuroleptic or ECT can be used. Inhaling solvents has led to cerebral edema and cardiac arrhythmias, which require specialized medical treatment.

Addiction and Withdrawal

Tolerance to these substances does develop, and there are reported cases of severe withdrawal symptoms, including cramps, headache, chills, hallucinations, and delirium tremens, although severe withdrawal is uncommon. Chronic inhalation of these substances may lead to blindness; bone marrow suppression with anemia; fatty degeneration of the heart, liver, kidneys, and adrenals; dementia; cardiac arrhythmias; and thesaurosis (a pneumoconiosis), all depending on which substance has been abused. Chronic users who have sickle-cell anemia may develop aplastic anemia. Some efforts at prevention have included stringent requirements on the sale of these substances to minors, and additives which are irritating to glue sniffers, but not to people using these substances for their original purposes. The results of these efforts are not known.

Hallucinogens

Names

There are over 200 hallucinogenic substances, but only a limited number are popular. These include D-lysergic acid diethylamide (LSD), 2,5-dimethoxy-4-methyl amphetamine (DOM, STP), O-phosphoryl-4-hydroxy-N-dimethyltryptamine (psilocybin), N,N-dimethyltryptamine (DMT), N,N-diethyltryptamine (DET), 3,4,5-trimethoxyphenylethylamine (mescaline), methylene dioxyamphetamine (MDA), and Δ-3-tetrahydrocannabinol (THC, marijuana and hashish).

Intoxication

Patients usually experience hallucinations, in any sensory modality, with visual hallucinations being most common. Kaleidoscopic visual hallucinations may occur. Illusions and synesthesias (perceptions mixing two sensory modalities, such as smelling a color) have been reported. Secondary delusions may occur. The entire gamut of moods may be experienced, and occasionally a patient may be irritable, combative, or terrified.

With the exception of tetrahydrocannabinol, all of the above mentioned hallucinogens are classified as adrenergic. This means that when the patient is intoxicated, he will experience elevations beyond his baseline level of blood pressure, pulse, and possibly body temperature, and his pupils will be dilated. With tetrahydrocannabinol the blood pressure, pulse, and possibly the body temperature may be slightly elevated, but the pupils are typically normal in width. Interesting findings associated with tetrahydrocannabinol intoxication include conjuctival injection lasting up to 2 years after the last use of the drug, hypoglycemia with a craving for sweets, and impaired ability to gauge time. Interesting features of the other hallucinogens occur as well. Mescaline frequently causes vomiting. LSD intoxication can be associated with lacrimation and salivation.

The dosage of LSD necessary to produce hallucinations is 35 mg, and the average street dose is between 50 and 350 mg. Because the dose necessary to produce hallucinations is markedly different from the hypothesized fatal dose (14,000 mg injected intravenously), death due to LSD overdose has never been reported. Tolerance can develop rapidly with LSD, but it disappears several days after the first day of abstinence. Because of the small doses, LSD is not detectable by most hospital toxicology labs.

Weeks and months after the last intoxication with any of the hallucinogens (rarely over a year), the patient may experience spontaneous recurrence (a "flashback") of some or all of the aspects of an earlier intoxication.

These can be pleasant or unpleasant, and the frequency is variable, with a maximum of perhaps 5-10 flashbacks in a day. The cause of flashbacks is unknown. They are most commonly associated with LSD use.

Patients intoxicated with hallucinogens should be "talked down" in a safe, supportive setting. A benzodiazepine can be used if the only sign is unremitting anxiety. If psychosis is present and does not start resolving as the hours go by, the patient can be given a neuroleptic or electroconvulsive therapy. Neuroleptics should be withheld if there is reason to suspect that the patient has taken an anticholinergic substance. There is no medical treatment for flashbacks, but supportive conversation is recommended.

Addiction and Withdrawal

These substances are not addicting.

Phencyclidine (PCP)

Names

This is an anesthetic, animal tranquilizer, and hallucinogen known alternately as PCP, Sernyl, "angel dust," and often misrepresented as tetrahydrocannabinol. It is described separately from the other hallucinogens because of unique, potentially disastrous and long-term effects and because of its recent popularity.

Intoxication

Signs of behavioral toxicity include hallucinations, delusions, mutism, catatonia, analgesia, panic, excited states, and combativeness. Flashbacks are common. Systemic toxicity is frequent and may be serious, since the substance has sympathomimetic and other autonomic effects. Sympathomimetic effects include tachycardia, hypertension, and increased deep tendon reflexes. Other effects of PCP include sweating, drooling, skin flushing, and meiosis. In cases of severe toxicity, the patient may experience status epilepticus, a hypertensive crisis, coma, respiratory arrest, and cardiac arrest. In very mild cases, treatment consists of observation. Acidification of the urine may help. Some patients prefer to be left alone in their hospital rooms. Occasionally, the patient will have to be restrained or secluded. α-adrenergic-blocking agents, such as phentolamine (Regitine) can be given for severe hypertension.

If agitation or psychosis does not resolve as the hours progress, or if combativeness occurs, haloperidol or electroconvulsive therapy (ECT) may be used. Not all patients eventually recover [16].

Volatile Nitrites

Because these substances have recently become popular as drugs of abuse, a short discussion is in order. Amyl nitrite and other nitrites are commonly used as room deodorizers, and are used in certain industrial manufacturing processes as well. When inhaled, they produce peripheral vasodilatation, perineal vasodilatation, and possibly but uncommonly, hallucinations. As drugs of abuse, they are often used during sexual intercourse to heighten the pleasure. Their effects are demonstrably transient, and are believed to result from a drug effect on the brain stem, not on the cortex. They have not yet been shown to be addicting, and their toxicology has not yet been studied in detail.

TREATMENT, PREVENTION, AND PROGNOSIS OF DRUG ABUSE IN GENERAL

Treatment of Drug Abuse in General

Just as for alcoholism, there are no controlled studies which demonstrate that any long-term treatment of drug abusers is significantly better than no treatment. The modalities which have been employed include the following:

Relaxation

Modalities used to produce relaxation, when the subject feels anxious, include the following: (1) Electrosleep, which is the application of low-voltage (below the voltage used for ECT) current to the patient's head; (2) biofeedback; and (3) other relaxation modalities—these include meditation, hypnosis, desensitization, and progressive relaxation.

Narcotic Antagonists

These are potentially useful for opioid addicts only. The patient takes a narcotic antagonist such as naltrexone or cyclazocine on a daily basis. He learns that if he does this, ingesting or injecting an opioid substance will not produce a "rush" or "high."

Behavior Therapy

The patient is given positive reinforcement (rewards) for abstinent behavior, and no rewards, or punishments, for drug-seeking or drug-taking behaviors.

Individual, Family, or Group Psychotherapy

Detailed discussion of these modalities are beyond the scope of this book.

Religious Conversion

This operates on the principle that the addict has his best chance to become abstinent if he develops a "cause" that supersedes pleasure-seeking behaviors. The Black Muslims claim good results for some converts to their faith.

Therapeutic Communities

These include Phoenix House, Gateway House, and other residential communities, where the key treatment modalities are group meetings, group encounter sessions, and the development of responsibility-taking on a progressive, graded basis.

Legal Constraints

Harford, Underer, and Kinsella [17] studied addicts in several treatment programs, some of whom were self-referred and some of whom were instructed to seek treatment by the court. They found that the addicts who were court-referred did not do better as a group, and sometimes did worse, than the self-referred addicts. Vaillant [18], in a 20-year followup study of 100 New York opioid addicts originally admitted to the Lexington (Kentucky) federal treatment center, found that the best results occurred in individuals who spent over 9 months in jail followed by over 12 months parole supervision.

Methadone Maintenance

For opioid addicts with a long-term failure to be abstinent, a daily dose of dolophine is used as a "substitute addiction,"employing 40-100 mg dolophine per day. At first, addicts are given their daily dose under supervision, and as they demonstrate reliability, the frequency of supervised doses is decreased.

Prevention

Weaver and Tennant [19] found that a group of eighth-graders, given a special drug education program, demonstrated an increased knowledge of drug abuse, but no actual change in drug use, as compared with a control group.

Long-Term Prognosis

For 20 years, Vaillant [18] followed a group of 100 opioid addicts originally admitted to the Lexington federal treatment center in 1952. After 20 years, 23% of this group had died, mostly of unnatural causes, 25% were still known to be using drugs, 10% were in "uncertain" states, and 35-42% had achieved stable abstinence.

REFERENCES

1. Callan, J., and Patterson, C. Drug abuse among military inductees. *Am. J. Psychiatry* 130:260-264 (1963).
2. Woodruff, D., Goodwin, D., and Guze, S. *Psychiatric Diagnosis.* Oxford, New York (1974).
3. Zinberg, N., and Jacobsen, R. The natural history of chipping. *Am. J. Psychiatry* 133:37-40 (1976).
4. Westermayer, J. *A Primer of Chemical Dependency.* Williams and Wilkins, Baltimore (1976).
5. Freedman, A. Opiate dependence, in *Compresensive Textbook of Psychiatry,* 2nd ed. A. Freedman, H. Kaplan, and B. Sadock, eds. Williams and Wilkins, Baltimore (1975).
6. Grant, I., and Judd, L. Neuropsychological and EEG disturbances among polydrug abusers. *Am. J. Psychiatry* 133:1039-1042 (1976).
7. Acord, L., and Barker, D. Hallucinogenic drugs and cerebral deficit. *J. Nerv. Ment. Dis.* 156:281-283 (1973).
8. Stefanis, C., Aris, L., Boulagouris, J., Fink, M., and Freedman, A. Chronic hashish use and mental disorder. *Am. J. Psychiatry* 133:225-227 (1976).
9. Guze, S. *Criminality and Psychiatric Disorders.* Oxford, New York (1975).
10. Beaubrun, M., and Knight, F. Psychiatric assessment of 30 chronic users of cannabis and 30 matched controls. *Am. J. Psychiatry* 130:309-311 (1973).
11. Weissmann, M., Sloberly, F., Prusoff, B., Merzrity, M., and Howard, P. Clinical depression among narcotic addicts maintained on methadone in the community. *Am. J. Psychiatry* 133:1434-38 (1976).
12. Hofmann, F., and Hofmann, A. *A Handbook on Drugs and Alcohol Abuse: The biomedical aspects.* Oxford, New York (1975).
13. Shader, R., Caine, E., and Meyer, R. Treatment of dependence on barbiturates and sedative-hypnotics, in *Manual of Psychiatric Therapeutics.* R. Shader, ed. Little, Brown, Boston (1975).
14. Post, R., and Kopanda, R. Cocaine. Kindling and psychosis. *Am. J. Psychiatry* 133:627-634 (1976).
15. Post, R. Cocaine psychosis. A continuum model. *Am. J. Psychiatry* 132:225-231 (1975).

16. Allen, R., and Young, S. Phencyclidine-induced psychosis. *Am. J. Psychiatry* 135:1081-1084 (1978).

17. Harford, R., Underer, J., and Kinsella, K. Effects of legal pressure on prognosis for treatment for drug dependence. *Am. J. Psychiatry* 133:1399-1404 (1976).

18. Vaillant, G. A twenty year followup of New York narcotics addicts. *Arch. Gen. Psychiatry* 29:237-241 (1973).

19. Weaver, S., and Tennant, F. Effectiveness of drug education programs for secondary school students. *Am. J. Psychiatry* 130:812-814 (1973).

12

Behavioral Medicine

FREDERICK SIERLES

INTRODUCTION

To me, the term behavioral medicine is preferable to the term psychosomatic medicine, for the latter implies that the "mind" and the body are somehow different or separate. Behavior is the product of brain function; brain functions and the functions of the rest of the body are inextricably intertwined. The brain is an organ which functions under the same laws of nature as the kidney, liver, and lungs. A number of phenomena support this conclusion.

All significant brain function and dysfunction has systemic manifestations.
There are numerous examples of this, only some of which will be presented. Anxious people often show tachycardia, increased systolic blood pressure, hyperventilation, sweating, diarrhea, and urinary frequency. Anxiety often produces changes in galvanic skin resistance (an indirect measure of sweating), and decreases the clotting time in blood donors [1]. Prior to speeches, public speakers show increased blood levels of norepinephrine, triglycerides, and free fatty acids [2]. Before income tax deadlines, the serum cholesterol of accountants rises [3]. Pilots flying a plane have greater corticosteroid responsivity than their radio personnel [4], and higher pulse rates than their copilots [5]. If the copilots take over the controls, the copilots' pulse rates exceed those of the original pilots [5]. Prior to exams, the skin free fatty acid levels of students with acne rises [6]. People who are anxious about their sexual "performance" may experience transient sexual dysfunction. [7].

Strong pleasant or unpleasant emotions affect the secretion of all hormones [8]; for example, sexually stimulating or frightening films produce increased adrenal steroid secretion [9].

In the interpersonal sphere, the heart rates of psychotherapists and their patients are positively correlated [10], and medical students who like or dislike each other show higher galvanic skin resistance than students having neutral attitudes towards each other [11]. In social primates, testosterone levels vary depending on a primate's place in the dominance hierarchy.

Endogenously depressed patients often show anorexia, weight loss, and alterations of the hypothalamic-pituitary axis with high levels of cortisol secretion [12], altered diurnal cortisol level variations, and impaired dexamethasone suppression [12]. Patients with acute psychotic episodes show increased serum creatine phosphokinase [13].

Employing biofeedback techniques, people can alter visceral functions such as pulse, blood pressure, and brain wave rhythms [14].

The brain plays a principal role in processing the sensory inputs emitted from diseased organs; for example, the degree of dyspnea experienced by asthmatic patients is correlated to only a limited degree with the actual amount of airway resistance [15,16].

The brain controls behavioral response to systemic illness. All significant illness evokes behavioral response. There are many possible responses to the symptoms and diagnosis of medical illness, and the responses may vary independently from the degree of tissue pathology. A patient may or may not report the symptoms to a doctor, dramatize the symptoms, comply with the doctor's orders, and function effectively once the illness has subsided. Twenty percent of patients who have had myocardial infarctions, when asked about the illness several weeks later, say they never had a heart attack [17]. One-eighth of patients who have myocardial infarctions become unemployed for preventable psychiatric reasons [18].

In systemic disease, the brain can be affected at the same time that other organs are being affected; uremic encephalopathy and hepatic encephalopathy are two of a myriad of examples.

Treatment of brain and other organ dysfunctions may itself cause brain dysfunction. Anticholinergic delirium, reserpine-induced depression, steroid psychosis, and digitalis delirium are four of a huge list of examples, the number being so vast that an entire book [19] has been written on the subject.

PSYCHOANALYTIC THEORIES

Psychoanalytic theory has had a major influence in the field of behavioral medicine, with the work of Alexander [20], Benedek [21], Bruch [22], Dunbar [23], Pollack [24], and Silverman [25] required reading in many training programs. Important psychoanalytic concepts include explanations of the cause of conversion reactions and psychophysiological disorders (see Chap. 14), the specificity hypothesis, the X-factor concept, the theory of somatic identification and "sensitized organs," and the notion of primary and secondary gain.

The specificity hypothesis posits that specific psychophysiological disorders are associated with specific unconscious conflicts (e.g., duodenal peptic ulcer and unmet dependency needs) [20] or with specific personality types [23] (e.g., type-A personality and coronary atherosclerosis).

The X-factor concept [26] posits that for a psychophysiological disorder to manifest itself, there must be a congenital predisposition (the X factor) as well as an unconscious conflict. For example, the X factor in people with duodenal peptic ulcer is that they are congenital hypersecretors of pepsinogen.

The somatic identification and sensitized organ concepts [25] hold that an organ is most vulnerable to disease if a relative or friend of the patient had an affliction of that organ (somatic identification) or that the patient had a previous illness of, or particular concern about, that organ (sensitized organ).

Primary gain is defined as the reduction of anxiety that the illness itself produces by resolving unconscious conflicts. Secondary gain refers to the benefits (e.g., not having to go to work, getting attention) that accrue to the patient by virtue of his being ill.

LIAISON-CONSULTATION PSYCHIATRY

Definitions

Consultation psychiatry, like medical or surgical consultation, means performing consultations on patients who are being treated by physicians outside of one's own specialty. *Liaison psychiatry* adds the dimensions of providing consultation to the service as a whole (e.g., "Observe your patients early in the day for subtle signs of delirium"), making rounds and attending conferences on that service, and identifying patients with susceptibility to, or early signs of, behavioral disorder. In the terminology of preventive medicine, liaison psychiatry is a means of providing primary and secondary, as well as tertiary, prevention.

Hints for Consultants

The following recommendations to consulting psychiatrists apply to physicians in all branches of medicine.

Respond promptly to requests. Usually, the sooner you arrive, the sooner the problem can be handled, the less ill or frustrated the patient will be when you arrive, and the less annoyed the physicians and nurses will be. If you cannot come promptly, specify exactly when you will come, or who can substitute for you. *Don't give the requesting physician a hard time.* Consultants who do not enjoy their work, or feel inadequate to handle a situation, often try to evade or postpone the consultation, usually by implying or stating that the consult is "inappropriate." *Don't trouble the requesting physician with the intricacies of your specialty.* The consultation request usually can be translated as "What's wrong and what are *you* going to do?" Writing extensive histories, physical exams (including mental status), and etiologic theories make for fine medical records if you have the time, but the requesting physician is primarily interested in getting these two questions answered clearly, directly, and specifically, either in person (preferably) or in writing (if he isn't around). Avoid using technical jargon where possible. Recommendations for treatment followup should be so precise that a second phone call or consultation request is unnecessary. For example, if the patient is to be referred to your outpatient clinic, specify the clinic name, the hours that it is open, its phone number, the registration procedure, and names of the clinic personnel who can expedite matters.

Specific Liaison-Consultation Areas

Surgical Patients

The Preoperative Mental Status Kimball [27], Abram [28], Kennedy [29], Kilpatrick [30], and Tufo [31] independently demonstrated that the better the patient's preoperative mental status, the better his postoperative medical prognosis. Kimball's study of open-heart surgery patients showed that those who were preoperatively depressed, or anxious without admitting to anxiety, had a higher postoperative morbidity and mortality. This occurred independently of the severity of the preexisting heart disease or the extent of surgery.

Several studies on psychological support prior to surgery indicates that supportive efforts on the part of physicians and other staff reduce the incidence of postoperative complications. Lazarus and Hagens [32] compared patients who received active, supportive preoperative care with a control group who received minimal preoperative support. The incidence of postoperative delirium was 14% for the former group, 33% for the latter. Egbert [33], an anesthesiologist, demonstrated that if patients are given clear explanations of their upcoming anesthesia, surgery, and postoperative state, and their questions are answered, their hospital stays will be shorter and they will make fewer requests for postoperative pain medication.

Surman [34] lists behavioral characteristics of patients who are good surgical risks:

1. They are intellectually intact.
2. They cope well with stress.
3. They have low-to-moderate preoperative anxiety.
4. Their anxiety relates to knowledge of the risks of surgery.
5. They are confident of a favorable outcome.
6. They are motivated to get well.
7. They have realistic expectations of the surgery.
8. They are not depressed.

There are a number of characteristics of patients who are prone to developing postoperative delirium [35,36]. They are: (1) previous or current emotional illness, including alcoholism, depression, coarse brain disease, or psychosis; (2) preoperative insomnia; (3) advanced age; (4) retirement adjustment problems; (5) "functional" gastroenterological disturbance; and (6) low socioeconomic status. The risk is also increased if there is a family history of psychosis. Finally, the longer the procedure and the more blood needs to be transfused, the greater the risk [35,36].

Based on the preceeding discussion, the following preventive measures are in order [35-37]:

Screen. The preoperative history and physical exam must include questions designed to elicit behavioral pathology if present.

Explain. The physician (and other staff members, if necessary) should explain the procedures, anticipate the commonest problems, answer the patient's questions, and respond to the patient's feelings. Most patients do not like being "surprised" with a nasogastric tube or catheter postoperatively, and would prefer to know that postoperative bleeding does not mean that "the cancer is still there."

Relax and sedate. Anxiolytic agents and hypnotics can be prescribed routinely for a day or two prior to surgery. Supportive conversation can be equally anxiolytic.

Consult. Psychiatric consultation can be requested if the patient manifests significant psychopathology.

Postpone. If indicated and possible, elective surgery should be postponed if the patient shows depression, unexplained or reversible coarse brain disease, signs of alcohol withdrawal, any poorly controlled severe psychiatric illness, or "predilection to death" (see Chap. 24).

Treat. All signs of alcohol withdrawal should be treated immediately and vigorously (see Chap. 11). Alcoholics who do not have withdrawal signs should receive 100 mg thiamine daily and 100 mg chlordiazepoxide (Librium) or 40 mg diazepam (Valium) daily, along with a multivitamin. Patients with *endogenous depression* should be treated with electroconvulsive therapy. Patients with *reactive depression* can be treated with supportive psychotherapy, behavior modification, or monoamine oxidase (MAO) inhibitor. For patients with *coarse brain disease*, the cause should be ascertained and, if it is reversible, appropriate treatment should be instituted.

Patients with coarse brain disease should be given extra attention and orienting, supportive conversation. For patients with *insomnia*, the underlying cause should be sought and treated (see Chap. 7).

Anesthesia Budd and Braun [38] found that when nurses provide cardiotomy patients with a specific postoperative reorientation procedure, the incidence of postoperative delirium is diminished.

Psychiatric complications associated with anesthesia itself include prolonged drowsiness, sleep disturbances including nightmares, and hallucinations, all of which are transient. Mostert [39] reports that the anesthetic ketamine is itself a hallucinogen, and that the hallucinations can be prevented if the patient simultaneously receives a benzodiazepine drug.

Levenson [40] reported that some patients recall statements made by others in the operating room while the patient was under anesthesia. Lewis et al. [41] could not reproduce this finding. Surman [34] writes that since this "awareness during surgery" is a possibility, operating room personnel should be cautious about what they say.

Delirium The commonest serious postoperative neuropsychiatric complication is delirium, which is characterized by diffuse intellectual dysfunction (some of which may be due to decreased concentration), with a minimental state score below 22, changing levels of consciousness and alertness, tachycardia, pallor, hallucinations, illusions, secondary delusions, and electroencephalogram slowing [40]. Any condition which can diffusely impair brain functioning can cause delirium.

Postoperative delirium is especially common in patients who have undergone open-heart surgery, neurosurgery, and bilateral eye surgery [42]. Delirium associated with bilateral eye surgery is called "black patch delirium" [43], and anticholinergic toxicity [44] and sensory deprivation (due to the bilateral eye patching) have been implicated. Where feasible, eye surgery should be done one eye at a time. Delirium is common in other settings as well. For example, close to 100% of hospitalized burn patients develop delirium [42].

The treatment of delirium is the following: *Seek and treat the underlying cause.* Cassem and Hackett [45] provide this checklist* for the workup of a delirious patient:

---

*From N. Cassem and T. Hackett (eds.). The setting of intensive care, in *Massachusetts General Hospital Handbook of General Hospital Psychiatry*. The C.V. Mosby Co., St. Louis (1978), with permission (Ref. 45).

1. Drug withdrawal states (alcohol, sedative-hypnotics, and anxiolytic agents)
2. Drugs (especially steroids, L-dopa, amphetamines, digitalis, lidocaine, and anticholinergics)
3. Temperature
4. Blood pressure
5. Hematocrit, mean corpuscular volume, vitamin B-12, folic acid
6. Erythrocyte sedimentation rate
7. Lupus erythematosus (LE) preparation
8. Sodium potassium, chloride, magnesium, calcium, phosphates
9. Triiodothyronine (T3) and thyroxine (T4)
10. Blood urea nitrogen
11. Fasting blood sugar
12. Arterial pO2 and pCO2
13. Liver function tests and ammonia
14. Veneral disease report
15. Electrocardiogram
16. Electroencephalogram
17. Skull x-rays
18. Brain scan
19. Lumbar puncture
20. Computerized tomography scan

Much of this information can be obtained within several hours, during which time other measures are being taken.

Provide *frequent supportive conversation* with explanation, reassurance, and orientation. Speak *simply*, slowly, and *clearly* to the patient. Make only one request at a time and don't present abstract concepts. A *clock* and *calendar* should be visually accessible to the patient. A *radio or TV* may be helpful. Ideally, all hospital rooms would have these routinely present, but this is often not the case. *Keep the lights on*, but dimly. Letting the patient keep familiar items by the bedside may be helpful. *Encourage relatives to visit*, and tell them that delirium is usually transient. Frequent brief visits are preferable to infrequent long visits.

If the patient is uncooperative or combative, he may have to be *restrained*. If anticholinergic toxicity and drug withdrawal have been ruled out and there is no problem with gastrointestinal motility, he can be given intravenous or intramuscular *haloperidol*. If he is properly sedated, restraints can be removed. If there are no signs of increased intracranial pressure, and the above measures don't work, electroconvulsive therapy (ECT) can be very helpful.

Plastic Surgery In the past, plastic surgery was stereotyped as useful for three categories of people—those with severe congenital or acquired deformities, wealthy vain people, and people with very large noses. Now while wealthy people still have greater access to plastic surgeons, it is well accepted in the medical community that considerable psychological relief can be provided by plastic surgeons to larger numbers of people, including many with deformities that are not especially conspicuous [46]. In the latter case, it is the patient's perception of, and response to, the deformities which is most important [46].

Despite the notable benefits, there are certain relative contraindications which include [46]: (1) when the request for plastic surgery is made by the patient under pressure from others, (2) when the patient is not able to give a clear description of his deformity, (3) when the patient disregards more prominent deformities, (4) when the patient is dissatisfied with previous competent plastic surgery, (5) when the patient has an unrealistic expectation of others radically changing their attitude towards him postoperatively, (6) when concern about the deformity is recent and in the context of significant personal stress (here one is advised to wait), and (7) acute serious psychiatric illness.

Mastectomy and Hysterectomy While these are both major surgical procedures, some authors have written that psychological distress [47,48] and postoperative visits to psychiatrists [48] are more frequent than when patients have most other procedures (e.g., cholecystectomy) [48], equal in both duration and surgical trauma. This is in part due to these procedures being perceived, by some patients and their husbands, as seriously impairing their "worth" or their "femininity," and in part because the surgery is often done for cancer, with its attendant concerns. Preoperatively and postoperatively, considerable dialogue between surgeon and patient (often including the spouse) are in order, with particular attention paid to the issues of self-esteem, support from the spouse, and bereavement.

Amputation Preoperatively, the patient should usually be made aware of the phantom limb phenomenon, which occurs in about 99% of patients in the immediate postoperative period, and 89% of patients 1 year after surgery [49]. This is the experience of sensations perceived as coming from the limb as if it were still present.

Patient Noncompliance

In over one-third of compliance studies, over half the patients fail to comply with the treatment regimen [50]. According to Gillom and Barsky [50], the following factors are associated with noncompliance:

Annoying side effects
Complicated treatment regimen
Treatment requiring considerable effort
Treatment that isolates the patient socially
The patient doesn't trust the doctor.
The patient is poor or unemployed.

Another obvious factor is brain dysfunction.

Some measures can be taken to increase compliance. In selecting drugs, the frequency and discomfort of side effects must be taken into account; for example, in treating anxiety states, MAO inhibitors have fewer annoying side effects than tricyclic antidepressants [51]. The frequency of doses is also important: For example, drugs, like neuroleptics, with a long half-life can be taken in once-a-day or twice-a-day dosages, which mean that a patient needn't bring medication to work.

The physician can minimize the complexity of a treatment regimen by giving careful explanations, using diagrams if necessary, and answering all reasonable questions. For example, in explaining paper bag breathing to a patient with hyperventilation syndrome, the physician can breathe into a paper bag and then have the patient do the same. Regimens which permit the patient to continue with his usual social and occupational activities will usually be better accepted. Here is an example:

A middle-aged divorced man is suffering from an endogenous depression. He requires electroconvulsive therapy, which is usually administered to hospital inpatients. However, he alone is responsible for supervising his 10-year-old son, doesn't have a friend or relative who can substitute, and he doesn't want to miss work if possible. Since he is fully cooperative and reliable, and not suicidal, he is given electroconvulsive therapy on an outpatient basis.

Many physician-related factors enter into a patient's trust of a physician. My list includes:

Prior successful treatment of the patient by the doctor
The doctor's comprehension of the patient's condition
Skillful performance of procedures
Intelligence
Responsiveness to patient's psychological needs
Respectfulness
Honesty
Reliability
Availability
Credentials satisfactory to patient

Some of these correlates of trust are learnable and some are achievable by the simple comprehension of their importance. The patient's own capacity to trust, which can be impeded by brain dysfunction, is of course another factor.

Intensive Care Units

Although intensive care units (ICU) are necessary because they are geared towards the treatment of urgent and high-risk conditions, from a behavioral standpoint there are significant problems [52].

    1. An alien environment with unfamiliar people and distortion of the usual day-night sequence

    2. Overstimulation in terms of unit routine, with busy staff moving about, monitors beeping, tests being conducted

    3. Sensory monotony, because much of the stimulation is impersonal and not thought-provoking

    4. Physical discomfort due to disease

    5. Side effects of medical drugs

    6. Crowding and lack of privacy

    7. Illness and death of other patients

Table 1 is a list of reasons for psychiatric consultation in coronary care units, surgical intensive care units, and respiratory intensive care units.

Table 1   Frequency of Consultation Requests According to Intensive Care Setting

Coronary care unit	Surgical ICU	Respiratory ICU
1. Anxiety (80%)	1. Delirium	1. Depression
2. Depression	2. Depression	2. Anxiety weaning from
3. Management of behavior	3. Anxiety weaning from	respirator
(signing out, dependency)	respirator	3. Management of behavior
4. Hostility		(drug dependency,
5. Delirium (26%)		dependency)

Source: From N. Cassem and T. Hackett (ed.). The setting of intensive care, in *Massachusetts General Hospital Handbook of General Hospital Psychiatry*. The C.V. Mosby Co., St. Louis (1978), with permission (Ref. 45).

Regarding the coronary care unit, Cassem and Hackett [45] are even more specific (see Fig. 1): On the first two days after admission, anxiety and fear are the commonest reason for psychiatric consultation; from the third to sixth days, depression is most frequent. Problems stemming from chronic personality traits, while not as frequently a source of referrals as depression, are most likely to occur on the fourth day.

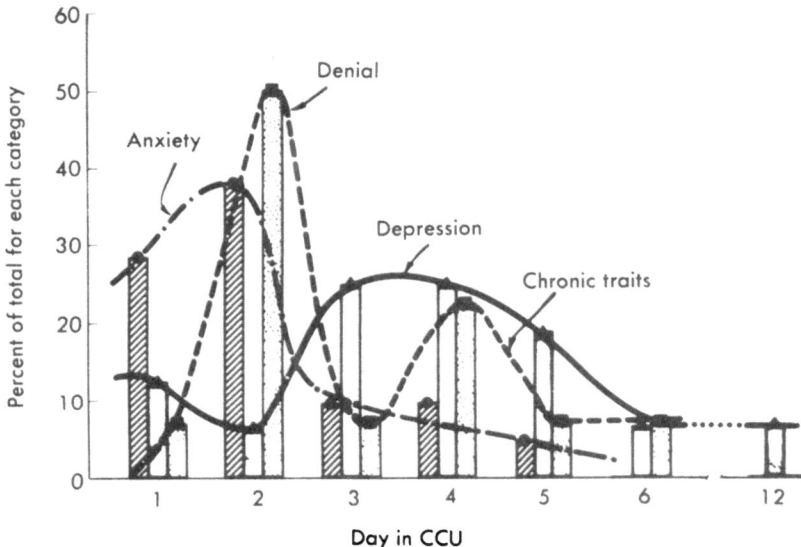

FIG. 1. Hypothetical sequence of emotional and behavioral reactions of a coronary care unit (CCU) patient, derived from the frequency of psychiatric consultation for each category of reaction. (From N.H. Cassem. What is behind our masks? AORN J. 10:79-92, 1974, with permission.)

Despite the many problems of intensive care units, most ICU patients are quite resilient. Hackett and Cassem [42] found a high rate of acceptance by patients of receiving last rites, and good tolerance for seeing others experience cardiac arrest. In the latter situation, patients (logically) perceived that the patients experiencing the arrest were sicker than they [42].

Many patients who survived their own cardiac arrest had some emotional turmoil afterwards, often in the form of nightmares, but it was usually transient. Two-thirds had no memory of the period of the arrest. The incidence of serious psychiatric sequelae was low; of them, Cassem [45] writes: "In general, the literature supports the emotional adaptability of survivors of cardiac arrest."

The question of the protective value of denial in these situations is an interesting and important one. Hackett [42,45] found that patients who were not at all worried about their situation ("major denial") had a better prognosis, supporting a conclusion that denial may have a protective function in coronary care patients. The survival value of denial in other medical situations, particularly when there is no myocardial irritability, is uncertain. Both Kimball [27] and Janis [53] wrote that denial in a preoperative patient is correlated with poorer prognosis; on the other hand, Kennedy and Bakst [29] concluded that blocking out of fear improved prognosis.

Whatever measures are taken, the intensive care unit will continue to be a high-risk setting. Nevertheless, certain manipulations may be helpful. Some patients should have access to reading material, radio and television, a clock and a calendar. Visiting should be encouraged, and there should be a high frequency of staff-patient contact with supportive conversation. Explanations of procedures should be provided, frequently experienced emotions should be anticipated, and questions should be answered. There should be mobile room dividers or mobile curtains to increase privacy when needed, and staff members should announce their presence before entering a room.

The staff should be vigilant for common psychiatric complications, and psychiatric consultation should be readily available. The prevention and treatment of delirium, and the treatment of anxiety and depression, are discussed earlier in this chapter.

The period when a patient is transferred from the intensive care unit, or weaned from a respirator, is often an anxious one. Serum catecholamine levels are elevated on the day of discharge from a coronary care unit (CCU) [54]. The patient should be told that although his care will no longer be as intense, he is well enough to handle this transition. This may be a good time to discuss the illness and its potential effect on the patient's future. Anxiolytic agents may be prescribed.

Hackett [42] writes that one problem faced by staff in respiratory ICUs is the intubated patient's inability to speak, requiring that he either write or communicate nonvervally. This is frustrating to those members of the staff who want an instant response; Hackett suggests that the frustration may be less if the staff member, as well as the patient, communicates by writing.

Cardiology

Coronary Arteriosclerosis   Coronary arteriosclerosis is one of the leading causes of death in the United States, and we rank second in the world (Finland is first) in prevalence of this condition.

Cardiologists Friedman and Rosenman [3,55] found a high correlation of coronary arteriosclerosis in patients with a type-A personality, which is characterized by being hard-driving and ambitious, having a sense of time pressure, and being preoccupied with numbers and accomplishments. They recommend that type-A people "reengineer" their lives by adhering to guidelines such as the following:

> Eliminate as many events and activities as possible that do not contribute directly to your socioeconomic well being.

Never waste time responding to a letter if your secretary or someone else can do it for you.
Learn the fine art of discerning quickly and accurately those whose words have no value of any kind for you. [55]

While following recommendations such as these may increase our efficiency, favorable results of this reengineering have yet to be demonstrated.

Regarding drugs in patients with myocardial pathology, propanthelene (Pro-Banthene), which doesn't cross the blood-brain barrier, should be considered as a substitute for atropine, which does cross it, in the treatment of elderly patients with bradycardia [56]. Electroconvulsive therapy is more benign, as well as more clinically effective, than tricyclic antidepressants for the treatment of endogenous depression [57]. Of the neuroleptic drugs, if one must be used, haloperidol is least likely to produce postural hypotension, arrhythmia, or anticholinergic delirium.

Hypertension Cobb and Rose [58] found that air traffic controllers have 4 times the prevalence of hypertension than "second class airmen." However, they did not determine whether this difference was a consequence of the job or of some characteristic of the individuals in the jobs. Kasl and Cobb [59] found that men who were laid off from work had blood pressure elevations until they were established at their new jobs. Blacks have a higher incidence of hypertension than whites.

Regarding drugs and hypertension, neuroleptic drugs and tricyclic antidepressants negate the hypotensive effect of the potent antihypertensive agent guanethidine (Ismelin). The antihypertensives alphamethyldopa (Aldomet) and reserpine (Serpasil) are associated with an increased incidence of depression.

Pulmonary Medicine

Bronchial Asthma In addition to the previously stated relationship between dyspnea and airway resistance in asthmatics, there are other studies which show that brain function is important in asthma. Asthmatic patients given placebos, and told the placebos are allergens, experience an increase in airway resistance [15,16]. Asthmatics shown pictures of allergens may have asthma attacks [60]. Patients given a placebo and told it was isoproterenol (Isuprel) experienced bronchodilation [15,16]. Allergens sprayed into patients' hospital rooms, unbeknownst to the patients, failed to produce asthma attacks [61].

Hyperventilation Syndrome Some patients who experience severe anxiety hyperventilate, which causes a "blowing off" of CO_2 with a consequent respiratory alkalosis. Then, they may have palpitations, chest pain, pares-thesia, tetany, headache, and fainting. This can easily be confused with cardiopulmonary disease. During a hyperventilation episode in the hyper-ventilation syndrome, the patient should breathe in and out of a paper bag cupped around the nose and mouth (a closed breathing system), and receive 5-10 mg diazepam or 25-50 mg chlordiazepoxide orally, deeply intramuscu-larly, or intravenously. Calcium gluconate should *not* be used. The patho-physiology should be explained to the patient at a level that he can under-stand. Followup should include treatment of the original cause of the anxiety, which is often a chronic anxiety state like anxiety neurosis or a phobia.

Smoking   There is a strong relationship between smoking and most of the severe pulmonary diseases. Smoking remains extremely common; in 1973, 4 out of 10 adult men were regular smokers. There are no surefire treat-ments for smoking; of people who seek treatment to discontinue smoking, the minority are abstaining at 1- and 2-year followups. Nevertheless, huge num-bers of people do quit smoking; Mausner [62] estimated in 1973 that 29 mil-lion Americans had quit smoking. He wrote that people stop smoking be-cause they have an expectation of immediate benefits from stopping, not be-cause of a fear of long-term consequences. Physicians treating smokers should bear this in mind.

Obstetrics and Gynecology

Teenage Pregnancy   Adolescence is the only age group with an increase in pregnancy and parenthood in the last decade. This is especially significant because the maternal and neonatal mortality rate is higher in this group than for any other. Teenage pregnancy is often repetitive; one study [63] of preg-nant teenagers found a statistical likelihood of three succeeding pregnancies prior to legal or common-law marriage. A study of boyfriends of pregnant teenagers [64] showed that most of the boyfriends continued to see their girl-friend, to be interested in her well-being and the baby's well-being, and to be available to discuss the situation if a medical caretaker takes the lead.

Almost by definition, physicians have postponed many of their own gratifications, so many do not approve of teenage pregnancy. And often the families of pregnant teenagers, and the teenagers themselves, view the preg-nancy as "a mistake." Despite this, most experts state or imply that a judg-mental approach is useless, and advocate a tolerant, reflective posture. The most commonly recommended attitude is that the physician be an ally whose primary concern is that the girl and her boyfriend make educated choices about whether or not to have sex, to use contraception, to have an abortion, and to give the baby to an adoption agency. Using the "emancipated minor" concept, a physician may treat a pregnant teenager or teenage mother without consent of the teenager's parents. For a teenager who is not an emancipated minor, education and discussion of matters of sex can take place under the aegis of discussion of prevention of venereal disease, which can be discussed without parents' consent in many states.

Psychosis Associated with Pregnancy Taylor and Levine [65] found that if a woman became psychotic while pregnant, the odds favored that the baby would be female, and if the woman became psychotic postpartum, the odds favored that the baby would be male. They hypothesized that fetal androgens might have an antipsychotic effect for the mother.

Neurology

Temporal Lobe Epilepsy Particular attention must be given to temporal lobe epilepsy, since it is common and can mimic many psychiatric syndromes. The commonest causes of this syndrome are Ammon's horn (hippocampal; sclerosis and tumors, the former associated with birth injury or recurring febrile seizures in childhood. The temporal lobe motor seizure lasts for a few minutes at most, and can present automatisms (reflexive, stereotyped, automatic behaviors like chewing and making sucking movements) or staring episodes. Preceeding the motor seizure or during it, there may be hallucinations, obsessions, pains, dysmegalopsia, "déjà vu," "jamais vu," "jamais pensé," depersonalization, derealization, and various moods [66].

The interictal (between-seizure) behavior of temporal lobe epileptics has aroused great interest. Bear and Fedio [67] describe interictal personality characteristics that are common in temporal lobe epilepsy: These are religiosity, pseudoprofundity, humorlessness, hypergraphia, "stickiness," dependency, and obsessiveness. Hypersexuality, hyposexuality, emotionality, and aggressiveness may also be seen. Circumstantial or adhesive speech may occur. Flor-Henry [68] writes that there is a high frequency of a schizophrenia-like syndrome in temporal lobe epileptics with dominant hemisphere disease, and an increased incidence of a mania-like syndrome in patients with nondominant hemisphere disease. Diphenylhydantoin (Dilantin) is used for the motor seizures, carbamazepine (Tegretol) is used for associated behavioral dysfunctions, and small doses of neuroleptic drugs have been useful in treating the schizophrenia-like and mania-like syndromes.

Brain Tumors "Mental" (behavioral) changes are the commonest (94% of cases) symptom or sign of brain tumors, commoner even than headache (86%), vomiting (38%), and seizures (37%) [69]. Sometimes the patient is aware of the behavioral change, and sometimes it is noted only by a relative or the patient's physician. The behavioral change can be the first sign, the only sign, or the most noticeable sign, of brain tumor.

Dermatology

Histamine Response Schizophrenic patients show a decreased wheal-and-flair in response to the intradermal injection of histamine [70] and people experiencing anxiety have a decreased wheal-and-flair response to histamine [71]. The mechanism of this is unknown.

Hyperhydrosis People have different physiological manifestations of anxiety; some hyperventilate, some feel depersonalized, and some sweat excessively—the latter group have hyperhydrosis. Some patients with hyperhydrosis become afraid of sweating, a fear which can acquire phobic intensity. The excessive sweating itself can be minimized by the prophylactic application of topical high-concentration aluminum hexahydrate (Drysol) once daily. If this does not itself alleviate the anxiety, the patient should be treated like any patient with an anxiety state, as discussed in the chapter on psychopathology (Chap. 8).

REFERENCES

1. Macht, D. Influence of some drugs and of emotions on blood coagulation. *JAMA* 148:265-270 (1952).
2. Taggart, P., Carruthers, M., Somerville, W. Electrocardiogram, plasma catecholamines and lipids, and their modifications by oxyprenolol when speaking before an audience. *Lancet* 2:341-346 (1973).
3. Rosenman, R., and Friedman, M. The central nervous system and coronary heart disease. *Hosp. Prac.* 87-97 (1971).
4. Miller, R. Secretion of 17-hydroxycorticosteroids in military aviators as an index of response to stress. A review. *Aerosp. Med.* 39:498-501 (1968).
5. Responsibility brings jump in pulse. *JAMA* 201:23 (1967).
6. Kraus, S. Stress, acne and skin surface free fatty acids. *Psychosom. Med.* 32:503-508 (1970).
7. Masters, W., and Johnson, V. *Human Sexual Inadequacy.* Little, Brown, Boston (1970).
8. Mason, J. A review of psychoendocrine research on the pituitary-adrenal cortical system. *Psychosom. Med.* 30:516-607 (1968).
9. Brown, W., and Heninger, G. Cortisol, growth hormone, free fatty acids, and experimentally evoked affective arousal. *Am. J. Psychiatry* 132:1172-1176 (1975).
10. DiMascio, A., Boyd, R., Greenblatt, M., and Solomon, H. The psychiatric interview. A sociophysiologic study. *Dis. Nerv. Syst.* 16:2-7 (1955).
11. Kaplan, H., Burch, N., Bloom, S. Physiological covariation and sociometric relationships in small peer groups, in *Psychobiological Approaches to Social Behavior.* P. Leiderman and D. Shapiro, eds. Stanford, Polo Alto (1964).
12. Carroll, B., and Mendels, J. Neuroendocrine regulation in affective disorders, in *Hormones, Behavior and Psychopathology.* E. Sachar, ed. Raven, New York (1976).
13. Meltzer, H., and Crayton, J. Subterminal motor nerve abnormalities in psychotic patients. *Nature Lond.* 249:373-375 (1974).
14. Miller, N., Barber, T., Dicara, L., Kamiya, J., Shapiro, D., and Stoyva, J. *Biofeedback and Self-Control.* Aldine, Chicago (1973).

15. Luparello, T., Lyons, H., Blecker, E., and McFadden, C. Influences of suggestion on airway resistance in asthmatic subjects. *Psychosom. Med.* 30:819 (1968).
16. Luparello, T., Leist, N., Laurie, C., and Sweet, P. The interaction of psychologic stimuli and pharmacologic agents on airway reactivity in asthmatic subjects. *Psychosom. Med.* 32:509 (1970).
17. Croog, S., Shapiro, D., and Levine, S. Denial among male heart patients. *Psychosom. Med.* 33:385-397 (1971).
18. Wynn, A. Unwarranted emotional distress in men with ischaemic heart disease. *Med. J. Austria* 2:847-851 (1967).
19. Shader, R. *Psychiatric Complications of Medical Drugs.* Raven, New York (1972).
20. Alexander, F. *Psychosom. Med.* Norton, New York (1950).
21. Benedek, T. *Psychoanalytic Investigations.* Quadrangle, New York (1973).
22. Bruch, II. *The Golden Cage.* Harvard, Cambridge (1978).
23. Dunbar, F. *Mind and Body: Psychosomatic Medicine.* Random, New York (1947).
24. Pollack, G. *Psychosomatic Specificity.* Univ. Chicago, Chicago (1963).
25. Siverman, S. *Psychological Aspects of Physical Symptoms.* Appleton-Century-Crofts, New York (1968).
26. Mirsky, J. Physiologic, psychologic and social determinants in etiology of duodenal ulcer. *Am. J. Dig. Dis.* 3:285 (1958).
27. Kimball, C. Psychological responses to the experience of open heart surgery. *Am. J. Psychiatry* 125:348 (1969).
28. Abram, H., and Gill, B. Predictions of postoperative psychiatric complications. *N. Engl. J. Med.* 265:1123 (1961).
29. Kennedy, T., and Bakst, H. The influence of emotion on the outcome of cardiac surgery. A predictive study. *Bull. N.Y. Acad. Med.* 42:311 (1966).
30. Kilpatrick, D., Miller, W., Allain, A., Huggins, M., and William, L. The use of psychological test data to predict open heart surgery outcome. A prospective study. *Psychosom. Med.* 27:62 (1975).
31. Tufo, H., Ostfeld, A., and Shetielle, R. Central nervous system dysfunction following open-heart surgery. *JAMA* 212:1333 (1978).
32. Lazarus, H., and Hagens, T. Prevention of psychosis following open heart surgery. *Am. J. Psychiatry* 124:1190 (1968).
33. Egbert, L., Battet, G., Welch, C., and Bartlett, M. Reduction of postoperative pain by encouragement and instruction of patient. *N. Engl. J. Med.* 270:825 (1964).
34. Surman, O. The surgical patient, in *Handbook of General Hospital Psychiatry.* T. Hackett and N. Cassem, eds. Mosby, St. Louis (1978).
35. Morse, R., and Litin, E. Postoperative delirium. A study of etiologic factors. *Am. J. Psychiatry* 126:388 (1969).
36. Morse, R. Psychiatry and surgical delirium, in *Modern Perspectives in the Psychiatric Aspects of Surgery.* J. Howells, ed. Brunner/Mazel, New York (1976).
37. Murray, G. Confusion, delirium and dementia, in *Handbook of General Hospital Psychiatry.* T. Hackett and N. Cassem, eds. Mosby, St. Louis (1978).
38. Budd, S., and Brown, W. Effect of a reorientation technique on post-cardiotomy delirium. *Nurs. Res.* 23:341 (1974).
39. Mostert, J. States of awareness during general anesthesia. *Perspect. Biol. Med.* 19:68 (1975).
40. Levinson, B. States of awareness during general anesthesia: preliminary communication. *Br. J. Anesthesiol.* 37:544 (1965).
41. Lewis, S., Jenkinson, J., and Wilson, J. An EEG investigation of awareness during anesthesia. *Br. J. Psychiatry* 64:413 (1973).
42. Hackett, T., and Cassem, N. The psychology of intensive care. Problems and their manage-

ment, in *Psychiatric Medicine*. G. Usdin, ed. Brunner/Mazel, New York (1977).

43. Weisman, A., and Hackett, T. Psychosis after eye surgery. Establishment of a specific doctor-patient relationship in prevention and treatment of black patch delirium. *N. Engl. J. Med.* 258:1284 (1958).

44. Summers, W., and Reich, T. Delirium after cataract surgery. Review and two cases. *Am. J. Psychiatry* 136:386-391 (1979).

45. Cassem, N., and Hackett, T. The setting of intensive care, in *Handbook of General Hospital Psychiatry*. T. Hacket and N. Cassem, eds. The C.V. Mosby Co., St. Louis (1978).

46. Olley, P. Psychiatric aspects of cosmetic surgery, in *Modern Perspectives in the Psychiatric Aspects of Surgery*. J. Howells, ed. Brunner/Mazel, New York (1976).

47. Maguire, P. The psychological and social sequelae of mastectomy, in *Modern Perspectives in the Psychiatric Aspects of Surgery*. J. Howells, ed. Brunner/Mazel, New York (1976).

48. Raphael, B. Psychiatric aspect of hysterectomy, in *Modern Perspectives in the Psychiatric Aspects of Surgery*. J. Howells, ed. Brunner/Mazel, New York (1976).

49. Parkes, C. The psychological reaction to loss of a limb. The first year after amputation, in *Modern Perspectives in the Psychiatric Aspects of Surgery*. J. Howells, ed. Brunner/Mazel, New York (1976).

50. Gillum, R., and Barsky, A. The diagnosis and management of patient noncompliance. *JAMA* 228:1563-1567 (1974).

51. Sheehan, D. Extreme manifestations of anxiety in the general hospital, in *Handbook of General Hospital Psychiatry*. T. Hackett and N. Cassem, eds. Mosby, St. Louis (1978).

52. Kimball, C.: Psychosomatic theories and their contributions to chronic illness, in *Psychiatric Medicine*. G. Usdin, ed. Brunner/Mazel, New York (1977).

53. Janis, J. *Psychological Stress*. Wiley, New York (1958).

54. Klein, R. Transfer from a coronary care unit. Some adverse responses. *Arch. Intern. Med.* 122:104-108 (1968).

55. Friedman, M., and Rosenman, M. *Type A Behavior and Your Heart*. Knopf, New York (1974).

56. Bernstein, J. Medical-psychiatric drug interactions, in *Handbook of General Hospital Psychiatry*. T. Hackett and N. Cassem, eds. Mosby, St. Louis (1978).

57. Abrams, R. A suggestion concerning ECT. *Psychiatr. Opinion* 16:11-15 (1979).

58. Cobb, S., and Rose, R. Hypertension, peptic ulcer and diabetes in air traffic controllers. *JAMA* 224:489-492 (1973).

59. Kasl, S., and Cobb, S. Blood pressure changes in men undergoing job loss. *Psychosom. Med.* 32:19-38 (1970).

60. Dekker, E., and Groen, J. Reproducible psychogenic attacks of asthma. A laboratory study. *J. Psychosom. Res.* 1:5-8 (1956).

61. Lamont, J. Which children outgrow asthma and which do not?, in *The Asthmatic Child*. H. Schneer, ed. Hoeber, New York (1963).

62. Mausner, B. An ecological view of cigarette smoking. *J. Abnorm. Psychol.* 81:115-126 (1973).

63. Sarrel, P., and Davis, C. The young unwed primipara. A study of 100 cases with 5 year followup. *Am. J. Obstet. Gynecol.* 95:722-725 (1966).

64. Pannor, R. The teenage unwed father. *Clin. Obstet. Gynecol.* 14:466-472 (1971).

65. Taylor, M., and Levine, R. The interactive effects of maternal schizophrenia and offspring sex. *Biol. Psychiatry* 2:279-289 (1970).

66. Ervin, F. Brain disorders associated with convulsions (epilepsy), in *Comprehensive Textbook of Psychiatry I*. A. Freedman and H. Kaplan, eds. Williams and Wilkins, Baltimore (1975).

67. Bear, D., and Fedio, P. Quantitative analysis of interictal behavior in temporal lobe epilepsy. *Arch. Neurol.* 34:454-467 (1977).

68. Flor-Henry, P. Schizophrenic-like reactions and affective psychoses associated with temporal lobe epilepsy. Etiologic factors. *Am. J. Psychiatry* 126:400-404 (1969).

69. Paal, G. Mental changes as indicators of brain tumors, in *Modern Perspectives in the Psychiatric Aspects of Surgery*. J. Howell, ed. Brunner/Mazel, New York (1976), pp. 140-161.
70. Lipinski, J., and Matthysse, S. Biological theories of schizophrenia, in *Biological Basis of Psychiatric Disorders*. A Frazer and A. Winokur, eds. Spectrum, New York (1977).
71. Cormia, R. Experimental histamine pruritus. *J. Invest. Dermatol.* 19:21 (1952).

Part II

General Theories of Behavior

13

Psychoanalytic Theory

FREDERICK SIERLES

INTRODUCTION

Psychoanalysis,* fathered by Sigmund Freud during the last decade of the 19th century and the first decade of the 20th, is a theory of personality development, a method of behavioral investigation, and a treatment for certain mental disorders. There are two concepts which are the underpinnings of psychoanalysis [1]: The first, *determinism,* posits that behaviors are never random — they are caused by underlying mental processes that originated in past events. The second, a belief in the *unconscious,* posits that what we think about at a given time represents only "the tip of the iceberg" of our mental processes, that there are enormous quantities of mental energy attached to processes outside of our awareness. These processes continually affect our behavior even though we may not be aware of them.

TOPOGRAPHY AND STRUCTURE OF THE MIND [1-5]

According to psychoanalysts, the mind is organized in two ways. *Topography* refers to the accessibility of mental processes to conscious awareness. *Structure* refers to a theoretical division of the mind into several functional units. These entities have never been linked to specific anatomic localizations in the brain.

---

*When the term psychoanalysis is used in this article, it is meant to apply to Freudian, or "classic" psychoanalysis, as opposed to Adlerian, Jungian, Sullivanian, Kleinian, or other schools of psychoanalysis.

Topography

The *conscious* is a like a complex sense organ; it consists of whatever we are aware of, or perceive, at a given point in time. The *preconscious* is those thoughts or mental processes that can be made conscious by a simple act of will. High-level, abstract, and complex thinking occurs at this level. The unconscious is those mental processes which cannot reach awareness no matter what we do; these mental processes can only be inferred through indirect means.

Structure

The *id* is a person's reservoir of innate (sometimes referred to as infantile) drives, which are arbitrarily divided up into *sexual* and *aggressive*. It is entirely unconscious. Many psychoanalysts believe there are more than sexual and aggressive drives. The *superego* is a person's internalized sense of right and wrong. It has conscious, preconscious, and unconscious components. Breaching its "code of ethics" may lead to *guilt*. The *ego ideal* is a person's internalized sense of ideal performance and behavior. It also has conscious, preconscious, and unconscious components. Failing to live up to its "standard of performance" may lead to *shame*. Some authors consider the ego ideal to be part of the superego.

The *ego* is usually defined by its functions. These are:

1. Perception
2. Affects and emotions
3. Intelligence
4. Learning and memory
5. Insight
6. Reality testing
7. Motor activity
8. Defense mechanisms
9. Object relations
10. Impulse control
11. Mediation between the other structures (id, superego, and ego ideal) and the outside world

Reality testing is the ability to decide what is real and what is not. *Object relations* are relations with other people. *Impulse control* is self-control. Ego function 1 is called the ego's *perceptual function*. Functions 3-5 are called the ego's *integrative functions*. Function 6 is called the ego's *reality-testing function*. Functions 7-11 are called the ego's *executive functions*. The ego has conscious, preconscious, and unconscious components.

The *defense mechanisms* [6] of the ego are ways of decreasing or minimizing severe *anxiety* which, in turn, results from fear of one's own drives, fear of punishment or injury, or fear of abandonment. Some of the common defense mechanisms are:

1. *Sublimation:* The channeling of unwanted impulses into socially acceptable behaviors.
A former thief becomes a professional baseball player and leads his league in stolen bases.
2. *Suppression:* The conscious relegation of an unwanted thought into the unconscious.
A doctor worries about the health of a critically ill patient after he comes home from work. Finally, he says, "I've just got to push this case out of my mind, because I'm not paying attention to my family," and does so.
3. *Identification:* The process of "becoming like" another person, including the taking on of one or more of that person's characteristics.
A resident in psychiatry starts using interviewing techniques and idiosyncratic gestures that are identical with those of an attending physician on his service.
4. *Regression:* The return of a person, usually only in a very partial sense, to an earlier state of thinking, feeling, or functioning.
Hospitalized medical patients are expected, during the acute phase of their illness, to give up their usual control over their daily schedules, to dress in pajamas, robes, and gowns, to lie in bed, not to conduct their usual daily business, and generally to let themselves "be taken care of." For a few days, many patients enjoy this part of their illness.
5. *Displacement:* The experience of a thought and its accompanying affect directed at one person or object when the thought was originally directed, but unacceptably so, at another person or object.
A student, angry at an attending doctor, becomes irritated with his friends and inexplicably tells them "to stop bugging" him.
6. *Repression:* The unconscious relegation of an unwanted thought into the unconscious.
A young woman, attending the funeral of her boyfriend, experiences a murderous feeling towards the dead boyfriend, then suddenly "forgets" the feeling (repression) while simultaneously becoming blind (*conversion*).
7. *Reaction formation:* The turning of an unwanted thought into its opposite, e.g., unconscious hate into conscious love.
A mother becomes smotheringly overprotective of a retarded child she unconsciously doesn't want to care for.
8. *Intellectualization:* The use of complex, impersonal, and abstract ideas instead of dealing with painful or unwanted thoughts and feelings.
Many people think in, and employ, complicated, stilted language when they are dealing with subjects which are sensitive and painful to them. A

patient stated that he had never once been angry during the past 15 years. He did, however, say that he sometimes felt "pleasantly assertive."

9. *Dissociation:* The phenomenon whereby certain of an individual's mental processes are not functioning in concert with his other mental processes.

A physician drives home alone from the hospital, intently rehashing the care of a difficult patient. She is startled to find herself halfway home, thinking that she had not had any perceptions of the highway and the traffic; in fact, other cognitive functions were "guiding" the trip home.

10. *Rationalization:* The giving of a superficial reason for an action, believing it to be the best explanation, when another reason is the actual one.

A physician on call to an emergency room, asked to see a patient with a problem that he is fearful of treating, tells the emergency room physician, with no willful duplicity, that the call is an inappropriate one and that a consultant in another specialty should be sought.

11. *Fixation:* The retention of some childish behavior patterns, with partial impairment of development of more mature behavior patterns to take their place.

An alcoholic man's main gratifications include drinking heavily and chain-smoking cigarettes *(oral fixation)*.

An obsessive-compulsive man, whose parents were very rigid and controlling, has been controlling, orderly, punctual and meticulous since his childhood *(anal fixation)*.

12. *Projection:* The attributing to another person (or other people) of one's own unwanted thoughts.

The husband of a woman being treated on an ENT ward starts believing incorrectly that the otolaryngologist is having an affair with his wife after visiting hours. Before he and his wife were married, he had an affair with her while she was married.

13. *Denial:* The complete rejection of readily available and unmistakable, but unwanted, information about oneself or others.

A patient with extensive metastatic carcinoma states, "They tell me I've got metastases all over, but I think I'd get well if only they'd discontinue the medication they're giving me."

PSYCHOSEXUAL DEVELOPMENT

According to psychoanalysts, in addition to physical, motor, and cognitive development, there is a kind of development called *psychosexual* development, so-called because it parallels changes in relative prominence of *erotogenic* (pleasure-giving) zones, which are zones of physical pleasure associated with psychological investment. Some psychoanalysts believe that this *libido theory* is either incorrect or overemphasized. The periods of psycho-sexual development are as follows:

The Oral Period (Birth to 1½ years)

The infant derives considerable pleasure from, and spends considerable time at, sucking on breast, bottle, and nipple. During the early part of this period, the id is predominant "structure." This is the period where *basic trust* [7] (an attitude that the world, and its people, is fundamentally, although never completely, safe) develops, if it is going to develop.

During the first 2 or 3 months of this period, there is the phase of *primary narcissism*, where the infant has no sense of himself as separate or distinct from the world around him. With the appearance of the *social smile,* which is a smil-ing response to a human face that starts at 2 or 3 months, the child is as-sumed to start sensing others as separate and distinct from himself. This is considered an important early stage in ego development. [8,9].

The Anal Period (1½-3 years)

The anus, rectum, and urethra are prominent erotogenic zones at this time. There is considerable motor and cognitive development, and the tod-dler wants and needs to be allowed some degree of control in his activities. There is considerable ego development.

The Oedipal Period (3-7 Years)

The genital area is the prominent erotogenic zone and masturbation is common. The Oedipus complex occurs: The child falls in love with the parent of the opposite sex, and wants to marry and have children with this parent. Also he wants to kill the parent of the same sex, and consequently fears retaliation by the same-sex parent. This complex resolves if the parent of the opposite sex isn't seductive, and if the parent of the same sex acts lov-ingly and nonthreateningly. This is the initial period of superego develop-ment, with much of the superego consisting of internalized values originally conveyed by the child's parents. If the Oedipus conflict does not resolve well, the patient retains an unconscious fear of mutilation or castration, which may result in various types of psychopathology, such as neurosis or sexual perver-sion.

Latency (7 Years to Puberty)

Sexuality is far less prominent, and a lot of wishes and feelings are sublimated into learning at school, competing at games, and playing with chums. Superego development continues here, and there is considerable identification with adults and peers.

Adolescence

Along with anatomic and physiological changes (puberty), there is an upsurge of sexual feelings, and a number of tasks to be mastered. These include becoming *independent* from parents, establishing an *identity* [10] (a sense of sameness and continuity over time), seriously considering *career choices*, and developing relationships with members of the *opposite sex.*

Adulthood

According to psychoanalysts, this is the genital phase of psychosexual development. Most psychiatrists feel that significant development continues to take place during this time, even though character patterns are well established. This is discussed in Chapter 22.

PSYCHOPATHOLOGY

Psychoanalysts believe that the above phenomena play a part in the development and manifestations of mental illness. Some common psychoanalytic explanations of some "mental conditions" are described here.

Psychoses

These are considered by psychoanalysts to be associated with major problems in the ego, with *ineffectiveness of reality-testing,* turning away from reality (as in hallucinations and delusions), ineffectiveness of usual defenses, use of very primitive defenses (like denial and projection), and very prominent regressions.

Some psychoanalysts believe that in some cases the initial event in *schizophrenia* is a profound *regression to the phase of primary narcissism,* where the patient experiences a *world destruction fantasy,* in which all borders and boundaries between himself and other people are broken down and all that is perceived is an amorphous nothingness [11]. Delusions and hallucinations are believed to be an attempt to bring back structure, meaning, reality, and boundaries (*restitution*). Some of the delusions are based upon *unconscious homosexual wishes,* which are transformed by reaction formation and projection into delusions of persecution and delusions of grandeur [11]. Other analysts believe that schizophrenia is primarily associated with the patient having very pathological models for identification. Still others feel that family pathology, such as the excessive presentation of confusing (e.g., *double bind*) messages to the child or a parental need for the child to be ill (*psychosis wishes* of the parent for the child), has a major influence.

Some analysts believe that in *depression* there is *guild about unconscious anger at an ambivalently loved (loved and hated) object (person) who is figuratively introjected (taken within) into the depressed person's ego* [12]. Other analysts believe that, either associated with the above, or separately, there is a significant *loss of the depressed person's self-esteem* [13].

Some analysts believe that *manic episodes* are a defense against depression, where there is a transient suspension of superego functioning, leading to diminished guilt about previously-unacceptable thoughts and behaviors [3].

Neuroses

These are considered to be the result of *unconscious conflicts which produce anxiety*. This necessitates the use of ego defense mechanisms, which represent the symptoms themselves. The unconscious conflicts often, but not always, center around the Oedipus complex.

Example: A 16-year-old school boy is brought into an emergency room with paralysis of both lower extremities; there are no signs of upper or lower motor neuron disease. As he is telling the examining physician about how he wants to kill his father, who has just beaten him, the paralysis resolves.

Personality Disorders (Character Disorders)

There are *life-long maladaptive behavior patterns*. Explanations include the following:

1. Parental deprivation, selfishness, or cruelty may lead to malfunctions of object relations (such as excessive mistrust, excessive selfishness [narcissism] and excessive dependency) and impaired impulse control.
2. Parental overprotection may lead to immaturity and excessive dependency.
3. Parental overcontrol may lead to a characterological need to control others and to be in control of everything one does.
4. Instead of developing a symptomatic neurosis (*symptom neurosis*) like a phobic or obsessional neurosis, a person experiencing an unconscious conflict develops a *character neurosis*, where chronically maladaptive behavior patterns are chronically employed to ward off anxiety.

Psychophysiological Disorders

These are conditions involving structural and/or physiological changes in *viscera* and the autonomic nervous system, and there is a *measurable pathophysiological disturbance* or an *observable lesion*. These are distinguished from conversion reactions, which involve the voluntary musculature, the somatic nervous system, and organs of special sense. Also, there are no structural changes in conversion reaction [14]. According to some psychoanalysts, examples of psychophysiological disorders are migraine headache, essential hypertension, bronchial asthma, duodenal peptic ulcer, thyrotoxicosis, diabetes mellitus, rheumatoid arthritis, and ulcerative colitis. According to some psychoanalysts, patients with psychophysiological conditions have all of the following characteristics:

1. A congenital predispositon (e.g., duodenal peptic ulcer patients are congenital hypersecretors of pepsinogen) [15].

2. A significant life stress (e.g., the stresses listed in the "life change units" scale in Chap. 25).

3. Excessive unexpressed anger and/or excessive unfulfilled dependency needs [14]. Examples include an asthma attack explained as a symbolic "cry for help," a duodenal peptic ulcer attributed to insufficient psychological and alimentary "feedings" associated with excessive psychological and alimentary "needs" and secretions; migraine headache and essential hypertension linked to a vascular "fight-and-flight" reaction when excessive unexpected rage is built up.

Example: A 36-year-old maintenance man suddenly became comatose from hypertensive encephalopathy. This occurred minutes after his being inappropriately and incorrectly criticized for sloppiness at work. Once he recovered, he told his doctor that he experienced no anger, either while he was being criticized, or immediately afterwards.

Sexual Perversions

These include exhibitionism, transvestitism, fetishism, and sexual sadomasochism. Psychoanalysts believe that in many cases, when these occur in males, they are often the product of an unconscious fear of punishment by castration.

Example: A 35-year-old Army sergeant, who felt "like I'm not much of a man," exposed his penis to a woman in a public place on several occasions. He said that each time this happened, he waited until the woman looked startled or surprised, and experienced considerable pleasure when this happened. As he began feeling more "like a man" over the course of time, this behavior stopped.

PSYCHOANALYSIS AS PSYCHOTHERAPY

Psychoanalysis is a form of psychotherapy which takes place 4 or 5 times a week for several years at least. The therapist *(the psychoanalyst)* is a physician or other professional who has been certified by a *psychoanalytic institute,* and who has, himself, been psychoanalyzed. Most analysts believe that the patient *(the analysand)* should either be neurotic or have a neurotic character disorder in order to benefit from psychoanalysis.

The patient lies on a couch and the analyst sits behind him, out of view. The patient talks about whatever comes to his mind *(free association),* with minimal interruption from the analyst [2]. The goal is to uncover, and thus make conscious, the patient's *unconscious fantasies.* In order that this occur, the analyst must remove the patient's *resistances* [2] to doing this. One type of resistance is called *transference* [2], where the patient unconsciously transfers, onto the analyst, thoughts and feelings that he has towards other people in his life, present and past, especially his parents or parent-substitutes.

Good clues to the content of the patient's unconscious fantasies come from, among other sources, *slips of the tongue* and dreams [16]. Most dreams are disguised *wish fulfillments,* which have several components: The *latent content* contains the undisguised unconscious wishes. The *day residue* consists of details, from recent events, which will be incorporated into the dream. The *dream censor* (ego or superego) combines aspects of the latent content with aspects of the day residue to produce the *manifest content,* the dream itself.

When the analyst helps to explain an unconscious fantasy or a resistance, it is called an *interpretation.* When the analyst acts differently from a pathogenic way in which the aptient thinks he was treated in the past, it is called a *corrective emotional experience* [3]. This helps to foster the *therapeutic alliance* between doctor and patient, diminish unnecessary resistances, and open to question previously held attitudes towards people. The ultimate goals are sustained symptom relief, insight, and personality change. The analyst must become aware of, and hence avoid acting upon, his *countertransference* feelings, wherein he transfers, onto his *patient,* thoughts and feelings which he has towards other people in his own life. Blindness to his countertransference feelings could significantly decrease his objectivity.

Psychoanalytically oriented psychotherapy is a briefer, less intensive variation of psychoanalysis, where patient and therapist sit face to face.

RESEARCH ON PSYCHOANALYSIS

While clinical information on psychoanalytic treatment has been gathered and reported for decades, the reports have generally taken the form of case examples and anecdotes; there has been a relative paucity of sophisticated statistical analysis of the data. Nevertheless, some statistical analysis does exist, and is reported and discussed in publications by Kline [17], Fisher and Greenberg [18], Silverman [19], Vaillant [20], Gunderson and Kolb [21], and Bergin and Garfield [22], among others. But much more remains to be done.

PSYCHOLOGY OF THE SELF

One of the newer developments in psychoanalytic theory has been Kohut's controversial theory which he calls the "psychology of the self" [23]. Basically, just as the content of the mind can be divided into conscious, preconscious, and unconscious on one level of abstraction, and into id, ego, superego, and ego ideal on another level, a third level of abstraction, which cross-cuts the other two, is also possible. Here, the content of the mind is divisible into that which pertains to oneself (called the *self*) and that which pertains to others (called the *objects*). In infancy, some of this mental content takes the form of idealized, archaic images of oneself (the *grandiose self*) and idealized, archaic images of projections of oneself onto others. Projections of oneself onto others are referred to as *self-objects;* the idealized, archaic images of the self-objects are referred to as *parent images.*

As normal development continues, the mental energy attached to the grandiose self and the parent imagos becomes transformed into energy attached to more realistic images of the self and of others. For some people, because of lack of parental empathy due to parental narcissism, these archaic images persist into adult life, leading the development of the *narcissistic personality disorder*, mentioned briefly in Chapter 9 but beyond the scope of this chapter.

REFERENCES

1. Brenner, C. *An Introduction to Psychoanalysis.* Doubleday, New York (1974).
2. Freud, S. *A General Introduction to Psychoanalysis.* Washington Sq. Press, New York (1968).
3. Alexander, F. *Fundamentals of Psychoanalysis,* Norton, New York (1963).
4. Zetzel, E., and Meissner, W. *Basic Concepts of Psychoanalytic Psychiatry.* Basic Books, New York (1973).

5. Holtzman, P. *Psychoanalysis and Psychopathology*. McGraw-Hill, New York (1970).

6. Freud, A. *The Ego and the Mechanisms of Defense*. Int. Univ., New York (1966).

7. Erikson, E. *Childhood and Society*. Norton, New York (1963).

8. Spitz, R. *a Genetic Field Theory of Ego Formation*. Int. Univ., New York (1959).

9. Spitz, R. *The First Year of Life*. Int. Univ., New York (1965).

10. Erikson, E. *Identity: Yough and Crisis*. Norton, New York (1968).

11. Freud, S. Psychoanalytic notes upon an autobiographical account of a case of paranoia, in *Three Cases Histories*. Collier (MacMillan), New York (1968).

12. Rado, S. The problem of melancholia, in *The Meaning of Despair*. W. Gaylin, ed. Science, New York (1968).

13. Fenichel, O. *The Psychoanalytic Theory of Neurosis*. Norton, New York, (1945).

14. Alexander, F. *Psychosomatic Medicine*. Norton, New York (1950).

15. Mirsky, I. Psysiologic, psychologic and social determinants in the etiology of duodenal ulcer. *J. Dig. Dis.* 3:4 (1958).

16. Freud, S. *The Interpretation of Dreams*. Basic Books, New York (1956).

17. Kline, P. *Fact and Fantasy in Freudian Theory*. Methuen, London (1972).

18. Fisher, S., and Greenberg, R. *The Scientific Evaluation of Freud's Theories and Therapy*. Basic Books, New York (1978).

19. Silverman, L. Psychoanalytic theory. The reports of my death are greatly exaggerated. *Am. Psychol.* 31:621-637 (1976).

20. Vaillant, G. *Adaptation to Life*. Little, Brown, Boston (1977).

21. Gunderson, J., and Kolb, J. Discriminating features of borderline patients. *Am. J. Psychiatry* 135:792-796 (1978).

22. Bergin, A., and Garfield, S. *Handbook of Psychotheraphy and Behavior Change*. Wiley, New York (1971).

23. Kohut, H. *The Analysis of the Self*. Int. Univ., New York (1971).

14

Conditioning

FREDERICK SIERLES and BERNHARD E. BLOM

INTRODUCTION

Conditioning is the process by which we learn new behaviors, maintain them, or discontinue old behaviors. Conditioning falls into two categories: There is *classic* (*respondent* or Pavlovian) conditioning, developed by the Nobel prize-winning Russian physiologist *Pavlov*, and *operant* (*instrumental*, Skinnerian) conditioning, developed by the American psychologists *Watson, Thorndike,* and *Skinner*.

The difference between classic and operant conditioning is as follows: In classic conditioning the behavior under study is *elicited* as a response to a stimulus which *precedes* it. It is associated most closely with *reflexive* responses. For example, meat presented to a dog elicits salivation. When a bell is paired with the meat, the bell will begin to elicit salivation even in the absence of the meat.

In operant conditioning, the behavior under study is *emitted* in anticipation of an occurrence called a *reinforcer* (or *reinforcing stimulus*) which will follow it in time. For example, students study hard in order to get knowledge, a high grade, and a diploma. Thus, operant behavior has an initiating, active quality about it, and respondent behavior has a passive, reflexive, or responsive quality about it. Nevertheless, control or shaping of behavior is occurring in both instances.

OPERANT CONDITIONING

There are two predominant forms of operant conditioning. In the first, *reinforcement*, a desired behavior is *increased* in its frequency, magnitude or duration by following it with a "rewarding" stimulus. In reinforcement learning the reward can occur in two ways. In *positive reinforcement*, something desired or needed is *presented* to a person. For example, a child is given a lollipop by a doctor after the child receives an examination. This reinforces the child's willingness to partake in a behavior which enhances his health. In *negative reinforcement*, an *aversive* stimulus, which is a stimulus that produces discomfort, is *removed* or avoided as a consequence of the desired behavior. For example, a person can't hear in his left ear because of an accumulation of cerumen. He therefore goes to a doctor who removes the cerumen, and then he can hear again. Here, the deafness due to the cerumen is the aversive stimulus, and its alleviation is negative reinforcement for coming to the physician's office. There are two kinds of negative reinforcement, *escape* and *avoidance*. In escape, a behavior *terminates* an *ongoing* aversive stimulus, as in the case where the ENT doctor restores hearing to an ear which had been occluded by cerumen. In *avoidance*, an aversive stimulus is *prevented* from occurring because of a behavior. For example, an alcoholic patient taking disufiram (Antabuse) will choose abstinence (i.e., avoids drinking) instead of drinking, for he knows that if he drinks a severe, highly undesirable reaction will ensue; thus the patient's abstinence behavior prevents an unpleasant physical reaction and a desirable behavior (abstinence) is learned.

The second kind of operant conditioning, *punishment*, is aimed at *reducing* the frequency, magnitude, or duration of an undesired (maladaptive) behavior. Here, an aversive stimulus is presented to, or a desirable stimulus is removed from, a person as a consequence of the behavior which is *not* desired. For example, a patient is discharged from the hospital against his will as a consequence of flagrant violation of hospital rules, or a child is spanked as a consequence of misbehaving.

A number of general principles, or laws, apply to both operant and respondent conditioning. The *law of magnitude* holds that the more powerful the stimulus, the more likely it is that the behavior will occur. For example, all things being equal, patients are more apt to seek medical attention because of severe pain or discomfort than they are for mild pain or discomfort. And all things being equal, physicians are more apt to work hard for a high fee than for a low fee.

The *law of practice*, also known as the law of frequency or repetition, holds that the more frequently a stimulus and response are associated (e.g., behavior is reinforced) the more effectively the response will be learned. For example, the more times a physician sees intramuscular penicillin cure diplococcal pneumonia in his patients, the more likely it will be that he will prescribe penicillin for diplococcal pneumonia.

The *law of recency*, also known as the law of contiguity, holds that the more closely a behavior is followed in time with a reinforcing (or punishing) stimulus in time, the more likely that the behavior will be learned (or "unlearned"). For example, in teaching interviewing technique, it is best for the instructor to present feedback to the student interviewer immediately after the interview, not days later. Or when a 2-year-old child runs into the street, the child's parent should spank him immediately after rescuing him from the street, not hours later.

The *law of contingency* holds that a behavior is most likely to be learned when the person is able to make a direct connection between the behavior to be shaped and the consequent reinforcing or punishing stimulus. For example, physicians are able to make a direct causal connection between the administration of antibiotics and the control of infections. Every time an antibiotic is administered, an observable reduction in signs and symptoms of infection occurs. This causal connection is known as a contingency relationship. Patients learn to make causal connections between their health-enhancing responses and the consequent rewards of feeling relief from discomfort, pain, or illness. They learn that relief from discomfort is contingent on seeking medical help.

The *law of effect* summarizes operant conditioning in simple terms; it holds that any behavior followed by a positive consequence (reward) is likely to be repeated and any behavior followed by an aversive consequence (punishment) is *not* likely to be repeated. For example, if a patient wishing to be admitted to the hospital is admitted to the hospital every time he complains of hallucinations or suicidal ideation, he may present these symptoms whenever he seeks entry into a hospital, even when these symptoms are minimal or nonexistent. Or, if every time a physician tells a certain joke to a patient the patient laughs, the more likely it is that the physician will tell the joke again to another patient. Similarly, if a patient is severely berated by his physician after seeking consultation for a health problem, that patient will be less likely to approach the physician with future health problems.

There are, however, occasional exceptions to these laws. For example, if a patient develops a near-fatal urticaria with laryngospasm as a result of eating a certain food, and is told of the relationship of the laryngospasm to the food, he will not need or want to have another experience with the food in order to learn to refrain from eating the food. In this instance of *one-trial conditioning*, the laws of practice and recency do not really apply, for the laws of magnitude and contingency are sufficient to produce learning and behavior change.

As you can see, conditioning is occurring continuously in our lives, whether or not we are aware of it. In fact, we all participate in elaborate formal operant *schedules of reinforcement*. There are four basic reinforcement schedules.

In *fixed-ratio schedules*, rewards are presented each time we perform a behavior a specific, fixed number of times. Factory piecework schedules are good examples. Another example is the payment-by-fee system for for physicians; every time the physician sees a patient, he is eligible to receive a fee. The latter is an example of a 1:1 fixed ratio schedule, otherwise known as *continuous reinforcement*. Continuous reinforcement is a highly useful method of teaching very young children a new behavior. For example, every time a child says "cup" the cup comes. Moreover, parents are likely to present the child with lavish praise (social reinforcers) for saying the word cup. Unfortunately, continuous reinforcement, just as continuous supervision of very young children, is very tedious and demanding. As the child grows older, different schedules can be effectively employed.

In the *variable ratio schedule*, varying frequencies of behaviors sometimes not known to the person being influenced, are required before rewards are presented. For example, the first reward may be presented after 5 instances of the behavior, the second reward presented after 2 instances of the behavior, and the third after 16 instances of the behavior. This is the schedule which usually applies in gambling situations, such as roulette, card-playing, lotteries, betting pools, "one-armed bandits," and investing in the stock market. The occurrence of compulsive gambling attests to the effectiveness of this schedule; behaviors are maintained for long periods at high frequencies because the person cannot "predict" when the payoff will occur.

In the *fixed-interval schedule*, the reward is presented after a certain predictable amount of time has elapsed. Examples of this schedule are payment of a fixed monthly salary to employees and election year-nonelection year cycles for politicians. The productivity of people on the fixed interval schedule tends to peak just prior to the time that the rewards are to be presented, for employees and politicians are aware that employers and voters tend to make "reward" decisions based on the most recent events. Because behaviors early in the fixed interval are not immediately followed by rewards, there tend to be few of them. The graph of productivity against time in the fixed-interval system gives a "scalloped" picture, as presented in Figure 1.

A medical example of proper application of a fixed interval schedule is in the treatment of postoperative pain. When considerable pain can reasonably be expected in the postoperative situation, it is preferable to prescribe narcotics at regular (fixed) time intervals, as opposed to an "as-needed (PRN) for pain" basis. This is because narcotics have a positively reinforcing, rewarding quality, and to give them as needed for complaints of pain would be to reward the experience of pain and increase the frequency of its occur-

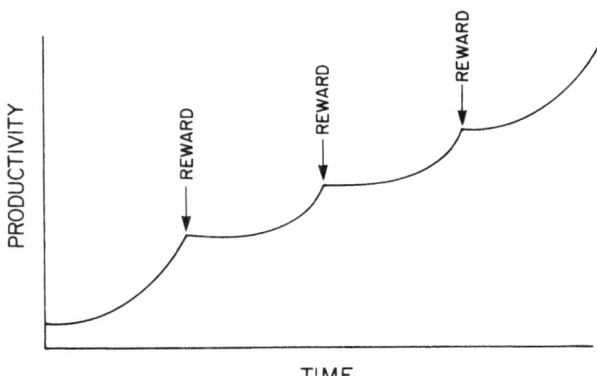

FIG. 1.   Productivity versus time in the fixed-interval system.

rence, as well as the frequency of the pain behaviors (symptoms, complaints) even when there is no severe pain present.

In the *variable interval schedule*, the elapsing of variable (unpredictable) periods of time pass before rewards are presented. Real estate brokers and business owners are subject to the variability of economic cycles; business may thrive for a time and then become poor for another, indeterminate interval. Another example of a variable-interval schedule is a patient trying to reach a busy doctor by phone.

The abovementioned schedules are relatively simple. More complex schedules can be designed and can occur naturally. *Compound schedules* require conformity to two or more schedules concurrently. For example, in the *conjunctive schedule* a response will only be reinforced if the requirements of both a fixed-interval and fixed-ratio schedule are met.

Many of the more complex behavior sequences learned by humans and animals alike have to be taught as simple individual components first. Such complex behaviors have to be shaped. Shaping is the practice of systematically rewarding successive approximations to the final desired complex behavior pattern.

Thus parents intuitively reward a toddler with praise for taking his first stumbling steps; they do not wait until the complex act of fully coordinated locomotion occurs in its final form. Rewarding the child for its first awkward "approximations" to walking, and all the successive (not necessarily successful) approximations, is an example of shaping.

Extinction occurs when the frequency of a behavior diminishes as a result of cessation of reward (i.e., no reinforcers are presented following the behavior). For example, a child has temper tantrums, where he lies on the floor and screams, and this causes his parents to pay extra attention to him, which is reinforcing. The doctor suggests that the parents consistently ignore the tantrum, removing the reward for the tantrum, and the tantrums cease (become extinct). The rapidity with which a learned behavior can be extinguished is one measure of the strength of learning and of different schedules used in the learning process.

In general, ratio schedules are harder to extinguish than interval schedules and variable schedules produce stronger learning than fixed ones. One exception to this rule is the continuous (fixed-ratio 1:1) schedule, which is the easiest of all schedules to extinguish, because it becomes rapidly apparent to the subject that the reward schedule is not going to be maintained.

Punishment, while not a form of negative reinforcement, is a conditioning method whereby control employing aversive measures is used. Punishment is often not as effective as positive reinforcement for a number of reasons. It tends to make people angry and resentful. For example, a physician is not notified that there has been a switch in an on-call schedule, and thus doesn't appear for work on a day he is supposed to be on call. This comes to the attention of the hospital administrator who fines the doctor and sends him a letter of reprimand. The letter is a source of humiliation for the doctor who, until the episode, was a paragon of enthusiasm, and after the episode begins feeling that he will do only what he has to do and not put out any extra effort. Another problem with punishment is that it has to be contingent, immediate, frequent, and powerful to be effective, and has to be employed whenever the undesirable behavior occurs, virtually requiring a continuous (1:1 ratio) schedule. Thus, many criminals continue their criminal activity even after one or several episodes of arrest and imprisonment, because they realize that much of the time they will not be arrested and imprisoned, and the instances of reinforcement for criminal behavior greatly outnumber those of punishment.

There are other aspects of conditioning that merit some discussion. Some learning will occur as a result of watching someone else perform an activity which followed with that person getting rewards or punishments. This is referred to as *imitative learning* (modeling). For example, some aspects of the interviewing and physical examination style of a senior physician may be adopted by residents on that physician's service. Of course, once a modeled behavior is adopted, the manner in which it continues to be reinforced will help determine the extent to which it is maintained.

Sometimes learning may occur as a result of a behavior coincidentally being followed by a positively reinforcing stimulus, where the behavior and the stimulus were truly independent of each other (i.e., noncontingent). Despite the complete coincidence of the two events, the person believes that the events are causally related, so he continues the behavior, expecting positive reinforcement to follow. This is the mechanism of *superstitious behavior*. An example of this occurs when a pediatrician prescribes an antibiotic for what turns out to be a viral pharyngitis. The child recovers rapidly, his parents feel that the antibiotic cured him, and ask for the antibiotic again the next time the child becomes ill. Another example is when a medical student wears a certain sweatshirt for several final examinations, scores well in those examinations, and feels compelled to wear the same sweatshirt on all future examinations.

Thus far, we have presented conditioning as a fairly straightforward, one behavior-one reinforcing stimulus phenomenon. Usually the situation is somewhat more complex, and a number of concepts merit some discussion.

Discriminative Stimuli

In operant conditioning, behaviors are emitted prior to, and in anticipation of, a reinforcing stimulus. Simultaneous with or preceding the emission of the operant behavior, a discriminative stimulus is often present. This is a stimulus which will not itself elicit the behavior, but will increase the likelihood of the behavior occurring if it had accompanied the behavior in the past when it was reinforced. A discriminative stimulus serves as a cue which allows a person to predict that a certain behavior is likely to be followed by a reward (or punishment). For example, if you run into one of your patients at a party, he will not necessarily be very spontaneous in conversing with you. However, in the privacy of your office (the discriminative stimulus), he is much more likely to speak spontaneously about himself and his health (the operant behavior) in anticipation of you listening to him and showing concern (the positive reinforcing stimulus).

Response Chaining

A response chain occurs when a series of behaviors occur which are related to stimuli that serve as both reinforcing stimuli and discriminative stimuli. A patient interview serves as an example.

Doctor: "What is the problem?" (discriminative stimulus—a *cue* or precondition for the patient to begin)
Patient: "My ear hurts." (operant behavior—emitted in anticipation of reinforcing stimulus)
Doctor: "Tell me about the pain." (reinforcing stimulus—concern and clarification *plus* discriminative stimulus—a *cue* for the patient to continue talking)

Discrimination Learning

We do not only learn to identify a stimulus; we can also learn to make distinctions between gradations and variations of the stimulus. The ability is a discriminative capacity. For example, while a medical student is first taught to identify a heart murmur and is rewarded for it, later in his career he will be able to distinguish a systolic from a diastolic murmur, and a mid-systolic from a holosystolic murmur. This results from correct (e.g., "this is a systolic murmur") responses being positively reinforced by a supervisor, and incorrect responses not being reinforced at all. We all have discriminative capacities that remain untapped for lack of motivation and reinforcement.

Generalization Learning

Just as we can learn to make fine distinctions between cues that resemble each other, so can we also learn to "overlook" such distinctions. This enables us to use similar cues in differing environments as predictors of forthcoming rewards or punishments for a particular behavior; for example, a child that has had to take unpleasant-tasting medication from a bottle may refuse to take another (perhaps pleasant-tasting) medication from a similar-looking bottle. This child has generalized from one stimulus (the first bottle) to all other similar-looking stimuli (other medication bottles).

Generalization learning can be adaptive as well as maladaptive: A patient with a history of positive or rewarding consequences for visiting one physician's office is much more likely to generalize his consultation-seeking responses to other physicians than a patient with negative experiences.

Topography of Responses

We not only learn to engage in a behavior; we can also learn to perform it in a certain specified way. For example, medical students are taught to palpate a patient's abdomen for tenderness, masses and enlarged organs. However, only if they palpate the abdomen from the patient's right side, and with their right hand, will the supervisor give positive reinforcement. Topography refers to the physical characteristics of the behavior performed, which is a step beyond simply whether or not the behavior is performed.

Motivation and Attention

To learn a desired behavior, the individual must be motivated to do so, and this is determined in large part by the nature and timing of the reinforcement which follows. In addition, the individual must be paying attention to the learning process, and must also learn to pay attention to the relevant aspect of a discriminative stimulus which sets the occasion for a desired behavior. *Supraordinate stimuli* inform the person of those aspects of a stimulus to which he should pay attention. For humans, words are the most common supraordinate stimuli. For example, in teaching auscultation of the lungs, the instructor will say, "Listen for crackling sounds, like the crackling of a piece of cellophane. Those sounds are called 'rales'." That informs the student what to listen for.

CLASSIC CONDITIONING

As we stated before, in classic conditioning the behavior under study is *elicited* as a response to a stimulus which precedes it, and it is most closely associated with reflexive responses governed by the autonomic nervous system. The response to the stimulus is referred to as a *respondent*. The learning takes place when a neutral *conditioned stimulus* (such as a bell rung in a dog's cage) is repeatedly paired with a biologically, innately effective *unconditioned stimulus* (such as meat when the dog is hungry) to elicit the *respondent* of salivation. Eventually, the dog will salivate when presented with the sound of the bell alone. To be categorized as *unconditioned respondent*, the response must be one that all members of the same species would make. For example, a bright light of a certain strength shone into a person's eyes at a certain distance will evoke approximately the same amount of pupillary constriction in all neurologically intact humans who are not taking drugs known to affect pupillary constriction.

Respondents are vulnerable to *habituation*, which means the gradual decrement in the strength of the respondent after a course of repeated elicitations. For example, we are initially anxious when we see a cadaver, or a person having a seizure, but after hours in an anatomy lab, or months working in a neurosurgical service, the respondent of anxiety (which can be defined in terms of complex physiological changes as well as subjective discomfort) diminishes considerably.

Sensitization may also occur during classic conditioning. The frequent or rapid presentation of a series of unconditioned stimuli produce a condition of overreactivity, or sensitization, where the organism is primed to respond to any stimulus which follows, be it an unconditioned stimulus or a conditioned stimulus. Thus, when an experimenter observes a respondent following the presentation of a conditioned stimulus, he or she must be sure that true conditioning or learning has occurred and that the respondent was not the product of sensitization.

In classic conditioning, there cannot be reinforcement schedules, since the respondents are elicited, not emitted. Nevertheless, the selection of intervals at ratios in which the unconditioned stimuli and conditioned stimuli are presented in classic conditioning is analogous to that in operant conditioning schedules. *Extinction* will occur when the conditioned stimulus is presented a number of times without the unconditioned stimulus.

There are a number of other parallels between classic and operant conditioning, but we will not discuss them here. Despite the fact that we all continually respond to unconditioned stimuli, and that classic conditioning can occur in humans, operant conditioning plays a more important role than classic conditioning in planned and naturally occurring behavior modification in humans.

BEHAVIOR MODIFICATION

Behavior modification is the process of altering undesired behavior and diminishing symptoms and signs by employing conditioning principles. Although we have cited a number of examples where the shaping of behavior occurs in an unplanned, albeit useful fashion, behavior modification typically refers to the planned or formal process of behavior change.

In general, in working with patients it is best to provide positive reinforcement for desired behaviors, and no reinforcement (only rarely should punishment be employed) for unwanted behaviors. For example, one advantage of periodic checkups is that the attention and concern of the physician constitute a positively reinforcing experience for the patient's operant behaviors of preventive health care and the state of being well. Thus, the patient needn't rely on the presentation of symptoms (illness behaviors) as the only means of receiving attention and reward from the doctor. For patients who are used to getting physician attention by dramatizing signs and symptoms, the physician can respond rather neutrally to the dramatizations, and be more responsive to the patient's discussions about his family, his accomplishments, and his taking steps to get well. For patients who are lax or negativistic about following the physician's instructions, the physician can reward, with enthusiasm, praise, or attention, any initial approximations or efforts of the patient toward following treatment instructions. After the first few times, when the desired behaviors start occurring regularly, the positive reinforcement should become intermittent in nature, since behavior learned on continuous reinforcement extinguishes rather rapidly. In addition, the physician should attempt to establish in the patient's mind that the good health which is expected to follow from following instructions has immediate rewarding qualities of its own. Berating the patient (punishment) and explaining to the patient that his health will be much better 20 years from now (no immediate reward) is rarely useful.

For patients with certain disorders, formal behavior modification programs are in order. These are typically conducted by psychologists, although some psychiatrists have formal training in behavior modification and can perform it competently. Behavior modification (or behavior therapy) differs from other forms of psychotherapy because it is typically briefer and hence less expensive, and because finding the cause of the symptoms is less important than (or not important at all) eradicating the symptoms. Finally, behaviorists have been more vigorous than other groups of therapists in scientifically studying the therapeutic utility of their treatment programs.

Monosymptomatic phobias are treated by a process called *systematic desensitization*, developed by the psychiatrist Joseph Wolpe. It is based on the principle of *reciprocal inhibition*, which holds that relaxation and anxiety cannot occur simultaneously. Thus, the patient is first taught a deep muscular relaxation procedure. Then he develops, with the behavior therapist, a list (hierarchy) of phobic situations, progressing from the mildest to the most fearful. He is then encouraged to imagine himself in the mildest situation in the hierarchy and then directed to relax, utilizing the method he has just learned. For each step in the hierarchy, he learns to relax in place of being anxious.

Flooding (implosion) is another way of attacking the same problem. Here, the patient is directed in the first therapy session to imagine and experience the most frightening situation possible and this is repeated in subsequent sessions, with a reduction in anxiety associated with each succeeding session. Extinction of the anxiety respondents occurs because of the absence of both classically conditioned (phobic) stimuli and operantly conditioned rewards (e.g., attention or concern from others for the anxiety attack).

Token economies employ a system of rewards (e.g., use of a telephone, canteen privileges) for desired behaviors. This reward system has been used for increasing the socialization and communication of withdrawn, chronically hospitalized psychiatric patients, for increasing the self-control of school children, and for teaching self help skills to retarded children.

Assertive training is employed for excessively meek people or for people who angrily overreact to slights from others. The patient practices expressing angry feelings, with the therapist playacting the role of the person at whom the patient gets angry. The patient learns not only to express anger, but also to express it constructively and in socially acceptable ways so that the object of his anger can receive some useful feedback. The classically conditioned components of anxiety and anger (respondents) diminish due to extinction, and the desirable operant behavior of assertive, nonaggressive, nonanxious behavior is systematically rewarded by the therapist with praise and the avoidance of anxiety.

Metronome speech retraining has been used in the treatment of stuttering. Some stutterers become more fluent when they are taught to pace their speech. The pacing is first learned to the beat of a metronome, which serves as a discriminative stimulus for the rate and flow of speech.

In *negative practice*, otherwise known as *paradoxical intention*, a patient is instructed to repeat an undesired behavior, such as a tic, thousands of times in brief training sessions perhaps 5-10 times per week. This has been shown to decrease the spontaneous frequency of the undesirable behavior once the negative practice sessions are terminated.

Aversion therapy has been used for the treatment of sexual deviations such as fetishism or pedophilia. Like other forms of therapy, this must be done with the patient's informed consent. The person receives a mild but unpleasant electric shock every time he experiences pleasure (e.g., an erection) when presented with the stimulus (e.g., the fetish) which typically provokes the undesirable response.

SELECTED BIBLIOGRAPHY

American Psychiatric Association Task Force on Behavior Therapy. *Behavior Therapy in Psychiatry*. Aronson, New York (1974).
Ferinden, W. *Classroom Management Through the Application of Behavior Modification Techniques.* Remediation Assoc., Linden, N.J. (1970).
Reynolds, G. *A Primer of Operant Conditioning.* Scott, Foresman, Glenview, Illinois, 1975.
Wachtel, P. *Psychoanalysis and Behavior Therapy.* Basic Books, New York (1977).
Wolpe, J. *The Practice of Behavior Therapy.* Pergamon, New York (1973).

Part III

Verbal and Nonverbal Communication

Part III

Verbal and Non-verbal Communication

15

Interviewing Techniques

FREDERICK SIERLES

INTRODUCTION

Other than the physical examination, the interview is the only medical procedure you will perform during virtually all your patients' visits. Its goals are to obtain data, to begin the inspection portion of the physical exam, to establish and maintain rapport, to increase or maintain patient comfort, and to educate the patient. Therefore, the essence of interviewing lies in the examiner's ability to obtain pertinent data while simultaneously responding to the patient's behaviors. Many of the techniques employed in the medical interview are also applicable to other interview situations, such as administrative interviews (e.g., screening a candidate for membership in your department). Interviewing skills can be learned and are not an all-or-nothing, "you've either got it or you don't" phenomenon.

Although interview situations, patient's clarity, openness, and spontaneity, and the personal styles of interviews vary, there are hints that are applicable to most interviews. These hints are not axioms; they are options available to you to increase your repertoire of responses.

There is a spectrum of interview styles that ranges from the structured to the semistructured to the unstructured (open-ended) interview. Most medical interviews fall somewhere in the middle of this spectrum. In the structured interview, all the questions, and the order in which the questions are asked, are spelled out beforehand. This style is most useful in research where there are numerous interviewers and where interrater reliability may be more vulnerable. It is rarely applicable in usual medical situations because it does not permit much responsivity to what the patient is saying. In the semistructured interview, you have a fairly fixed set of questions that must be answered, but the order of the questions, and the form of each question, are largely determined by what the patient is communicating verbally and non-verbally. The majority of medical interviews employ some form of the semi-structured interview.

In the unstructured (open-ended) interview, the primary determinant of what you say next is what the patient is communicating. Certain areas of questioning will be overlooked, but you may be able to go into greater depth about what the patient is thinking and feeling at the time of the interview. This form of interview is employed by psychoanalysts in initial interviews and therapy sessions, and may be employed at the beginning of an interview when an articulate patient, familiar to you, offers a chief complaint that "There's something I've just got to get off my chest." It is typical of conversations in life in general.

Interview styles vary from physician to physician, vary within a given interview, and vary from situation to situation. Your style should vary to some degree for each patient. When the patient is open, articulate, organized, honest, and insightful, your responses will not be the same as when the patient is guarded, inarticulate, disorganized, or confused.

PREPARATION FOR THE INTERVIEW

Often you have an opportunity to prepare a patient for an interview; for example, you do this when you refer a patient to a consulting physician, or when you explain a demonstration interview to be performed by yourself or by a colleague. Proper preparation is invaluable. The difference between whether or not the patient is prepared for an interview is like the difference between visiting someone as an invited guest and dropping in uninvited (or even unwelcome). You should explain the purpose of the interview and an-swer any questions the patient has about it.

> *Example:* A pediatrician tells the parents of a 16-month-old boy, "I'm un-able to determine the cause of your son's cyanosis, and I'd like to refer you to Dr. Jones at the University Hospital. Dr. Jones will once again take your history and form her own impressions. In addition, she has access to a number of tests not available in my office. She and I will keep in close touch, and I'd like to continue treating your son once a diagnosis is estab-lished. Have you any questions?"

CONVERSING IN THE WAITING ROOM

It is inadvisable to begin the interview formally until you and the patient are sitting comfortably in the office or at the patient's bedside. It is important that you be comfortable, and your office should be designed with your comfort as well as the patient's in mind. If you are going to converse at all before beginning the interview, you should not ask "How are you doing?" because this question is universally associated with superficiality. Also, if the patient were to say "fine" in response to that question, your logical response might be: "If you really felt that way, you wouldn't have come here," and that would make an awfully awkward beginning. Empathic comments are sometimes useful en route to the examining room.

> *Example:* An emergency room consultant is working in a busy emergency room with a long waiting period. After greeting a patient, the first question he asks is "How long have you been waiting?" Upon hearing an angry "About four hours" from a seemingly alert patient, he says "That can be infuriating." In this interchange, he has learned that the patient is appropriately angry, and oriented to the waiting time. In turn, he has tried to turn a resentment-inducing situation to his best advantage.

THE INTRODUCTORY STATEMENT

If you and the patient have never spoken before, one effective way of beginning is to make an introductory statement, one or two sentences long, which includes (1) your name, (2) the referral source and reason for the interview, (3) a phrase or two about what you know about the patient, and (4) an open-ended request for the patient to begin talking about his present problems.

> *Example:* "Hi, I'm Dr. Green, and I'm going to be your doctor while you're here. I've looked at your chart, but a chart can't explain as much as a patient can, so perhaps we could start by you telling me what's been the problem."

Since you don't usually know in advance how articulate a patient is going to be or exactly what's troubling him, your opening remarks usually have to be rather stereotyped. However, a "standard" introduction must be dispensed with under certain circumstances.

> *Example:* A psychiatrist is called in to consult on a patient who is talking incomprehensibly because of delirium. As he approaches the patient, the patient is muttering at the ceiling and paying him no attention. The psychiatrist approaches him by entering his field of vision, and begins in an exaggeratedly friendly, loud fashion: "Mr. Gray, I'm Dr. Williams, how

are you?" If he were to say much more, it might further confuse this already confused patient.

THE MAIN PHASE OF THE INTERVIEW

Although it is important to have considerable knowledge of the conditions that are problematic for the patient, a useful interview can be conducted even if you are not an expert on pathology. This is another way of saying that the form of an interview is as important as its content. Even freshmen medical students, asked to interview patients before they have had a course in pathology, can get a reasonable history.

Facilitating Techniques for Interviewing Open, Articulate, and Insightful Patients

I believe that the majority of adult medical and surgical patients are reasonably open, articulate, and insightful. The following hints apply to this majority.

1. Try to employ a *judicious balance between open- and closed-ended questions.* Usually you begin with general, open-ended questions and proceed to closed-ended questions if the open-ended ones are producing insufficient information. An open-ended question is typically answered in several sentences or a paragraph, more than just a word or two. Examples of open-ended questions include "What is the problem that brought you here today?" "Could you tell me some more about that?" "Tell me about the health of your parents." "Explain that." and "Could you elaborate on that?" Closed-ended questions can be answered in a word or two. Examples are "How old are you?" "How many days have you been in the hospital? and "Have you ever had diabetes?"

The frequency with which you will ask open-ended questions is proportional to the degree to which the patient presents the history articulately and gives you the diagnosis "on a silver platter." Here is an analogy: If you are lost, and drive into a gas station, you will likely begin by asking the attendant something like "How do I get to Chicago?" and not "Do I make a left or a right turn out of this station to get to Chicago?" If the attendant's directions are crystal-clear, you don't have to ask much more. If they are not clear, you may have to ask several closed-ended questions. The patient is like the gas station attendant, and you try to ask the right questions to get the "route" to his diagnosis.

2. *Listen to the patient.* Don't interrupt unless he is clearly being irrelevant or avoiding crucial issues, or unless you're in a hurry. Being a good

listener demands considerable self-control on your part. Of course, some patients are extremely meticulous and compulsive and feel continuously compelled to present every little detail. In this situation, both you and the patient can benefit from frequent interruptions; you won't have to listen to unnecessary details, and the patients will appreciate not having to be so precise and perfect.

> *Example:* In presenting her history, a schoolteacher begins narrating, in the most extensive detail, a series of hostile encounters she has had with her principal. After hearing the details of two such encounters, the interviewer reaches the conclusion that the patient doesn't trust the principal, and that further examples will probably not enhance the interview. He interrupts at the end of a sentence, and says "I realize that your relationship to him is quite important to you, but there's certain additional information I need to have," and changes the subject.

3. *Stick with the subject the patient is talking about* as long as what he is saying seems relevant and important. I feel that most of the time patients talk about matters which are of importance both to them and to you, and that most patients don't like to be interrupted. Sometimes changing the subject reflects your own anxiety about the subject, and this in turn can increase the patient's anxiety.

> *Example:* A middle-aged patient keeps referring to having "been in trouble with the police" and how he feels "very badly" about it. The interviewer, thinking this would cast aspersions on the patient's morality, avoids asking him what kind of trouble he was in, and what he means by "feeling badly." The interview remains awkward, the patient continues to convey discomfort, and insufficient data is gathered. The interviewer's supervisor, who was present during the interview, then asks the patient "What sort of trouble are you in ?" The patient responds very directly and with feeling, and presents a history of having stolen machinery from his boss' office while he was experiencing a severe depression, and that he feels extremely guilty about it. In presenting this information, key pieces of information are obtained and the patient appears much more comfortable.

Also, the more times the subject is changed, the less spontaneous and free-flowing the interview. Of course, if a patient is being redundant or evasive or if you are in a hurry, the subject should be changed. And some patients are more at ease when the doctor gives the interview a definite structure. One way of encouraging a patient to elaborate on a subject is to select an interesting and potentially revealing word, phrase, or sentence he has just spoken and either repeat it with emphasis, or ask an open-ended question about it.

Example: A patient with extensive metastatic cancer, in discussing his feelings about the cancer, says "I feel I've been cheated," and stops talking for the moment. The doctor looks at him more intently and says with emphasis *"Cheated?"*

What happens if a patient is talking about one subject and makes a reference to a significant new subject? Do you stick with the original subject and return to the significant new subject later, or do you direct the interview towards the new subject? At least *some* subjects must be developed fully without interruption, so you will often stick with the original subject. However, if the new subject is presented with a great deal of feeling, or is especially revealing of symptoms, this subject could be dealt with right away. If *you* want to bring up an entirely new subject or a new line of questioning, it is sometimes useful to make an empathic transition to the new subject. For example, if the interview is drawing to a close and you feel that it is vital that certain data can be obtained before the end of the interview, you can wait until the end of a sentence and then interrupt with a statement like: "The interview is drawing to a close and there is certain additional information I msut have, so I'm going to change the subject." This lets the patient know that the interviewer is aware of having interrupted him.

4. *Try to do something about impediments to the progress of the interview.* If a patient is not being open and spontaneous, and you think he is capable of being open and spontaneous, this should be discussed. If you don't resolve impediments, they will usually continue to impede the interview.

Example: A physician is called to see a patient who has recently taken an overdose of pills. The patient is fully alert and in no obvious distress, and her relatives say she is "quite a talker when she gets started." The physician begins by saying "I'm Dr. White. I was told by the nurse that you took an overdose of pills. Tell me how you're feeling now." The patient looks at the physician sullenly and doesn't answer. The physician then says "I need to know more about what's going on in order to properly treat you." The patient then says "Do I have to talk to you?" The physician says "Not necessarily, but an overdose is an urgent situation, and you must be treated for it. It will be easier for me and safer for you if you talk with me." The patient then proceeds to present a clear history.

If the patient is experiencing distress, you may need to take measures to alleviate the distress or at least to empathize with it.

5. *Make empathic comments.* Although there are a number of exceptions, identifying what a patient is feeling often puts him at ease. This may give him the feeling that someone else understands him, or it may help him to under-

stand his mood and how it is perceived by others. Comments like "You seem blue," or "You look angry," if correct, can increase rapport. If the patient appears upset but you cannot identify his mood, you can say "You seem upset." The patient's nonverbal communication provides cues about his mood. For example, anxiety is revealed by chain smoking, hand tremor, fidgeting, sweating, exophthalmos, and lip-licking, and anger is revealed by visible tensing of muscles, clenching of fists, and explosiveness or loudness of speech.

Hints for Interviewing Patients Who Are Not Open, Articulate, and Insightful

There are many exceptions to the use of the facilitating techniques we have just discussed. These exceptions include interviews of patients who are either guarded, disorganized, or confused. Many of them have significant brain dysfunction—this includes patients with delirium and dementia, receptive aphasia, acute mania, and catatonia.

Some severely mistrustful patients will answer questions while simultaneously communicating indirectly that they don't want to be in a hospital and don't want to be interviewed. But if they are directly confronted with this, they may refuse to answer further questions. By avoiding such a confrontation, the interviewer will usually be able to complete the interview satisfactorily.

Open-ended questions are often not useful for patients with significant brain dysfunction. Often, empathic comments are useless or confusing, and periods of interviewer silence are useful only for the purpose of detecting a formal thinking disorder. For people with severe brain dysfunction, you should employ simple, direct, clear closed-ended statements and questions that demand minimal reflection and abstraction. Remember, the patient with significant brain dysfunction often does not comprehend much and often feels confused and threatened by lack of clarity in the interview situation.

Example: A physician, interviewing a patient with severe receptive aphasia, said things like "Now tell me what is the name of this finger," and if the patient answered correctly, he would smile and say "That's very good." As the interview progressed, it was apparent that this was the only way to maintain the patient's cooperation, for the patient could barely comprehend what the physician was saying. Thus, what would be patronizing and judgmental for another patient was appropriate for this one.

Example: Here is an example of a tactical error on the part of an inexperienced nurse. A hyperactive patient, with severe brain dysfunction, placed his hands around the nurse's neck. Her response was to ask gently "Why are you doing that?" He didn't release his grip. Another nurse, sensing the problem, called out firmly "Now you stop that right now!" and the patient released his grip.

Example: Here is an example of a tactical error on the part of an experienced physician. Another hyperactive patient, with severe brain dysfunction, barged into a conference in which the physician was talking to two staff members and another patient. The physician, thinking he was making himself clearly understood, said to the intruding patient "We're having a conference now." This didn't deter the intruding patient at all. As you can expect, one of his colleagues, thinking more wisely, called out firmly "You must leave here right now!" and the intruding patient walked out.

There is a technique called the Amytal (amobarbital) interview which is used for patients who are alert but mute, and where the interview may be critical for the diagnosis. Explain to the patient that you're going to give him some medicine which will probably help him to speak, and obtain his informed consent. Mix 500 mg sodium amobarbital powder in a syringe with 20 cc sterile water. Start an IV with 5% dextrose in water. Then, at a rate not to exceed 1 cc/min, inject the amobarbital mixture into a vein via the IV tubing. By the time half the amobarbital is injected, many patients who are mute due to catatonia or depression will give you a reasonable history which will reveal symptoms and signs of the underlying condition. Once the effects of the amobarbital have worn off, the patient will usually become mute again. If the patient has voluntary (elective) mutism or extensive coarse brain disease, the Amytal technique will usually not work.

THE ROUNDING OUT PHASE OF THE INTERVIEW

If important areas have not yet been covered and time is running short, make a transitional statement indicating that you will ask a number of questions rather rapidly, e.g., "We are running out of time, so I am going to have to ask a number of questions rather rapidly," and proceed to ask a series of closed-ended questions.

BRIEF CONCLUDING DISCUSSION

At the end of the interview, make a very brief statement which relates to or summarizes what has been said, and then make a recommendation if it is in order. For example, "Well, as you suspected, you do have a serious disorder and you will need to take the Dilantin. I recommend that you make once-a-week outpatient visits here at the clinic," or, "Although you do seem to be a lot more comfortable than you used to be, I still think that you should continue with your medications." After this wrap-up statement is made, let the patient respond briefly, respond to his response, say something like "Let's stop now," shake the patient's hand (if it's an initial interview), and stop the interview on a note conveying hopefulness and continuing concern for the patient's well-being.

SELECTED BIBLIOGRAPHY

1. Enelow, A. Programmed Interview Instruction. National Medical Audiovisual Center Films T2244X-T2255X (1970). Association Films, Atlanta, distributors.
2. Engel, G., and Morgan, W. *Interviewing the Patient*. Saunders, Philadelphia (1973).

16

Issues in Talking with Patients

FREDERICK SIERLES

In the preceding chapter, we discussed techniques for the initial interview. In this chapter, we will cover additional issues that arise in talking with patients, either in initial interviews or followup visits.

1. *"Put-downs."* Putting patients down (being critical, sarcastic, or contemptous) often makes them feel ashamed, guilty, or resentful, lessens the chance that they will reveal embarrassing symptoms to you in the future, and decreases the chance that they will comply with your recommendations.

> *Example:* A teenage male college student, who has just experienced a discoloring nitric acid facial burn in the chemistry lab, asks the doctor: "Will it leave a scar?" The doctor responds, sarcastically: "We should send you to the ladies' powder room, the way you're carrying on." The student seeks out another doctor's care for followup treatment.

> *Example:* An alcoholic patient comes to a hospital emergency room following a seizure. The intern ends the interview by saying "No wonder you're having seizures, you're just an alcoholic." The patient walks angrily out of the interview.

2. *Nonmedical Advice.* Doctors frequently have to give advice, but this should be limited to medically proven treatment regimens. Sometimes doctors overstep their medical bounds and advise patients how to run their lives in general.

> *Example:* A teenage girl, a high school senior, goes with her parents to the family's highly respected doctor and asks for some feedback about her tentative choice of medicine as a career. He responds by saying "It's really better for a girl to go into nursing." (This was in the 1960s.) She and her

family agree, and she winds up going to nursing school, becoming a nurse, and regretting her choice because it wasn't her first one.

There is no reason to believe that physicians have more wisdom than their patients about life in general, yet sometimes they feel compelled to offer advice about issues like deciding whether to get married, get a divorce, go to medical school, or get an abortion. This sets up a situation where if the advice is taken and works well, the patient may relinquish future decisions to the physician instead of making them himself, and if the advice does not work out well, the physician can be held legally responsible. You should reflect upon how often you truly respect and follow advice given to you by others.

3. *Gross reassurance.* Reassurance that is not based on solid data, and is given blindly to make the patient feel better temporarily, is a very risky business.

Example: A patient has a history of nine prior psychiatric hospitalizations with minimal improvement each time. After half an hour initial interview, she asks her new doctor, a first-year psychiatry resident, whether she will be cured. He responds by saying, "Yes, definitely." Her response is "You jerk, you don't know anything," and leaves the office. The resident may have been right, but neither he nor the patient knew it at the time.

Patients do need reassurance, but it should be based on solid data.

Example: A patient with endogenous depression is told "The chances are 80-90% that electroconvulsive treatments will alleviate this depression you are experiencing."

Also, reassurance can be given in an indirect fashion.

Example: A patient says to her doctor, "Are you sure it's safe for me to drive a car since I just had a fainting spell last week?" The doctor, who had already given consent to drive and given reasons for the decision, say "You seem to be having doubts about my judgment," and the patient smiles and says "No doctor, I was just testing."

4. *Expression of emotion by the patient.* Patients often express strong emotions, and sometimes this presents a problem for the physician.

Crying or anger: If the crying or anger are mounting in intensity, and this is getting the patient agitated and less able to participate in the interview, then you must intervene. However, this is the exception rather than the rule; more often when the physician allows the patient to express an emotion (without changing the subject or acting judgmental) the interview will be enhanced. Physicians sometimes become anxious when a patient expresses sadness or anger, and change the subject to avoid their *own* anxiety.

Laughter: Patients sometime laugh or joke. If the patient has said something which is funny because it is insightful, you certainly can laugh with him. However, when the joking or laughter is cruel or self-deprecatory, you should refrain from laughing.

5. *Personal questions.* Patients often ask questions about the physician's personal or professional life. If the questions are reasonable and appropriate, they should be answered briefly and honestly. If a patient asks such questions repeatedly, you should seek out the reason for questions. You should not let the patient "turn the interview around" (dominate the interview) by asking you a long series of questions.

6. *Stopping the Interview.* You should have in mind the amount of time you think the interview should last, and stick to that time unless there is an emergency. Occasionally, a patient will keep talking beyond the expected time. You should verbally or nonverbally (by standing up, walking to the door, and gesturing towards it) communicate the need to stop. This may seem callous, but in reality, you have schedules and people are in the waiting room. If you regularly extend interviews, you become vulnerable to being late for later appointments, being resentful of your long-winded patients, and having patients save their most interesting information for the end of interviews.

7. *Confidentiality.* This is discussed in Chapter 31. It is important to add that clarifying the ground rules about confidentiality may facilitate some interviews.

> *Example:* A medical student asks for an appointment with a faculty member and begins the appointment by asking, "Is this confidential?" The faculty member replies, "Yes, unless it's a life-and-death emergency." The student, appreciative of hearing the ground rules, presents a clear, self-revealing history.

> *Example:* A military physician, asked by headquarters to evaluate a soldier accused of having sex with his daughter, begins the interview by saying, "What you tell me is not confidential, so watch what you say." The patient, appreciative about the warning, seeks treatment from the physician after the legal case is closed.

8. *Adolescents.* Interviewing adolescents is sometimes different from interviewing adults. Adolescents are less likely to be open and spontaneous, and are therefore less likely to respond well to open-ended questions or to silence. Compared to interviews with adults, empathic comments by the physician are more likely to yield spontaneous responses. Declarative statements are sometimes more effective than questions. The physician is more likely to be

challenged to take a position and be self-revealing, and should do so if possible.

9. *Drug Abusers.* Interviewing alcoholics is covered in Chapter 10. In interviewing drug abusers, it is important to appear tolerant and nonjudgmental. If the interviewer feels at ease with drug culture "lingo," he can use it, e.g., "Do you *do* any drugs?" or "Ever *drop* acid?" instead of "Are you a drug abuser?" or "Are you an addict?"

10. *Families.* In cases where one or more family members have accompanied a patient with obvious brain dysfunction, it is useful to ask the patient and the family together whether they would prefer to be interviewed together rather than for the patient to be interviewed alone. If they agree, which is usually the case, the family interview serves several purposes: (1) If the patient is recalcitrant or mute, the family's history may be the only history you will get, (2) a separate meeting "behind the patient's back" may increase mistrust, especially if the patient hasn't given prior consent, and (3) your interview style may serve as a model for how to talk to the patient. In interviewing the family with the patient get all members to participate actively, because this takes some pressure off the patient (defocusing), and gives the family members a chance to express feelings and get questions answered.

11. *Convincing patients to come into the hospital.* In trying to get patients to consent to enter the hospital, it is helpful to offer reasons which are restatements of what the patient has already admitted is problematic, rather than to make a separate judgment that may not be congruent with the patient's view of the situation. For example, if a psychotic patient states he is very scared, it may be helpful to say "How would you like to come into the hospital to get some treatment *so you won't be so scared?*"

> *Example:* A patient with alcoholic hallucinosis comes to the emergency room and says "They are going to kill me with rays." The doctor, instead of saying "You're ill and you need hospitalization (which the patient likely would have rejected), says "If you come into the hospital, we'll do everything we can to keep anyone from getting you with rays. What do you say?" The patient, feeling relieved, signs right in.

Sometimes, it is better to put the initial recommendation for hospitalization in the form of a question, to give the patient some sense of control over, and responsibility for, the situation. If this does not work, the doctor will have to be more direct.

SELECTED BIBLIOGRAPHY

Enelow, A. Programmed Interview Instruction. National Medical Audiovisual Center Films T2244X-T2255X (1970). Association Films, Atlanta, distributors.

Engel, G., and Morgan, W. *Interviewing the Patient*. Saunders, Philadelphia (1973).

Ginott, H. *Between Parent and Teenager*. Macmillan, New York (1969).

Tarachow, S. *An Introduction to Psychotherapy*. Int. Univ. New York (1963).

17

The Phenomenologic Mental Status Examination

MICHAEL ALAN TAYLOR

INTRODUCTION

The mental status examination is part of the complete physical examination of every patient seen by a physician. No physician would think his examination complete unless he listened to the patient's heart and recorded the vital signs. The brain deserves just as much attention. Of all hospitalized acutely ill medical/surgical patients, 10-15% have brain dysfunction and consequent abnormal behavior secondary to their systemic illness [1-3]. Additionally, 15-20% of the general population may be at risk for psychiatric disorder [4,5]. The mental status examination is essential in identifying individuals with brain dysfunction.

The goals of the mental status examination are to (1) foster a reasonable doctor-patient relationship, and (2) thoroughly evaluate the patient's present behavior, both normal and abnormal. Historical information, although extremely important in diagnosis, does not belong in the mental status examination. The mental status exam deals only with "the here and now."

The mental status examination must not be haphazard; some structuring is important and questions and procedures should proceed in a logical pattern. But the questioning should also be responsive to the specific needs and behaviors of the patient. The examiner should be prepared to cover every area of the examination, and develop a facile, standardized manner of eliciting each form of psychopathology. Table 1 summarizes some of the basic characteristics of the mental status examination.

The phenomenologic mental status examination is an approach to the

Table 1   Desirable characteristics of the mental status examination

Manner	Warm, supporting, concerned, interested
Tone	Conversational, semi-informal
Strategy	Semistructured
Tactics	Follow rules of social interaction; relate questions to patient's complaints; do not challenge, but be truthful; respond to appropriate questions

mental status examination used in many parts of Europe and by some research groups in the United States. This approach is nontheoretical and provides the reliable clinical information necessary for valid diagnosis [6]. The basic principles of phenomenology are: (1) *Objective observation* of behavior, free from interpretation; (2) communication of these observations through *well-defined terminology*; and (3) separation of behavior *form* from behavior *content*. This is the descriptive approach to psychiatric diagnosis that is the basis of our present-day sets of research criteria [7-9].

Objective observation, well-defined terminology, and a standardized semistructured examination procedure are essential for reliability of diagnosis. Identification of behavior form is also essential to the diagnostic process, and observations should separate behavior form from behavior content. For example, what an hallucinated voice says is content; the clarity, duration, and location of the voice is form. What a person is talking about is content; the use of language and its syntax is form.

The phenomenologic mental status examination can be divided into *eight* broad areas of observation. These will be listed below, with phenomenologic terms and definitions associated with each observational area. The presence or absence of each listed behavior alters the probabilities of a given diagnosis. These behaviors have been discussed in greater detail by Jaspers [10], Fish [11,12], and other phenomenologists [13,14].

AREAS OF OBSERVATION

Appearance

Appearance includes body type (endomorphic, mesomorphic, ectomorphic, dysplastic), sex, race, and age. Observe also the patient's manner, nutrition, health, personal hygiene, and state of consciousness (e.g., clouded, fluctuating, dazed, fuzzy). Here are two examples:

This patient is a 32 year old, white, ectomorphic man who appears thin, stoop-shouldered, and dazed. He is unkempt, has nicotine-stained fingers, and moves in a slow, absent-minded fashion.

The patient is a short, stocky hirsute 25-year-old woman with greasy sweat, frozen face, and general bradykinesia.

Motor Behavior

Observations of motor behavior should include comments about gait, abnormal movements, rhythm or coordination, speed and frequency of gestures. Look for the following:

Agitation: Increased frequency of small motor behavior (small hand movements, jerks of head and shoulders, foot tapping). *Agitation refers only to the frequency of motor behavior.*

Hyperactivity: Increased frequency of gross activity which is goal-directed (e.g., talking to several people one after the other; going to one place, then another in quick succession).

Catatonia: Catatonia is a *syndrome* and is observed in several conditions [15]. At least 25% of catatonics have an affective disorder [15]. Mutism is not synonymous with catatonia [15,16].

Facial expressions: A flat expressionless face without eye-blinking is most characteristic of schizophrenia. Grimacing and other fixed facial postures can also occur.

Stereotype: Repeated nongoal-directed motor behavior (e.g., the patient knocks his forehead repeatedly with his knuckles).

Echopraxia: Repetitive copying of the interviewer's motor behavior.

Automatic obedience: Despite the examiner's instructions to the contrary, the patient moves a body part (e.g., arm) upon light pressure from the examiner.

Posturing: Assuming odd body positions (psychological pillow).

Catalepsy (waxy flexibility): The patient assumes or can be placed in odd postures which are maintained for long periods of time.

Affect

Affect is the emotional tone underlying all behaviors. *Affect has range, intensity or amplitude, stability, appropriateness of mood, relatedness, and quality of mood,* all of which will are discussed as follows:

Range: Variability of emotion over a period of time. Normal range can be compared to the variations and resonances of a musical piece. Range of affect tends to be restricted in depression and expanded in mania.

Intensity: Intensity of affect refers to the amplitude of emotions. It does not refer to variability. The psychomotor epileptic can shout and rage with great force, never varying his intensity, until overcome by exhaustion. His range is totally restricted but his affective amplitude is intense.

Stability: This refers to the rapidity of change in mood and affective intensity. Normal changes occur relatively slowly during the course of the day. Rapid shifts during the interview are pathological. Lability (instability) of affect is charactristic of mania and many coarse brain syndromes.

Mood Appropriateness: This refers only to the interview situation and is determined in part by the interviewer's own mental state and empathic understanding of the patient's behavior. In other words, what is appropriate to you is appropriate for the patient. Inappropriateness of mood (laughing in a sad situation) is not diagnostic, because it is present in many serious psychiatric illnesses; it should not specifically suggest schizophrenia.

Relatedness: This refers to the ability of the patient to express warmth and to interact empathically with the interviewer. Schizophrenics are notoriously unable to respond in this manner, and often appear cold and unfeeling. You might feel you are addressing a computerized voice.

Quality of Mood: This refers to expressions of anger, sadness, happiness, anxiety, and apathy. Mood is but a part of an individual's affectivity.

Thought Processes and Thought Content

Thought processes refer to the *form* of thoughts as expressed in speech, and can be examined in terms of rate, pressure, idiosyncracy of word usage, tightness of associational linkage, and form of associational linkage. *Thought content* [15] is what the patient is talking about; it is not the same as thought process. Thought content can suggest mood (e.g., depression, euphoria), but no matter how "bizarre" the content, it is never diagnostic of formal thought disorder. Proverbs are poor tests of thinking; they are never diagnostic and are so culture-dependent that they are useless in a mental status examination [17,18].

Rate of Speech

The rate of speech can be speeded, slowed, halting or dysrhythmic, the latter often seen in Huntington's chorea and multiple sclerosis. Rapidity of thoughts can be reported only by the patient, but it can be inferred from the rate of speech. Slow and/or hesitant speech is characteristic of depression, altered states of consciousness, and certain coarse brain diseases where the ability to select and/or express the proper words is defective (aphasia).

Pressure of Speech

Pressure of speech refers to the drive to talk. Rapid, pressured speech is a cardinal sign of mania.

Word Usage

Abnormalities of word usage include neologisms and word approximations. This is one type of "formal" thought disorder, and is frequently observed in dominant hemisphere coarse brain disease and in schizophrenia. Here are two examples of word approximations:

"The nurse came and took my thermometer (temperature) and said I had a heat (fever)."

"I need to sign some papers; may I use your writer (pen)?"

Tightness of Thought Linkage (Associations)

Loosening of associations refers to the disruption of meaningful connections between words or phrases. Loosening of associations is not pathognomonic of schizophrenia; in fact, mild loosening is most frequently observed when severe anxiety is present. *Word salad* refers to loosening between words so that consecutive words seem unrelated in meaning. An example is, "I, or what, what, the sky, he, me, she, she, she, she, cold, it." *Fragmentation of* thought refers to loosening between phrases and sentences. An example is, "Then going over the world, then coming down, I'm going to meet, riding and riding down; how's it coming, Johnny? Now, now, going home, going home." *Simple or mild loosening* refers to loosening of associations between paragraphs.

Form of Linkage

The form of linkage is the formal structure whereby associations are linked.

In *tangential thinking*, the linkage is tight but associations, formed in a straight line, never reach the goal of answering the question relevantly. Here is an example:

Doctor: "What kind of work do you do?"
Patient: "I'm a worker, alright. Been doing it for years."

In *circumstantiality*, the linkage is tight, but extra nonessential associations are added before the goal is reached. This is typical of the speech of chronic epileptics, alcoholics, and some passive-aggressive individuals: Here is an example:

Doctor: "What kind of work do you do?"
Patient: "I've been working all my life. It's been hard, but I've always worked. Now take this present job. I don't like the boss. He's the type who thinks they own the world. I'm not going to clean up for everyone. Not me. No sirree. That's how it is for us secretaries; that's what I am, a secretary."

In *verbigeration (palilalia, stereotypic speech)*, the linkage is tight, but some associations, particularly at the end of thoughts, are repeated in an automatic manner. This is often observed in catatonic states. An example:

Doctor: "What kind of work do you do?"
Patient: "I'm a doorman, man, doorman door, door man, man."

In *thought blocking*, the continuity of thought suddenly stops. If the patient begins a new train of thought after blocking, the process is called blocking with *derailment*. This does *not* refer to the "blocking" described in psychotherapeutic settings or conversations, when a person stopes talking at an emotionally laden moment, or forgets what he is talking about; it *does* refer to the sudden absence of all thought and activity, as occurs in petit mal epilepsy.

In *perseveration,* the linkage is tight, but certain stock phrases and words are continually repeated. There is often evidence of coarse brain disease. Here is an example:

Doctor: "What kind of work do you do?"
Patient: "I'm a doorman, what ho, what ho, I'm a doorman. Apartment building, what ho, what, what ho, what, I'm a doorman, in an apartment building."

In *rambling speech*, there are fragmented nongoal-directed associations. This is common in acute brain disease. Sometimes people who are very drunk speak this way.

In *driveling* (double-talk) the associations are better than for rambling speech, and the speech is fluent, but what is said makes little sense. This is frequently observed in persons with coarse brain disease, particularly with dominant temporal lobe dysfunction. An example:

"Put on the bag last night, and it bumped pretty cold. But then again, twenty-two, forty-nine."

With *nonsequiturs*, the linkage is tight, but the total thought is irrelevant to the question posed. This is common in schizophrenia as well as in coarse brain disease with aphasia. An example:

Doctor: "How old are you?"
Patient: "I ate a banana for breakfast."

In flight of ideas, association lines are broken, and the patient jumps from subject to subject; each shift in subject occurs in response to external stimuli. Flight of ideas is typical of mania. An example: "It is a beautiful day. The sky is blue. I have a nail in my shoe. I'm hungry. I have to get a new coat."

In *clanging*, associations are determined by the sound of words rather than their meaning. This is typically observed in mania. "Clanging, banging, hanging, danging" is one example.

Apophanous (Delusional) Phenomena

Delusional Mood (Atmosphere)

This is the "feeling" that something is wrong, "not right," or sinister. It may also be a feeling of being watched. This is akin to the self-consciousness felt by sensitive people entering a noisy room full of people who, for a moment, become quiet to observe the newcomer. Delusional mood can be observed in almost any psychiatric condition, and is not diagnostic.

Delusional Ideas (Notions)

Delusional ideas are fixed false beliefs not commonly shared. They may be *secondary* to other phenomena such as an altered mood, an hallucination, or a delusional mood. An example: A depressed patient, feeling he was a terrible person, believed he was causing all the illness in the hospital.

They may also be *primary* (autochthonous). Delusional ideas occur in a variety of conditions, and are no more diagnostically specific than an elevated sedimentation rate or white blood cell count.

Delusional Perception

Here, a real perception is suddenly personalized and becomes extremely significant to the patient. (see First Rank Symptoms.)

Perceptual Disturbances

Perceptual disturbances are frequently observed in psychiatric syndromes. *The content of these phenomena is never diagnostic. Only the form suggests specific conditions.*

Elementary Hallucinations: Examples of this include unformed lights, and unidentified noises, smells, and touches.

Incomplete Auditory Hallucinations: These are among the most common types of hallucination, and at least 50% of normal individuals experience them. They are characterized by lack of vividness. When they are voices, the voices are muffled, often experienced as coming from inside the head, and usually limited to a few words or phrases. While frequently experienced in schizophrenia, these phenomena occur as readily in many psychoses [10-12].

Functional Hallucinations: These occur only after actual stimulation, for example, when a real musical tone sounds like a voice calling the patient's name.

Extracampine Hallucinations: These are hallucinations which occur outside the realm of physiological possibility. For example, a patient *saw* a devil standing *behind* her.

Dysmegalopsia: Dysmegalopsia is the experience of seeing objects changing in size. They are often observed in epilepsy and in early stages of schizophrenia [10-14]. *Micropsia* refers to objects becoming smaller, and *macropsia* refers to objects becoming larger.

First-Rank Symptoms (FRS)

First-rank symptoms were first systematized by Kurt Schneider [13], who believed that the presence of any one of these was *decisive* (pathognomonic) in the diagnosis of schizophrenia. When present, the diagnosis of schizophrenia must be considered, but FRS can occur with coarse brain disorders and affective disease [19]. First rank symptoms include the following:

Thought Broadcasting

The patient's experiences that his thoughts are escaping audibly from his head into the outside world. This experience is a delusion, not an hallucination, and is often associated with delusional notions of telepathy or electronic surveillance.

A young black man came to a psychiatric emergency clinic on his 17th birthday, to see what could be done about "the machine" being used to "broadcast" his thoughts. In an interview with him and his parents, he felt foolish and patronized when asked to speak, as it was clear to him that we already knew what he was thinking. He frequently responded with "Come on . . . you know." It was a poignant example of empathic understanding: Both the interviewer and the patient's parents empathized with his severe distress, but neither psychiatrist-interviewer nor naive participant-observer could share his strange, frightening experience.

Experiences of Alienation

The patient experiences that his thoughts, feelings, impulses, or actions are *not his own*, but are those of some external force. Delusional notions explaining the nature of this external force are common, but secondary to this experience.

A 19-year-old patient complained of concentration difficulties resulting from unwanted thoughts which suddenly appeared in his stream of consciousness. They were "obviously" not his own. He insisted that "Someone keeps putting things in my head . . . and the pressure is too much." He spent hours cleaning the ward kitchen but insisted the cleaning activity was not part of him. He knew it was there while it happened, but the action was "disconnected" from his "self," like a "foreign body," and was attributed to the "actions of God."

Experiences of Influence

The patient experiences that his thoughts, sensations, feelings, impulses, and actions are imposed upon him by some external agency. He feels that he is "being controlled" and must passively submit to these experiences. Secondary delusional notions about the nature of this "control" may occur.

A frightened 19-year-old female student described her teacher as continually "sending energy waves" which made her think certain homosexual thoughts and which made her assume "certain sexual" body postures. The student "felt" the teacher "control" her body, "touching her genitals," while she remained still, unable to move or resist.

Complete Auditory Hallucinations

These hallucinations, occurring in clear consciousness, are experienced as clearly audible voices coming from outside the patient's head. They are in full sentences and often are like a running commentary about the patient's thoughts.

A 20-year-old in boot camp began hearing several people in his barracks discussing his homosexuality, and debating with his father (thousands of miles away) about the best way to kill him. These "conversations" were clear and persistent, finally forcing the patient to flee camp in hopes of escaping his tormentors.

Delusional Perceptions

These arise from real, normal perceptions, which lack special meanings for others, but which suddenly have special private meanings for the patient, often leading to an elaborate "delusional system." Here are two examples:

> A 21-year-old patient said his girlfriend was pregnant with three babies because he had to adjust his wristwatch 3 times that morning.

> A sailor saw a hawk fly over his ship and said that it meant his ship was in danger.

Intellect (Cognitive Functioning)

Intellectual functioning and memory can be evaluated only if the patient's ability to concentrate is intact. The *ability to concentrate* is often impaired by anxiety or fatigue. An altered mood (depression or elation) and intrusive thoughts or perceptions can also interfere. Tests include the *repetition of numbers forward* and *then backward* (six forward, four to five backward should be considered normal), and *serial subtraction* of 7 (or 3) beginning at 100 (normal is completion within 90 sec with no errors). Clinical tests of intellectual functioning include calculations, fund of information, vocabulary, and object similarities. A fairly reliable and valid test would be:

Q. What is the similarity between an orange and an apple?
A. They are both fruits.
Q. What is the similarity between an airplane and a bicycle?
A. They are both means of transportation.
Q. What is the similarity between paint and concrete?
A. They both must dry and harden to function properly.

Proper answers to the first two questions suggest normal intelligence. A proper answer to all three questions suggests above-average intelligence.

Memory

Memory is discussed on pages 18 and 19. Two abnormalities of memory are discussed here.

> *Confabulated ("made up") Memory* can be evaluated by suggesting false

events to the patient who may agree and elaborate. Confabulation is most frequently observed in Korsakoff's encephalopathy but "fantastic" confabulations can occur in mania [11,12,20] and with frontal lobe lesions [21].

Pseudomemories are not the result of memory impairment. They most frequently occur in patients with delusional ideas who are attempting to support their apophanous notions with "historical" evidence.

Judgment

Judgment is discussed briefly on page 16.

Global Orientation

Global orientation refers to the precise awareness of oneself and one's surroundings. "Orientation x 3" is redundant; if you write that a person is oriented, you mean oriented to time, place, and person. Responses to questions of orientation are often not diagnostic, but certain responses are suggestive. A response within a day or two of the actual date is usually accepted as normal. Strange responses (e.g., "this is another planet," "we're in the future") suggest a psychosis or hysteria. Presentation of precise but incorrect dates, employing the dates just prior to the onset of illness, suggests anterograde amnesia. Vague, incorrect, and mundane responses (e.g., "I'm home") suggest a coarse brain syndrome.

REFERENCES

1. Morse, R.M., and Litin, E.M. Post-operative delirium. A study of etiologic factors. *Am. J. Psychiatry* 126:388-395 (1969).
2. Wells, C. Chronic brain disease. An overview. *Am. J. Psychiatry* 135:1-12 (1970).
3. Wells, C. Delirium and dementia, in *Basic Psychiatry for the Primary Care Physician*. H. Abrams, ed. Little, Brown, Boston (1976).
4. Weissman, M., Meyers, J., and Harding, P. Psychiatric disorders in a U.S. urban community 1975-1976: *Am. J. Psychiatry* 135:459-467 (1978).
5. Goodwin, D., and Guze, S. *Psychiatric Diagnosis*, 2nd ed. Oxford, New York (1979).
6. Spitzer, R., Fleiss, J., and Endicott, J. Problems of classification. Reliability and validity, in *Psychopharmacology: A Generation of Progress*. M. Lipton, A. DiMascio, K. Killam, eds. Raven, New York (1978).
7. Taylor, M., and Abrams, R. The prevalence of schizophrenia. A reassessment using modern diagnostic criteria. *Am. J. Psychiatry* 135:945-948 (1978).
8. Feighner, J., Robins, E., Guze, S., Woodruff, R., Winokur, G., and Munoz, R. Diagnostic criteria for use in psychiatric research. *Arch. Gen. Psychiatry* 26:57-63 (1972).
9. Spitzer, R., Endicott, J., and Robins, E. Clinical criteria for psychiatric diagnosis and DSM-III. *Am. J. Psychiatry* 132:1187-1192 (1975).

10. Jaspers, K. *General Psychopathology.* J. Hoenig and J. Hamilton, trans. University of Chicago, Chicago (1963).
11. Hamilton, M. (ed.). *Fish's Clinical Psychopathology: Signs and Symptoms in Psychiatry.* Wright, Bristol, England (1974).
12. Hamilton, M. (ed.). *Fish's Schizophrenia.* Wright, Bristol, England (1978).
13. Schneider, K. *Clinical Psychopathology.* M. Hamilton, trans. Grune & Stratton, New York (1959).
14. Slater, E., and Roth, M. *Mayer-Gross Clinical Psychiatry,* 3rd ed. Williams and Wilkins, Baltimore (1969).
15. Abrams, R., and Taylor, M. Catatonia. A prospective clinical study. *Arch. Gen. Psychiatry* 33:579-581 (1976).
16. Morrison, J. Catatonia: Retarded and excited types. *Arch. Gen. Psychiatry* 28:39-41 (1973).
17   Andreasen, N. Reliability and validity of proverb interpretation to assess mental status. *Compre. Psychiatry* 18:465-472 (1977).
18. Reed, J. The proverbs test in schizophrenia. *Br. J. Psychiatry* 114:317-321 (1968).
19. Taylor, M., and Abrams, R. The phenomenology of mania. A new look at some old patients. *Arch. Gen. Psychiatry* 29:520-522 (1973).
20. Barbizet, J. *Human Memory and Its Pathology.* D. Jordine, trans. Freeman, San Francisco (1970).
21. Struss, D., Alexander, M., Lieberman, A., and Levine, H. An extraordinary form of confabulation. *Neurology* 28:1160-1172 (1978).

Part IV

Development

18

Ethology

GEORGEDA BUCHBINDER

INTRODUCTION

Ethology is the study of animal behavior. Classically, the word ethology applied to the behavior of animals in their natural habitats, but now it is used more loosely to include all animal behavior. Among other tasks, ethologists make *ethograms,* which are descriptions of the behavior of a species, a species being a population of organisms that share a common gene pool and are reproductively isolated from other populations. As a result of their common gene pool, members of a species share many behavioral as well as morphological and physiological characteristics. *Homo sapiens* differs from many other species in that much of its complex social behavior varies from one society to the next; that is, it is not panspecific.

We often assume that understanding animal behavior is relevant to understanding human behavior. But to what extent is such an assumption legitimate? As Hinde [1] noted, a scientist considering this question is pulled in opposite directions: Since he subscribes to the theory of evolution by natural selection, he must acknowledge that there are continuities between the behavior of animals and humans, and that the closer their relationship, the greater the continuity. However, since he also studies species differences, he knows that even closely related species have to adapt to different environments, and that these adaptations involve morphology, physiology, and behavior. Those who study nature are often awed by its diversity, and often exhibit humility when generalizing from one species to the next. This is why the central theories of sociobiology [2,3] (see Chap. 1) have generated such heated controversy.

The behavioral gap between other animals and humans is enormous:

Animals are inferior to humans in cognitive functioning, degree of foresight and awareness, and ability to reflect on their own behavior. Chimps can paint simple designs, but this is not art. Many animals live in complex societies, but the signals which integrate their social lives are very different from human language. Chimpanzees use tools, but this technology is dwarfed by our own. No animal has a culture involving values, beliefs, and norms of behavior which even approaches ours. To further complicate the issue, not only are there tremendous differences between animals and humans, but also there are differences among animal species and *among human societies*. These differences make generalization even more tenuous. Some of the differences between other animals and humans are exaggerated by the methods used to study animal behavior. As is the case for other scientists, the ethologist is forced to simplify; in order to describe behavior, he must delineate regularities, and in so doing he must gloss over irregularities. In making generalizations he must focus on the phenomena they encompass, and neglect other phenomena. In analyzing the behavior of a species he may ignore individual variation, so a bias towards simplification is thus built into his work. Therefore, the application of concepts derived from the study of relatively simple animals to the more complex human situation is even more tenuous, since the original concepts are themselves simplifications.

Thus it is clear that the study of animal behavior is limited in helping us to understand human behavior. But it can help in some ways, and many of these arise from the fact that other animals are in many ways simpler than people. The study of animals permits the development of methods that can be adapted to humans. This is commonplace in most medical sciences. Some of the behavioral analyses and treatments used in behavioral disorders were first developed with animals. The continuous stream of behavior of an individual must be broken down into its elements, and those elements must be classified before analysis can proceed. The experience of researchers in describing animal behavior has made the description of human behavior easier.

In addition, animals can sometimes be used for experiments which would be unethical if performed on humans. For example, monkeys have been used to study the effect of separating infants from their mothers, a subject in which planned experiments cannot be done in people. Of course, these findings must be extrapolated with caution, and assessed wherever possible in light of more direct evidence.

The study of animal behavior can provide data, principles, or generalizations whose relevance to humans can subsequently be assessed. Thus, one can study the use of nonverbal communication in animals, or the way in which experience influences aggressive behavior, or the nature of mother-infant interaction, and *then* see to what extent the findings apply to our own species.

The relative simplicity of animals permits the isolation of phenomena which might be shrouded in the complexity of the human case. Furthermore, it is possible to select for study species in which particular aspects of behavior are well developed or are more accessible for study than in humans. For example, infant monkeys spend nearly all their time clinging to their mothers, and the "contact comfort" they obtain from their mothers plays an important part in their development. Its study has lead to better appreciation of the importance of contact comfort for the human child.

Finally, comparative study of different species also gives us some understanding of the biological functions of behaviors and the ways in which they evolved to enhace survival and reproduction. To understand function one must study differences between organisms; we could make little progress if we studied only our own.

But, as we stated before, care is needed in generalizing the findings to humans. It is easy to select facts to fit theories and to neglect awkward cases. *Indeed animal evidence can be used to support almost any ethical, social, or political system.*

In summary, the study of animal behavior can give perspective to the behavior of humans. It emphasizes those features that are shared with lower forms, giving depth to our inevitably anthropocentric view, and it also highlights our uniqueness.

ANALOGIES BETWEEN HUMAN BEHAVIOR AND OTHER ANIMAL BEHAVIOR

The remainder of this chapter will be devoted to a discussion of some commonly cited analogies between human and other animal behaviors, and a consideration of some important ethological concepts and their application to human behavior.

Territoriality

This means that an individual animal, a mated pair and their offspring, or a larger social unit, identifies a specific site or location as its own, can find it at a distance, and may defend it against other conspecifics. Territories may be large, small, or virtually symbolic (e.g., the posts used as perches by sea gulls). They may be held exclusively by the individual or social groups (as in some birds) or overlap (as in many primate species). They may be permanent, seasonal, or shifting in relation to resource availability. Many animal species exhibit some form of territorial behavior, and a variety of human behaviors have been called territorial. These phenomena range from "personal space" to home-owning, neighborhoods, city limits, and national boundaries. Human territorial behavior shows much variation and is generally culture-specific rather than species-specific, raising questions about its "innateness." Americans and northern Europeans need more personal space than anyone. Australians insist on owning their own houses and gardens. Members of some cultures never travel more than a few miles from their place of birth, while there is a small subculture of "jet setters" who regularly travel enormous distances and feel at home almost anywhere. Ancient cities were walled, most modern ones are open, and natural boundaries can be relatively open or closely defined. Hunters and gatherers rarely have exclusive territories, while agriculturists do.

Dominance Hierarchies

This is a system of ranking of animals within a group, and occurs in many social species from barnyard fowl to baboons. Dominance may be associated with greater access to food, or nesting sites, or mates. It usually involves deference and submission rituals and in many species it may serve to lower levels of aggression. Dominance hierarchies among nonhuman primates may be stable over time, or may be quite labile and situational. Sometimes there is linear ranking within a troop, and sometimes coalitions form. Dominance behavior tends to be more pronounced when a troop is under stress, or when valuable resources are scarce. In many primate species, such as chimpanzees and baboons, the aggressive component of dominance behavior becomes more pronounced when animals are fed a preferred food in close proximity to each other, or when they are spatially restricted, as in zoos. Some human social behaviors such as class and caste resemble dominance hierarchies, but these behaviors are nonpanspecific, and have strong cultural determinants. For example, Eskimos and Bushmen appear totally egalitarian, while ancient Maoris ranked every person. Ranking among humans, when it occurs, may involve individuals or groups, may be based on birth or achievement, and may be fluid or fixed. Thus it remains to be proven that social classes are biologically inevitable.

Pair Bonding

This refers to continuous pairing with a mate for the purpose of reproduction. Animals exhibit as many variants of mating behavior as do humans, but generally each species other than *H. sapiens* exhibits only one kind. In *annual monogamy* a male and female are bonded for one year. This occurs in gibbons, swans, eagles, and many humans [3]. In *polygamy,* one male is bonded with several females. This is seen in flycatchers, red-winged blackbirds, fur seals, elk, baboons, and some humans [3]. In *polyandry* one female is bonded with several males. This is seen in rheas, jacanas, and some humans [3]. Some animals are *promiscuous,* like the grouse, bears, wildebeest, many monkeys, and some African apes [3]. This behavior, while permitted in some societies for adolescents, is rarely sanctioned when childbearing is the goal.

Other Analogous Behaviors

There are many other behaviors seen in humans which occur in other animal species. These include gift-giving, aggression, division of labor, homosexuality, complex communications, and incest prohibition. In order to assess the relevance of these behaviors to the human situation, they too must be analyzed in terms of their content, function, and frequency of occurrence.

OTHER ETHOLOGICAL CONCEPTS AND THEIR POSSIBLE RELEVANCE TO HUMAN BEHAVIOR

Deprivation of Attention and Affection

Harlow and his colleagues [4,5] provided monkeys with sufficient amounts of food in clean cages, but deprived them of contact with other monkeys (or other animals) for periods of either 3, 6, or 12 months. These monkeys, upon being returned to social life with other monkeys, showed decreased playfulness, excessive fearfulness combined with excessive aggressivity, rejection of sex when presented with ample opportunity for sex, and rocking movements. Harlow stated that these monkeys went through the stages of protest and despair that Bowlby [6] described for deprived human infants, but did not experience a comparable apathy phase. The abnormalities described in the deprived monkeys could be reversed by continuous placement with peer monkeys ("monkey therapists") [4,5].

Some of these abnormalities could be prevented by allowing the isolated monkeys to have contact with a cloth "mother surrogate," which provided *contact-comfort.* The abovementioned effects of deprivation could *not* be reversed by time alone, and could not be prevented by wire mother surrogates. These studies demonstrate a need for physical and/or emotional contact by monkeys. This can easily be extrapolated to the rearing of human children, with evidence in human studies (e.g., Spitz' [7] anticlitic depression) to "validate" the analogy.

An unanswered question is What is the essence of what is being deprived in experimental or accidental deprivation? Is it contact comfort, mental stimulation, empathy, affection, or some combination of these? Can one be effective without the others? Rosenzweig [8] demonstrated in animal experiments that stimulation causes an increase in size and convolution of the cerebral cortex. Whether or not more data come in, physicians will continue to advise parents to hold, stimulate, and be empathic with their infants and young children.

Instinctive and Learned Behavior

The term instinct implies innate biological tendencies and capacities. Some behaviors appear to be almost wholly instinctive: Praying mantids that have been hand-fed from the time they are hatched, and have never had to catch a fly, are able to catch flies effectively at the first opportunity [9]. Human infants will show sucking, rooting, and grasping behaviors automatically. A *fixed action pattern* is a behavior which is definitely instinctive and requires a specific stimulus, the *innate releaser*, to trigger it. To qualify as a fixed action pattern, a behavior must show the following [10]:

1. The behavior involved must occur in exactly the same way each time the stimulus is presented.
2. The behavior must occur at the first presentation of the releaser before there has been a chance for learning to take place.
3. The response must occur in all members of a species.
4. The response must occur in individuals raised in isolation from species members.

Many instinctive behaviors have an automatic *blind* character. For example, newly hatched chicks may follow, like a mother, the first object they encounter after hatching [10].

Many behaviors require a combination of instinct and training (learning). Lorenz' concept of *instinct-training interlocking* [11,12] "implies that the behavior of a particular organism is a continuous process of smooth integration of learned aspects of behavior with the instinctive components." For example, cats attack mice. However, not all cats attack mice; cats are more apt to attack mice if they have seen other cats attack mice, less apt to attack mice if they have not seen other cats attack mice, and less apt to attack mice if they have been experimentally reared with mice. Another example is sexuality: Sexual behavior appears to be an instinctive capacity of all animals, yet many primates and possibly humans are unable to mate if they have been reared in isolation.

Imprinting

Imprinting [9,11,12] is the concept that there are certain periods in an animal's development (e.g., right after hatching in the above example of Spaulding's chicks) where what is learned (e.g., to respond to Spaulding) is learned strongly, as if it were "imprinted" (stamped) on the animal's brain.

Action Specific Energy

Lorenz [11,12] spoke of a "reservoir" of energy associated with instinctive behavior. If a certain instinctive response is continually evoked by the appropriate stimuli, this reservoir will be temporarily depleted and the instinctive response will reappear only when new energy stores build up. If the appropriate external stimuli are not forthcoming, the instinctive response will occur spontaneously, as if the behavior were occurring in a vacuum. This kind of spontaneous expression of interest is referred to as *vacuum activity*.

Psychoanalytically oriented thinkers could offer this as support for libido theory, which includes the notion that unchanneled drives push compellingly for expression. Statistical data to support this theory in humans has not been forthcoming and the libido theory has been deemphasized in modern psychoanalytic theory.

Displacement

Tinbergen stated that when an animal experiences a conflict between two instinctive behaviors (e.g., an animal seeing food, which it ordinarily grabs, right near a rubber snake, which it avoids) will select a third behavior of little practical value. The choice of the third behavior is called displacement. This is in keeping with Masserman's model of experimental neurosis [13]. This model was derived from experiments such as the following: A cat is presented with a fish cake, but every time it reaches the fish cake, it is struck by a blast of air. After a while, it ceased to reach for the fish cake, and performs useless behaviors. In addition, the cat can be conditioned to be "alcoholic," with the alcohol giving the cat courage to seek out the fish cake. The conflict model is central to the psychoanalytic theory of human neurotic behavior, and has been propounded as playing a causal role in "psychosomatic" conditions such as a duodenal peptic ulcer.

Umwelt [10]

Uexkull is responsible for this idea that, of a series of stimuli, an animal will respond primarily to those stimuli which are relevant to its survival. For example, a woodtick will respond only to light, the scent of butyric acid, and a temperature of 37°C. The scent of butyric acid is given off by warm-blooded animals, which have a body temperature of 37°C and from which the woodtick feeds. Most patients will choose treatment that cures them or makes them more comfortable, although we know that many people engage in self-destructive behavior.

CONCLUSION

We can see that much can be learned about human behavior by the study of ethology, but we must be careful not to generalize too much nor to apply our knowledge of animal behaviors indiscriminately to human behavior.

REFERENCES

1. Hinde, R. *Biological Basis of Human Social Behavior.* McGraw-Hill, New York (1974).
2. Wilson, E. *On Human Nature.* Harvard, Cambridge (1978).
3. Barash, D. *Sociobiology and Behavior.* Elsevier, Holland (1977).
4. Harlow, H. *Learning to Love.* Ballantine, New York (1971).
5. Harlow, H. Ethology, in *Comprehensive Textbook of Psychiatry,* 2nd ed. A. Friedman, H. Kaplan, and B. Sadock, eds. Williams and Wilkins, Baltimore (1975).
6. Bowlby, J. Childhood mourning. *Am. J. Psychiatry* 118:481-498 (1961).
7. Spitz, R. *The First Year of Life.* Int. Univ., New York (1965).
8. Rosenzweig, M., Bennett, E., and Diamond, M. Brain changes in response to experience. *Psychology in Progress: Readings From Scientific American.* R. Atkinson, ed. Freeman, San Francisco (1975).
9. Chauvin, R. *Ethology.* Int. Univ., New York (1975).
10. Hess, E. Ethology in *Comprehensive Textbook of Psychiatry,* 2nd ed. A. Friedman, H. Kaplan, and B. Sadock, eds. Williams and Wilkins, Baltimore (1966).
11. Lorenz, K. *King Solomon's Ring.* Crowell, New York (1952).
12. Lorenz, K. *On Aggression.* Harcourt, Brace and World, New York (1966).
13. Masserman, J. Biodynamics, in *Comprehensive Textbook of Psychiatry,* 2nd ed. A. Friedman, H. Kaplan, and B. Sadock, eds. Williams and Wilkins, Baltimore (1975).

19

Child Development

P.S.B. SARMA

INTRODUCTION

Development refers to the step-by-step unfolding of the potential of the organism. It involves altered function resulting from the interaction between *growth* (increase in the number and size of the cells) and *experience* (the sum of all internal and external stimulation). The sequence of steps is not automatic; it depends on central nervous system growth and life experience. Within certain limits, a favorable environment can accelerate the progression from one stage to another, and an unfavorable environment can delay full progression. There is a lower limit for the appearance of each stage. The full blooming of one stage often depends on how the previous stages went—this is the *epigenetic* concept of development. In this chapter the main focus will be on the behavioral aspects of child development; most of the other areas will be covered only briefly, if at all.

COMPARATIVE ASPECTS

While the gestational period is about the same in apes and humans, the postnatal maturation is greatly prolonged in humans, leading to a longer period of dependency. This may be related to the fact that the human brain takes longer to develop fully. The brain weight of the infant chimpanzee is 170 g and that of the adult 375 g (2.2 times). The brain weight of the human infant is 350 g and that of the adult is 1,450 g (4 times). There is no homologue in other primates for the speech area in the human cortex.

COMPONENTS

Child development can be arbitrarily subdivided into physical, intellectual, and psychological development for didactic purposes. Factors influencing development are portrayed in Figure 1: *Physical development* refers to changes in size and function of the organs.

Intellectual development refers to changes in problem-solving ability; in early infancy, it is difficult to distinguish from motor and sensory functions. In later infancy and childhood, intellectual function is more readily measured by communicative skills and ability to understand, retain, and manipulate symbolic material.

Psychological development refers to the acquisition of (1) the capacity to experience and to handle affection, anger, sadness, anxiety, frustration, closeness, distance, pleasure, displeasure, trust, shame, and guilt in an age-appropriate manner; (2) the capacity to develop age-appropriate levels of perception, self-observation, and self-esteem; (3) the ability to form age-appropriate relationships; (4) a functioning conscience that helps to set limits on unacceptable impulses; and (5) a stable sense of "who I am" and "where I am going," which Erikson called *identity*.

Prenatal Factors

Prenatal care is crucial. There is a proverb, "when an infant is born, he is a year old." Intrauterine life is usually divided into two stages—embryonic and fetal. The embryonic period is the first 8-12 weeks of intrauterine life, during which the fertilized ovum differentiates rapidly into an organism which has most of the gross anatomic features of the human being. The 12-40

Table 1   Factors Influencing Development

Prenatal	Perinatal	Postnatal
Genetic	Prematurity	Nutrition
Sex	Anoxia/hypoxia	Infection
Hormones	Birth injury	Iatrogenic conditions
Nutrition	Hyperbilirubinemia	Toxins
Injuries	Postmaturity	Socioeconomic status
Infection	Birth rank	
Immunology		Stimulation
Metabolism		Sex
Maternal age		Parenting
Socioeconomic status		Birth order
Stress		Temperament

week fetal period is characterized by rapid growth and elaboration of function. In the following sections, we will discuss the prenatal factors that considerably influence development.

Genetic

Heredity is determined by the genes of the egg and sperm and mutations of these genes. The physiological potential of an individual is largely determined by genes. Personality characteristics are at least partially controlled genetically. In infancy, identical twins are more alike than fraternal twins in their tendency to smile and show fear of strangers [1]. Other studies have shown that basic personality traits like social introversion and inhibition are more similar in identical twins than in fraternal twins, suggesting a strong genetic component in these personality traits [2]. In intellectual functioning, identical twins reared apart are more similar than fraternal twins reared together [3].

The genetic makeup is itself influenced by biological and social factors. Age of the parent at conception and exposure to genetically noxious stimuli (e.g., irradiation) influence genetic makeup. People who are mentally ill often marry people who are mentally ill; this is an example of assortative mating.

While some genetically caused disorders are manifested in early infancy (e.g., radiation) influence genetic makeup. People who are mentally ill often fest until later. For example, Huntington's chorea may not appear until the fourth decade, and manic-depressive illness may not appear until the second or third decade.

Chromosomes are made up of genes, so when there are major abnormalities of chromosomes, development is often severely affected, as in Down's syndrome, Klinefelter's syndrome, and Turner's syndrome.

Sex

The sex of the individual has influences which go beyond sexuality per se. Statistically, newborn girls are 4-6 weeks more advanced than boys in skeletal age, and remain at 125% of male skeletal age until puberty [4]. During early development across species, males are more vulnerable to noxious influences such as trauma [5]. In one study, prenatal stress had little effect on female rat fetuses, but caused male fetuses to be demasculinized and behaviorally feminized, perhaps because of an influence on sex hormone levels [6].

Hormones

If androgens are present during specific periods of early embryonic development, masculinization and defeminization of morphology, reproductive physiology, and later behavior occur. In the absence of androgens, morphology and behavior remain feminized. Female children with virilizing adrenogenital syndrome participate more in rough-and-tumble play and show less interest in dolls. Boys who undergo prenatal exposure to female hormones are less aggressive and participate less in rough-and-tumble play [7]. Hormone deficiencies like hypothyroidism can affect development as well—untreated congenital hypothyroidism causes mental retardation.

Nutrition

Malnutrition in pregnant women leads to a high incidence of stillbirths or premature births. Calcium and protein in the maternal diet are related to bone structure and muscle mass in the newborn. Long-term undernutrition of the mother, extended into the period of conception and pregnancy, may be more detrimental for the fetus than an acute nutritional disturbance during pregnancy in a previously well-nourished mother.

Injuries

Injuries resulting from trauma, radiation, or noxious chemicals are detrimental to the developing fetus. Radiation, particularly in the first trimester, can be devastating. Therefore, before ordering an x-ray for a woman of childbearing age, inquire into probability of pregnancy, and rule out pregnancy when there is uncertainty.

Infection

Infections like syphilis, toxoplasmosis, and cytomegalic inclusion disease during intrauterine life can be devastating. Thus, it is important to perform a serological test for syphilis during pregnancy. Viral infection—most notoriously rubella (German measles)—in the first trimester can produce severe mental retardation and an autism-like syndrome.

Immunology

Immunologic disorders such as Rh incompatibility can be very damaging to the fetal development. Fortunately this is now preventable in new cases by the use of Rhogam.

Metabolism

Prediabetic and diabetic mothers give birth to large babies [8]. If a mother has high levels of blood phenylalanine, even a fetus without PKU will experience brain damage. In recent years, physicians have become aware of a fetal alcohol syndrome, which consists of a variable number of the following [9]: (1) Low birth weight, small size, and retarded postnatal growth, which may be permanent; (2) mental retardation with an average intelligence quotient (IQ) in the 60s; and (3) a variety of birth defects, including cardiac anomalies in almost 50% of the infants. The effects are believed to result from alcohol or its metabolite acetaldehyde acting on the fetal nervous system. This is further complicated by the effects of the heavy smoking, which is usual for alcoholics.

Maternal Age

Pregnant teenagers often do not seek good prenatal care. The children of women over 35 years have a higher incidence of Down's syndrome.

Medications

The use and abuse of prescription and nonprescription drugs by the mother, especially in the first trimester, can have adverse effects on fetal development. Heroin addiction in the mother produces a withdrawal syndrome in infants after birth.

Socioeconomic Status

Lower socioeconomic status correlates with a higher risk for disturbances in development in the prenatal, perinatal, and postnatal periods.

Stress

There is some influence on fetal activity by maternal emotional state, possibly through placental transfer of neurotransmitters [10]. The noxious effect of stress during the intrauterine period has been demonstrated in rats, and males are more vulnerable.

Perinatal Factors

Hypoxia

This may result from low maternal blood pressure, placental insufficiency, mechanical factors (e.g., mucus plug), injury to the brain, respiratory depression due to drugs administered to the mother during delivery, or convulsion from alcohol or drug withdrawal. The hippocampi of fetal brains are very susceptible to anoxia; the anoxia can cause gliosis and consequent epilepsy, often of the temporal lobe type. Children who have had a cerebral insult during delivery have a higher incidence of hyperactivity in later years [11].

Birth Injury

Besides the damage from anoxia or hypoxia, there can be birth injury from cephalopelvic disproportion, breech delivery, mid- and high forceps delivery, and prolonged labor. These can result in many types of injury, including subarachnoid hemorrhage and, especially in premature infants, intraventricular hemorrhage.

Birth Rank

When the maternal age is held constant, the firstborn has a higher risk of low birth weight. Lower birth weight is more common in multipara and there is a high risk of perinatal complications [12].

Prematurity

Prematurity (under 37 weeks gestation) and smallness for gestational age are frequently associated with intellectual, sensory, and motor deficits, convulsive disorders, and behavioral problems. The causes of prematurity include poor maternal health and nutrition, inadequate prenatal care, toxemia, and multiple pregnancies. Prematurity is more common in the lower socioeconomic classes. Minor degrees of prematurity have a reversible effect on development.

Postmaturity

Postmaturity (more than 42 weeks of gestation) is at times associated with placental degeneration and anoxia.

Postnatal Factors

Birth Order

First-born children usually have stronger consciences than second born [13]. In one study, when siblings were of the same sex and their age difference was less than 2 years, there were few personality differences between them [13]. It has also been reported that first-borns are more adult-oriented and achievement-oriented and represent a significantly high percentage of successful people [14,15]. Larger family size and later birth rank are associated with poorer cognitive ability [16]. This effect is less consistent in the higher socioeconomic groups.

The only child, even though labeled "spoiled brat" in early case studies, appears to be more complex and not necessarily impaired. In contrast to the first-born, the only child is high on aggression and low on anxiety. The only boy tends to be more feminine than other boys, and the only girl tends to be more masculine than other girls. The middle-born generally manifests less achievement and more aggression and is less popular than the first born, only child, and the youngest [17].

Iatrogenic Factors

Relatively recent developments in postnatal care have reduced the incidence of some medically induced conditions. The excessive administration of oxygen and vitamin K to premature infants, causing retrolental fibroplasia and jaundice respectively, is now rare. The deleterious effects of certain antibiotics (e.g., sulfonamides, chloramphenicol, and tetracycline) in infancy are well known.

Infections

Bacterial and viral infections of the brain can have profound effects on early development. For example, encephalitis in childhood often produces major neuropsychiatric sequelae. There are slow virus infections with serious behavioral consequences that may now show up immediately. For example, measles encephalitis may result in subacute sclerosing panencephalitis, prominent signs of which (e.g., convulsions and behavioral deterioration) may not appear until years later.

Nutrition

Combined prenatal and postnatal malnutrition can have a deleterious effect on development. Protein malnutrition in early infancy is particularly detrimental to brain function and cognitive development [18].

Parenting

Parenting is a term that refers to the activities of one or more consistent caretakers who minister to the needs of the child. Because it is usually the mother who fulfills this role, it is called "mothering" most of the time, even though it can be performed by any person or small group. The parent-child relationship has been under intensive scrutiny by researchers in the last 10-15 years. The child is not just a passive recipient in this relationship. From birth on, the baby scans the environment, sucks, cries and reacts to stimuli with increase or decrease of motor activity. A few weeks after birth the baby smiles and vocalizes. By 3 months of age he responds with a smile to familiar faces, clings, and is involved in a continuous interaction with his caretakers. The baby responds to stimuli that the parent emits, and emits cues to which the parent responds. This process can lead to the development of a progressive "fit" or "dissonance" in the interactions. There may also be fluctuations between fit and dissonance which can be very stressful for all concerned. To the extent that the parent perceives the child as an independent organism with its own needs and feelings, and experiences pleasure in meeting those needs, the baby usually develops nicely. If the parent has a soothing effect on the child, the child's responses may enhance the parent's sense of well-being. As the parent provides proper sensory stimulation for the child, the child utilizes his intellectual capacities to the fullest.

If the child is exposed to prolonged sensory deprivation, lack of human contact, restriction of activity, or prolonged cacophony, development is impeded. If the parent is anxious, restless, and given to activities which conflict with the child's rhythm, the child can become restless and unhappy. This in turn makes the parent feel less competent and more anxious, hurt, and angry. If the parent is depressed and does not respond to the needs of the child, the child, after an initial period of excessive crying, may become withdrawn and apathetic.

What the child needs from his parents changes over time. Parents who are enormously responsive to a 6-month-old are not necessarily highly responsive to the same child at 6 years. Because of this, it is extremely difficult to isolate the long-term effects of particular types of early parenting.

The child experiences a progressively increasing capacity for autonomy as the years unfold. He is able to move about more freely, to feed himself more nimbly, and to convey his needs through language and action. The child develops optimally if the parents can allow the child to enter (what is for the child) uncharted territory without their being too restrictive. The parents must at the same time introduce appropriate socialization, promote bowel and bladder control, promote the labeling and appropriate handling of feelings, promote self-observation and self-esteem, and promote the formation of a functioning conscience.

Parental psychopathology does not always adversely influence childrearing. Many psychiatrically ill patients are effective in meeting their children's needs, especially when the illness is under control. On the other hand, some parents who have no grossly apparent psychiatric illness, but do have personality disorders, impaired self esteem, selfishness, immaturity, or impulsivity can impede their child's development.

Single parent families   One out of every seven American children lives in a family headed by a single woman. The long-term effects of such a situation are not clear. However, most authorities agree that the presence of a father figure is important as a source of identification and catalyst for development of self-control, especially for boys between the ages of 3 and 6; boys and girls from fatherless families tend to have more emotional problems [15].

Parents with atypical sexuality   With a greater acceptance of homosexuality recently, there has been interest in children with a homosexual parent or parents. At the present time there is no evidence for major sexual identity or orientation problems in children, although there are some behavioral differences as compared with controls [19].

Sex

Girls attain verbal fluency earlier than boys and maintain this "lead" until adolescence. This is associated with earlier maturation of left hemisphere structures in girls [20]. Boys are larger than girls from birth to about 10 years of age, and also manifest greater aggression. Boys are generally superior in spatial-visualization tasks. The higher incidence of behavioral disturbances in males may be related to their relatively slower maturation. In studies of isolation in monkeys, males were more vulnerable and females were more likely to recover [21].

Socioeconomic Factors

Children from families of low socioeconomic status become ill more frequently and present at the doctor's office later in the illness than thoe who are better off financially. In one study, behavior disorders were found to be more common in urban industrial communities than in rural communities [22]. A prospective study demonstrated that the outcome of perinatal neurological damage was poorer in lower socioeconomic group children than in middle-class children [23].

Stimulation

Stimulation is necessary for development. A number of studies show that lack of stimulation at critical periods can lead to significant physiological and behavioral developmental lag. If, in the fourth and fifth weeks of postnatal life of kittens, we interfere with patterned vision by placing a translucent cup over one eye for 3-4 days, the covered eye on stimulation does not show visual placing or following reactions. There is atrophy of cells in the lateral geniculate body receiving projections from that eye [24].

Harlow showed that infant monkeys, isolated from birth to 6 months, develop self-stimulating and posturing behaviors, are extremely fearful, and are unable to relate when exposed to peer monkeys. This is similar to some of the behaviors seen in autistic children. If the isolation lasts less than 6 months, the monkeys recover slowly if the isolation is terminated. If it lasts for over a year, the impairments of social behavior are almost unchangeable [21,25].

The importance of producing social responsiveness in infants through face-to-face interaction with a consistent mothering figure was demonstrated by Rheingold [15,26]. The devastating effects of loss of the mother during infancy without replacement by an adequate substitute have been well documented by Spitz and Wolfe [27] as well as Provence and Lipton [28].

Temperament

A pioneering prospective study on temperament was performed in a sample of 141 children by Thomas, Chess, and Birch [29]. They categorized temperament on the basis of nine parameters: Activity level, quality of mood, approach-withdrawal reaction to new stimuli, rhythmicity (regular and irregular), adaptability, threshold of responsiveness, intensity of reaction, distractability, and attention span. They found fairly good correlation between temperamental profile in the first weeks of life and the profile at 2 years.

Another finding that emerged from that study was that 10% of the children, labeled "difficult babies" on the basis of temperamental characteristics, constituted a disproportionately large number (25%) of children with later behavior problems. These "difficult" babies had a low threshold of responsiveness irregularity, high intensity of reactions, and poor adaptability. If the parents were able to adapt to the child's difficult temperament, the outcome was better. If not, the basic difficult temperament snowballed into major behavioral problems.

Toxins

A deadly toxin, one that has affected a large number of children, is lead ingested from lead-based paint. It can produce brain damage, seizures, hemolytic anemia, and death if not treated properly. In general, accidental poisoning occurs more frequently when parents have not taken necessary precautions for keeping toxic substances out of the reach of young children.

ASSESSING DEVELOPMENT

Physical illness can at times affect emotional development, especially if the illness is chronic or serious. Delays in some aspects of development (e.g., intellect, endocrines, neurological maturation) often become manifest with associated behavioral problems. Behavioral problems at times complicate physical development (e.g., eating disorders like pica, bulimia, and anorexia nervosa). So physicians who treat children must be continually vigilant about all aspects of development.

Professionals in the Developmental Area

Psychologists are trained in administering tests of intellectual development and personality functioning; which tests are chosen depends on the child's age and the function to be assessed [30]. Child psychiatrists are physicians trained in assessing and treating behavioral dysfunctions. Speech therapists and audiologists assess speech and hearing, and provide rehabilitative therapy.

While these specialists are available for evaluating and treating difficult problems, the physician who treats children needs to be able to screen for developmental lags and disabilities and to make proper referrals, if necessary. The Denver Developmental Screening Test, presented in the Appendix at the end of this chapter, is very useful for this purpose. For the screening to reliable, it is important that the examiner be familiar with the manual for administration and scoring of the test [31].

Predictive Value of Early Assessment

While psychological tests and developmental measures are reliable and valid in assessing the infant and child, the predictive value of assessment of infants is limited. After age 3, when language is firmly established, there is relative stability in intelligence scores [32]. Girls develop more predictably than boys. Among those whose IQs change significantly, boys are more likely to gain while girls are more likely to lose [33]. This may be a reflection of the attitude of society toward female accomplishment. Children manifesting significant increases in IQ are more independent, competitive, and verbally aggressive than those with decreasing IQ. They also work harder in school and manifest stronger desire to master intellectual problems [34].

DEVELOPMENT MILESTONES

The Neonate (Birth to 30 Days)

At birth the head is about one-fourth of the total body length. The head/body ratio decreases with age. The neonate is remarkably alert once he begins to breathe, but he seems to pay attention to only one sensory channel at a time. His world may be made of single perceptions. When the human face is presented, the newborn focuses on the hairline and his attention seems to be attracted to contours. His brainstem activity predominates; higher centers modify responses by partial inhibition or facilitation. His pain threshold, high at birth, gradually decreases during the first week. He sleeps most of the time and rapid eye movement (REM) sleep constitutes 40-60% of sleeping time. Eagle and Brazelton report that small for gestational age (SMA) infants tend to have irregular sleep and waking rhythms, and oversensitivity to stimulation; they also tend to be "hard to reach" socially [35].

There are a number of reflexes that are present at birth and normally disappear at certain age periods:

The *Moro reflex* is elicited by extending the neck suddenly. The infant throws his arms laterally and extends his fingers and then brings his arms back toward the midline. This reflex generally fades by 6 months. In the *grasp reflex,* the infant grasps the examiner's finger when it is placed in the infant's palm and pressed. This generally fades by 3 months. The *Babinski reflex* (extension of the big toe on stroking the lateral aspect of the sole of the foot) disappears at about 2 years.

Infancy (Birth to 1 1/2)

Interpersonal Development

At about 2 or 3 months, the infant smiles when someone looks at him face-to-face. This is called the *social smile,* and is the first evidence that the infant may be able to identify a person in the environment as being separate from himself [36]. The social smile is an important part of an infant's greeting behavior, and the infant smiles differently for different people. However, between birth and about 8 months, the child makes minimal distinctions between family and strangers, and will respond to strangers and accept babysitters without becoming upset. At about 8 months, the attempt of a stranger to establish physical contact or eye contact with the child will evoke discomfort, crying, and screaming. This is called *stranger anxiety,* and is a milestone for the ability of the child to distinguish between people [36]. By 1 year, many children have a *transitional object,* an object (like a teddy bear, towel, or blanket) that comforts the child during his parents' absence, and with which the child has trouble parting [37].

Motor Development

At about 4 months the child can sit with support and raise himself on his elbows. At approximately 10 months, he can feed himself with his hands. At about 1 year, he can stand with support, and at about 15 months, he is able to walk.

Intellectual Development

Piaget calls this the *sensorimotor period* of cognitive development [38]. It has been demonstrated experimentally that at 1 week of age, learning and conditioning can take place. From birth to 4 weeks, the infant repeats simple acts for their own sake, rather than for their consequences. At 4 weeks, the child repeats responses that produce interesting results. When something is removed from a child's field of vision, he will not seek it out because what is "out of sight is out of mind." But between 28 and 32 weeks, *object permanence* is established; here, a child will push over a pillow to obtain a toy hidden under it, and out of sight is no longer out of mind. At 1 year, the child begins to notice more connections between events, speaks his first word, and prefers looking at complex visual patterns to looking at simple patterns.

Problem Areas

Profound mental retardation Profound mental retardation is usually discovered in the first year of life. It will be discussed in Chapter 20.

Infantile autism This condition may be discovered as early as the first year. The term autism refers to the child's inability to develop significant interpersonal relatedness. The incidence is 4:10,000 and it is commoner in boys than in girls [39]. The child is either mute or manifests a severe formal thinking disorder. The prognosis is very poor: 50% of autistic children (many of whom are also mute) must be permanently institutionalized.

Child abuse The majority of abused children are under the age of 5, and the problem is common: Many children brought to emergency rooms with injuries are victims of child buse. Often the abusing parent was abused as a child. The examining physician should be suspicious of child abuse in cases of multiple injuries, or injuries not in keeping with the history given by the parent. The physician is expected to act primarily as the child's personal physician/advocate in cases of definite or suspected abuse. Also in such cases, physicians are required by law to report the case to the local child protection agency, can be penalized in some states for not doing so, and have the right to hospitalize the child without parental approval. Physicians are exempted from lawsuits for the act of reporting in good faith a case of suspected child abuse.

Anaclitic depression This was described by Spitz, who studied institutionalized infants aged 6-8 months [36]. These infants lived in a prison nursery with a 1:8 nurse/child ratio, and were visited by their mother frequently. Spitz found that when the parents were unable to visit for periods of several weeks of more, the children developed a syndrome characterized by crying, weight loss, insomnia, impairment of development, apathy, and susceptibility to infection. If the parent resumed visiting within 3 months, the condition was reversible. After 3 months, some of the developmental impairment was irreversible. After 2 years, many of the children developed *marasmus* (severe malnutrition, cachexia, and apathy with susceptibility to infection and metabolic imbalance) and died. None of the infants whose parents continued to visit developed this syndrome.

Other Aspects of Infancy

This period of childhood is referred to by psychoanalysts as the *oral period*, so-called because the mouth, buccal area, and upper gastrointestinal tract appear to be the most important pleasure-giving (*erotogenic*) areas for the infant. Erikson, a psychoanalyst, said that the main developmental task at this time is the establishment of trust (*basic trust*) [40]. Spitz reported genital play in normal infants toward the end of the first year of life, and considered it normal. He found that it was lacking in children who were removed from the mother and in children whose mother alternated, unpredictably and frequently, between affection and hostility or rejection. Since it was not associated with erection or pelvic thrusts, Spitz did not consider it masturbation [36]. Galenson reported that the onset of genital play occurred earlier in boys (6-7 months) than in girls, and continued for months, while girls started late (10-11 months) and stopped within a few weeks. Galenson also reported that masturbation, as defined above, starts at 15-16 months of age. It continues in boys, while in girls there is cessations of manual genital manipulation and a changeover to indirect pathways such as thigh squeezing or rocking on a play horse [41].

Toddler Period (1½ to 3 Years)

Interpersonal Development

The toddler is developmentally miles apart from the newborn, and possesses considerable motor and cognitive capacities. Along with motor and cognitive development, the child develops a sense of separateness and individuality. He wants to do things on his own (to have *autonomy*), and not to obey his parents automatically. At around 18 months of age, *negative head shaking* appears, conveying the message "No, I don't want to do that." To establish his autonomy even further, the child may say no even when he wants to do what is asked of him (*normal negativism*). It is important for parents to recognize this, and to allow the child some autonomy, lest tenacious unproductive battles for control ensue.

Psychoanalytic Aspects of Toddlerhood

Psychoanalysts refer to this period as the *anal period* and also as the separation-individuation period. Erikson described the "normative crisis" of this period as being between *autonomy and shame and doubt*. Psychoanalysts feel that if toilet training is too strict and rigid during this period, an anal character pattern, or *anal fixation*, may develop later, characterized by miserliness, stubbornness, and excessive need to control others.

Motor Development

At 18 months of age, the child can throw a ball. Having begun walking at 15 months, he can run well by 2 years. Often his motor activity exceeds his judgment, and he "gets into everything," including drawers with poisons and medicines, and the house must be "childproofed" to some extent. However, some parents can go overboard in childproofing, and deprive the child of mental stimulation and a chance for self-control. Toilet training starts in this period. Regarding toilet training, three things should be borne in mind: (1) The child must be neurologically ready and the training should not proceed before the child has been walking for at least a year; and (2) The parent should not be too demanding, rigid, and controlling, lest he start a pitched battle with a child who has an equal need to control the situation.

Intellectual Development

The child has developed some degree of symbolic thinking, one example of which is the use of language. However, this symbolic thinking is still limited in comparison with future capacities. Although he sees himself as separate, he still has trouble comprehending his relationship with the world, and sees the world as centering about him (*egocentrism, centralism*). He sees his parents as very powerful in relationship to the world, a logical extrapolation of their considerable power in his life. *Animistic thinking* is prominent: Inanimate objects are endowed with human qualities; for example, rain may be seen as someone crying. By 2½ years, the child develops *gender identity*, a sense of being either boy or girl, which is irreversible after the age of 3 [42].

At 2 years, the child can copy a circle, and at 4 years, a cross. During this period, he is unable to conceive of death as permanent; he sees it as a transitory separation from loved people. Rules and concepts are not clearly established.

Problem Areas

Accidental poisoning   Because at this stage motor abilities exceed judgment, accidental poisoning is common. Toxic substances must be kept out of a child's reach.

Pica   This repeated ingestion of nonedible, dangerous substances like chipped paint from a crib, occurs most commonly among nutritionally deprived and culturally deprived children, and can lead to severe problems such as a lead poisoning.

Hospital stays   These are particularly difficult during this period, although difficulty with separation from parents is normal beginning at around 8 months and continuing well into childhood. If a child needs to be hospitalized he can be allowed to keep some favorite possessions in the hospital, and should be visited frequently by his parents. Some hospitals permit parents to "live in" in the child's room or an adjacent room. If the admission can be planned in advance, a preadmission visit to the hospital could be quite helpful.

Temper tantrums   Children usually pout or cry for a few seconds if they are frustrated. They may stomp their feet and say "Nobody loves me" or "I hate you," or make other angry statements. But some children, when they are frustrated, lie down on the floor, scream and kick their feet, or throw things around, and continue such behavior beyond a few seconds. Others run around the house screaming at the top of their voice, banging doors, and sometimes even hitting themselves. These behaviors are called temper tantrums and they can be extremely distressing to parents. These behaviors are often maintained because the parents unwittingly reinforce them by getting very upset and giving the child excessive attention, or by giving in (after initial refusal) to the demands of the child because of the tantrums. In the absence of major emotional deprivation or inconsistency in the family, the tantrums can generally be brought under control by isolating the child in a place, usually his bedroom, where he cannot do much harm, and by ignoring the tantrum. This approach should be combined with attention and affection when the child is *not* having a tantrum.

Thumbsucking   Persistent thumbsucking or sucking of other fingers usually fades by age 2. Many children continue to such their thumb for short periods when put to bed, as a way of soothing themselves to sleep. this usually disappears by the end of early childhood. Persistent thumbsucking, rocking, headbanging, or genital play generally requires an evaluation of the child and his environment, the latter which may promote such behavior by not providing normal outlets and stimulation or, knowingly or unknowingly, by reinforcing such behavior.

The Preschool Child (3-6 Years)

Interpersonal Development

The child is able to spend a morning away from home at preschool or kindergarten. In playing with other children, he truly interacts with them, as opposed to playing independently *(parallel play)* alongside them. Some normal children have *imaginary companions* at this age. Masturbation occurs in both sexes and there can be guilt about this. Psychoanalysts believe that there is an *Oedipus complex* where children fall in love with the parent of the opposite sex and feel competitive with the parent of the same sex. Whether this is frequent or universal remains unproven. One cross-sectional study showed that children preferred the parent who was the most responsive and available, *not* necessarily the parent of the opposite sex [43]. Of course, stated preference and actual romance need not be identical.

Motor Development

At 3 years, the child can ride a tricycle. By 6 years, she can perform complex motor activities such as ballet, swimming, ice skating, riding a two-wheel bicycle and playing catch, with considerable coordination.

Intellectual Development

At age 3, the child can speak in fluent sentences, and begins to learn numbers and letters. Between age 3 and 5, *ethnic identity* is established. At age 6, he has a few rudiments of adding, reading, and writing. Death is still not considered permanent, and is sometimes seen as an injury or mutilation. Transient fears (of dark, of death, or animals) are common and normal, as are occasional nightmares.

Problem Areas

Enuresis. This refers to repeated urinary incontinence after 3 1/2 years of age, not associated with seizures and not caused by a specific known neurological lesion that affects bladder control. It is commoner in boys than in girls. It may be related to delay in developing bladder control or to disturbances in previously acquired bladder control. Approximately 10% of children under 12 manifest occasional enuresis [44]. Of these, 80% children are *primary enuretics* who have not had stable bladder control for at least 3 months [45]. Treatment is mentioned on page 73.

Encopresis This is repeated fecal incontinence after 3 1/2 years of age, not associated with seizures and not caused by a specific neurological lesion known to affect bowel function. Like enuresis, it may be related to delay in developing control of bowel movements or it may be a disturbance following previously acquired bowel control. In one study, approximately 3% of children referred to a pediatric clinic manifested encopresis [46]. One situation that is confused with encopresis is the following: A child appearing to have diarrhea with incontinence might actually be severely constipated. The constipation may result in the formation of a functional megacolon and fecal impaction in a colon which loses its tone and water-absorbing capacity; the ensuing fecal leakage presents as diarrhea.

If there is no systemic illness causing and maintaining the disordered behavior, encopresis can be treated by behavior modification and bowel training [47,48].

Pavor nocturnus The child awakens screaming and it is difficult to bring him to reality for a few minutes. Unlike nightmares (where the child wakes from a frightening dream that he remembers) and fears of the dark, which are common, attacks of pavor nocturnus are not common. These occur in stage 4 sleep and are not associated with clearly remembered dreams. If frequent, these are treated with stage 4 sleep-suppressant medications.

Childhood psychosis Some children develop serious psychiatric disorders with onset after 30 months, manifested by impairment of relationships, with some of the following associated symptoms: Unusual relationships to objects; severe anxiety; obsessional preoccupations; speech disorders (echolalia, mutism, elective mutism); undersensitivity or oversensitivity to stimuli; abnormal motility (e.g., stereotyped movements or posturing); self-mutilating behavior; and severe compulsive and ritualistic behaviors. At times the child may have classic symptoms and signs of schizophrenia or mania. The exact prevalence of these disturbances is not known but they seem to be commoner in boys.

The diagnostic evaluation should consider disorders of the nervous system (e.g., temporal lobe seizures or degenerative disorders), endocrine disturbances, and primary psychosis in a parent reflected in the child. Treatment consists of treatment of the cause, management of symptoms with appropriate medications, counseling for patient and family, and behavioral programming. Removal from home or specialized educational programming for the child may be required.

The School Age Child

When adults are asked to think about their childhood, middle childhood is the period they remember most clearly and enjoyably. Most of early childhood is forgotten; what remains are bits and pieces of visual and auditory memories, both pleasant and unpleasant. Growth follows a cephalocaudal pattern in middle childhood. The head grows to its ultimate size earlier (by age 10) than do the extremities. Growth is slow and steady except for a pre-pubertal spurt in girls around 10-12 years and in some boys by age 12. The growth spurt in boys usually occurs at puberty.

Interpersonal Development

It is helpful to look at interpersonal development from the standpoint of three phases: Early (6-8 years), middle (8-10 years), and late (10-12 years).

Ages 6-8 Although at this age the child has become involved with friends who are important to her, she still needs the security and discipline of her parents. She enjoys telling her parents the jokes and riddles she learned in school. If the child of middle years has an older sibling, especially a teenager of the same sex, she may idolize and imitate this older sibling. If the older sibling is close in age, competition and bickering can be expected. If she has younger siblings of preschool age, she often sees them as a nuisance. A child of this age usually follows rules rigidly, and her value system is also rigid, probably because it is so recently established. The child is particularly attentive to the mechanics and rules of games; choosing up sides may be as involving as the game itself. Many children steal something to test what happens when prohibitions are violated. An identity regarding intellectual, physical, and social skills is forming. Children of this age get along well in twosomes and in larger groups, but when three get together, two generally side against the third.

Ages 8-10 At this age the child is keenly aware of his status in the group and tries very hard to be like others. Group pressure sometimes creates conflicts between him and his parents. The child might say "Mother, everybody else I know has a 10-speed bike" or "Everybody else can go swimming. Why can't I? You never let me do anything." At this age the child also begins to see his parents more realistically, in part because he has the opportunity and ability to compare them with his friends' parents. At times, he may feel embarrassed by his parents' old-fashioned ways or eccentricities, a feeling which may be even more pronounced in adolescence. He spends an enormous amount of time with other children, and learns a lot from them. Naturally, some of what he learns contradicts what his parents taught. From now on, parents will not hear many details of what occurs outside the home, for children are progressively continuing to detach themselves from their parents, a process which begain in infancy. Unless the parents are very involved in their children's life, and comfortably accompany them in some of their activities, they may actually not know much about their lives away from home. The only child and the youngest child are exceptions to this "rule." This is also the time when major problems outside of the home come to light, such as behavior problems, mild mental retardation, and learning disabilities. These are the commonest causes of referral to child psychiatry clinics, and middle childhood is the commonest age for referral. There is a lot of sexual curiosity, but it is discreet. Children generally stick to groups of their own sex, and avoid the opposite sex assiduously in public situations. There is a lot of teasing by the group if one of its members manifests any interest in a child of the opposite sex. Children form clubs or groups, in which they establish elaborate regulations. The child usually lists two or three best friends instead of just one. Alliances change frequently, and depend upon the activity in which the youngster is involved.

Age 10-12 Some 10 to 12-year-old children may already be experiencing pubertal changes. The age for menarche has been decreasing gradually over the decades. Now it is 9-11 years in girls [49]. Often there is a "turning inward" that occurs during this period, and the girl seems to withdraw from the adults in her family. Often during this period, especially among girls, intense friendships are formed. Some children, whose feelings for their parents become devalued and who do not have satisfactory peer relationships, construct a *"family romance fantasy,"* in which they believe they are not really the offspring of their parents, but rather the children of another family, often an exalted one [50]. This is an important period for the development of conscience, which is closely related to cognitive maturation. At the end of early childhood the child has rigid ideas of right and wrong that are related to fear of parental disapproval and punishment. During the period of 8-12 years, the child's ideas are tempered by experience. Even though he is still quite reliant on precepts of authority, he begins to be guided by *reciprocity*. After age 12, moral principles appear which are based on the uniqueness of the situation and on fairness. Of course, it is important to remember that the ability to articulate moral principles does not guarantee that they will be followed [51].

Sibling relationships Even though they are not as crucial for a child's development as are his parents, siblings play a pivotal role. When siblings are close in age, competitive feelings may be so strong that if a sibling has already established excellence in one area, the other child may strive for success in a different area. For example, an older child is hard-working in school, gets good grades, and is identified as bright by parents and teachers. Her younger sibling may stop trying to establish his identity in that area and become an average student, turn to sports or the social sphere for satisfactions and identity, or may become a "problem child" to establish his uniqueness. Children of this age are often given *nicknames* by other children which may be indicative of their unique characteristics and role in the group. In other families, especially those with many children, and where parents do not establish a close relationship, older siblings may become an inportant source of nurturance, support, and identification. This may be even more pronounced when parents give the older children major responsibility and authority in caring for and disciplining the younger ones.

Peer relationships   The child's contact with peers increases considerably during the middle years, and these interactions can have a marked effect on his self-esteem and self-image. In the last part of the middle years, the peers are often used as models.

Motor Development

There is a progressive increase in strength, coordination, and skill. The capacity for alternating movement increases, and the child of 7-8 years is able to suppress movements in other parts of the body while performing rapid alternating movements with one extremity [52]. Already learned skills are refined, and new ones learned, and this is aided by an increasing attention span and an attitude of diligence with a willingness to practice. Because of an emphasis on contact sports in some circles, with the associated risk of injuries, physicians are concerned about damage to ephiphyses, which can cause progressive impairment to the growth of the extremities. Thus, physicians often caution parents about involving young children in very strenuous contact sports such as football or hockey.

Intellectual Development

This is Piaget's period of *concrete operations* [53]. The child is able to handle complex school activities, such as doing multiplication and writing script. She can *categorize* and discern that an object can have more than one property. For example, a child is given some wooden beads, some of which are black but most of which are white. Then she is asked if there are more black beads or white beads, and she will answer "white." Then she is asked if there are more wood beads or white beads. A child in the previous stage of cognitive development (*preoperational,* ages 2-6) instinctively says "white," but the child in this stage will reflect and often say "more wood beads."

The child also possesses the cognitive skill called *conservation,* wherein a fixed quantity of a substance is seen as fixed in quantity regardless of the way it is distributed or the size of its container. For example, equal amounts of liquid are poured into two glasses of equal size, and the child identifies the amount of liquid as being the same in each glass. The liquid is then poured from one of the original containers into a cone-shaped container, and the liquid from the other original container is poured into a cylindrical container. The child in the stage of concete operations is able to say that the amount of liquid is the same in the cone-shaped container as in the cylindrical container. He is able to reverse computations; for example, if he figures out that 6 + 4 = 10, he can also reason that 10 − 4 = 6 *(reversibility)*. If he makes a mistake in a long problem, he is able to *backtrack*, rather than giving up in frustration or starting from the beginning. At age 7, he is able to copy a diamond shape. At age 8, for the first time he can see death as irreversible. Language becomes more complex. During the school years, children are quite fond of riddles and jokes. They are able to comprehend the rules governing language and are able to learn grammar. Their capacity for expressing ideas and manipulating concepts facilitates communication with children and adults.

Problem Areas of Middle Childhood

Minimal brain dysfunction—hyperactivity syndrome This is characterized by motor hyperactivity, decreased attention span resulting in inability to concentrate, secondary psychological problems and, at times, neurological signs. These include right-left disorientation, facial or body asymmetry, poor coordination, poor graphesthesia, or poor double simultaneous discrimination. Intelligence is usually normal, but there may be some deficits in patterns of learning (e.g., dyslexia, dysgraphia, dyscalculia). The treatment includes use of a stimulant (such as methylphenidate or dextroamphetamine), appropriate remedial educational programs, and counseling.

School phobia The child is fearful of going to school, makes excuses for not going, and sometimes refuses to go. Frequently, medical complaints are used as the reason, and this may be the way the child comes to medical attention. Sometimes, a parent covertly supports the child remaining home because of need to have the child at home. Although the physician should certainly do a medical evaluation if he suspects school phobia, it is preferable to do the evaluation on an outpatient basis because the major principle of treatment of this syndrome is to insist that the child attend school at least part-time (to the extent that the child is able to tolerate school without demoralizing anxiety), "because it is required by law," while dealing concurrently with the reason for the phobia.

Conduct disorders The child manifests various disordered behavior patterns (e.g., aggressive-impulsive behavior, withdrawal, running away, sexual promiscuity, truancy, stealing, drug abuse), but does not experience discomfort or suffering from these behaviors other than that caused by the reaction of the environment to his behavior. All of these are related to a lack of control of socially unacceptable impulses, At times, this behavior is reinforced and approved of by the child's peer group. Often there are biological predisposing factors (e.g., minimal brain dysfunction or learning disability) or problems in the child's immediate environment (family, school). In one study, a third of the children with conduct disorders manifested reading retardation [54]. Occasionally, a child struggling with intense psychological conflicts or depression may come to the attention of authorities because of conduct problems. Further evaluation will often reveal the underlying stress and unhappiness. Treatment of conduct disorders includes identification and remediation of the factors influencing the child behavior, provision of appropriate controls, and remedial education programs.

Adopted Children

Two to three percent of live-born infants become adopted children [55]. Because of the potential for problems in the development of attachment between parents and child, adoption placements ideally should be made before the infant establishes a strong bond to the first parenting figure (be it the biological mother or foster mother). Such attachment occurs by the sixth month of life. At the same time, there is some indication that adoptions of children between 5 and 12 yeas of age can work out nicely, provided (1) the child does not have significant behavioral problems; (2) the child has not had many foster home placements prior to the adoption (many placements may be a result of, or lead to, lack of bonding); and (3) the child does not retain a strong emotional attachment to the natural mother [56,57]. It is better that the child be told by his adoptive parents that he is adopted. When the parents do not present this information, it may come in an unexpected manner with resultant "shock" and distrust of the parents. Most adopted children are curious about their biological parents, and the family romance fantasy is intensified in these cases. Adopted children are referred for behavioral problems more than twice as frequently as are nonadopted children [58-60].

Puberty and Adolescence

Puberty refers to the physical changes initiating the sexual maturation of the individual. It starts with the increase in size of the ovaries and uterus in girls and the prostate and seminal vesicles in boys. For girls, the initial signs of the onset of puberty are changes in the size of the breasts and the appearance of pigmented pubic and axillary hair. For boys, the first changes are increase in the size of the testes and penis [61]. The onset of puberty has been occurring at progressively earlier ages in the last 50 years, though this may be leveling off. Generally the onset is at 9-11 years in girls and 12-14 years in boys. Onset of puberty before age 8 in girls or age 10 in boys is considered precocious. Delayed puberty in boys and girls refers to an onset after age 15. Puberty is associated with a growth spurt. In boys, just before the growth spurt, there is often an increase in the subcutaneous fat which is gradually lost over a year or two. The growth spurt in both sexes usually has the following progression: Legs start growing first; then there is an increase in trunk length and chest depth. Hips widen before shoulders; the lower jaw grows too. Last comes an increase in muscle mass and weight which continues after the increase in lengthy stops. The physical changes of puberty in boys usually have the following progression: Increase in size of genitalia, changes in pH and odor of sweat, pigmented pubic hair, axillary hair, enlargement of larynx and lengthening of vocal cords (deeper voice), and spermatogenesis. The physical changes of puberty in girls usually have the following progression: Budding of breasts, labial hair, axillary hair, pubic hair, menarche, and ovulation. With the onset of puberty there is an increase in resistance to minor upper respiratory infections. The frequency of masturbation for both sexes rises dramatically. Puberty is associated with, and caused in large part by, radical changes in hormone output. An increase in follicle-stimulating hormone (FSH) occurs, followed by an increase in luteinizing hormone (LH). FSH in girls shows a biphasic pattern before adolescence, with high levels in infancy, a "bottoming out" at 8 years, and another rise with puberty. In boys, FSH reaches adult levels by age 10. The level of urinary 17-keto-steroids during infancy and childhood is 3 mg/day. By 18 years in girls, the level is 4-9 mg/day, and by 18 years in boys, the level is 8-15 mg/day. Between 10-17 years in boys there is a 20-fold increase in plasma testosterone, which is probably responsible for the larger muscle mass in boys. In girls, by 6-9 months postmenarche, an adult menstrual rhythm in levels of estradiol appears.

Adolescence refers to the behavioral aspects of the extended period between the onset of puberty and the attainment of adulthood. It is a *second separation-individuation period* [62], the first being the toddler period. The goals of adolescence are: Achieving a stable sense of self (identity), achieving a relative emotional independence from parents, and achieving a comfortable adaptation to sexuality while establishing greater autonomy. Many psychoanalysts [3,6,62,63], considered normal adolescence to be associated with considerable turmoil, with much fluidity in the intrapsychic sphere. More recent studies [64-66] of middle-class teenagers reveal that youngsters can achieve emotional independence from parents gradually without significant turmoil. In other words, normal adolescence does not always mean "much ado" and "less sense." But what emerges from adolescence into the threshold of adulthood is not a finished product, as Chapter 21 will confirm.

Intellectual Development

Some observers state that ages 15-17 constitute the peak in learning ability, although actual fund of knowledge and application of knowledge improve well into the 30s and 40s. Adolescents are often proud of their reasoning abilities, and spend hours debating issues and concepts with their peers. They may argue in a like manner with their parents, and call attention to the parents' shortcomings.

According to Piaget [53], the *stage of formal operations* is well established as an individual becomes an adolescent. This stage of cognitive development is characterized by the capacity to consider possibilities that are beyond immediate reality, and the ability to evaluate one's decisions and conclusions. One of the important issues in terms of intellectual development is To what extent is intellect autonomous and not greatly influenced by the emotional state? It is futile to assess intellectual functions without considering the capacity for concentration.

Factors Influencing Adolescence

Physical growth   This is somehow related to social adjustment. Teenage boys who mature earlier physically were found to be more self-assured, matter-of-fact, socially poised, and able to laugh at themselves. Later maturers revealed more feelings of inadequacy, feelings of rejection, and rebellious feelings [65,66]. However, there does not seem to be a similarly clearcut picture with girls, as many late maturers become better interpersonally adjusted than many early maturers [66].

Family relationships   The development of adolescents is stressful for parents because it calls to mind the parents' earlier life problems and also highlights for parents that their most youthful years have passed. This may lead to reassessment of current reality in terms of past hopes and dreams. If the reality has fallen far short of earlier aspirations, sadness and frustration may result. If the parent cannot accept this reality and permits these feelings to contaminate the way the teenager is handled, problems may result.

If the marital relationship is not mutually satisfactory, the presence of a sexually mature young person in the home may activate a parent's unsatisfied urges. The parent either recognizes what is happening and deals with it realistically, or may follow maladaptive pathways. The parent may identify with the teenager, get vicarious gratification, and indirectly push the teenager to indulge in his impulses. The parent may project his unacceptable impulses onto the teenager and become very restrictive, or the parent may act on these feelings in extramarital relationships or incest. These maladaptive reactions of the parents can produce major problems in the parent-teenager relationship.

Peer relationships   Peers are also very important during this period because ties to the parents are loosening and there is an urgent need to find a replacement for earlier attachments. In our culture there is a separate "teen society" with its own styles of music, dress, and language. One way to understand this phenomenon is that because of the prolongation of adolescence in industrial societies, there is a need for the young to demarcate themselves from an adult society, which they are not permitted to join despite their physiological maturity. Another benefit may be that by establishing a group identity in these relatively superficial ways, adolescents do not have to be markedly different from adults in fundamental values and goals. Peer influence is reported to be less important than parental influence in areas of moral and social values and understanding of the adult world [15]. It is also reported that adolescents who are strongly peer-oriented are more likely to hold negative self-concepts as compared with adult-oriented adolescents [15]. The quality of the peer relationship is itself influenced by earlier role models (parents and older siblings) and by the adolescent's intellectual and social skills.

Problem Areas in Adolescence

Accidents   This is the leading cause of death in teenagers [61]. There is a 600 in 100,000 chance of a white U.S. male aged 15-19 dying from an accident.

Suicide   This is the third ranking cause of death in adolescence.

Anxiety   Anxiety is generally at a high level during this period and anxiety disorders occur. While many of the anxiety disorders can be treated easily (and are often self-treated by the adolescents through drug abuse), school phobia with first onset during adolescence is usually indicative of a more serious underlying disturbance.

Affective disorders and schizophrenia   Although the mean age of onset is well aboveteenage for these disorders,, they may become apparent in the teen years. Often an effective disorder in its earlier phases is misdiagnosed as an adjustment disorder because of the multitude of events that can be considered precipitants. A major change in the adolescent's behavior may be indicative of a serious disturbance.

Anorexia nervosa   This is an uncommon condition that frequently starts in adolescence. It is discussed in Chapter 8. Sometimes hypothalamic tumors produce a similar picture.

Drug abuse   In addition to the self-medicating aspect of drugs in anxiety and depression, to deal with boredom or to be accepted by peers, the adolescent unwittingly becomes a victim of, rather than master of, the drug. Aggressive psychotic states due to hallucinogen abuse may occur. *Alcoholism* is common, but major complications associated with long-term abuse are not seen frequently in teenagers.

Delinquency The term "delinquent" refers to a child or adolescent who is truant from school, who is out of parental control, or who engages repeatedly in illegal activities (e.g., shoplifting, breaking-in, stealing cars, selling drugs, prostitution). It has been reported that juvenile courts see caseloads equal to 10% of the teenage population, but this is an inflated statistic since many of the teenagers are repeaters. The current ratio of boys to girls is 3:1, but girls seem to be delinquent more lately. Delinquency rates are high in deprived and unstable communities. The majority of adolescent delinquents have a history of poor functioning from kindergarten to third grade and many were reported to have been hyperactive [15]. There is a high percentage of delinquents from broken homes, conflict-ridden family environments, or families characterized by apathy and indifference. The fathers of delinquents are more likely to be rated as cruel, neglecting, and inclined to ridicule their children. Middle class delinquents are likely to have been rejected by the peers, whereas lower class delinquents may either be popular or rejected.

Runaways These are common and more frequent among girls than boys [67]. Most runaways eventually reunite with their parent or guardian. There is a higher incidence of depression and venereal disease among runaways as compared with others. Runaways tend to lack the capacity to assertive and to express anger freely.

CONCLUSION

A knowledge of child development helps the physician to assess the development of the children who come to the office or hospital, and to identify those who need further evaluation and treatment. It also helps him or her to understand the emotional aspects of systemic illnesses, and the developmental influences on behavioral disorders. It is, therefore, a most worthy subject for study.

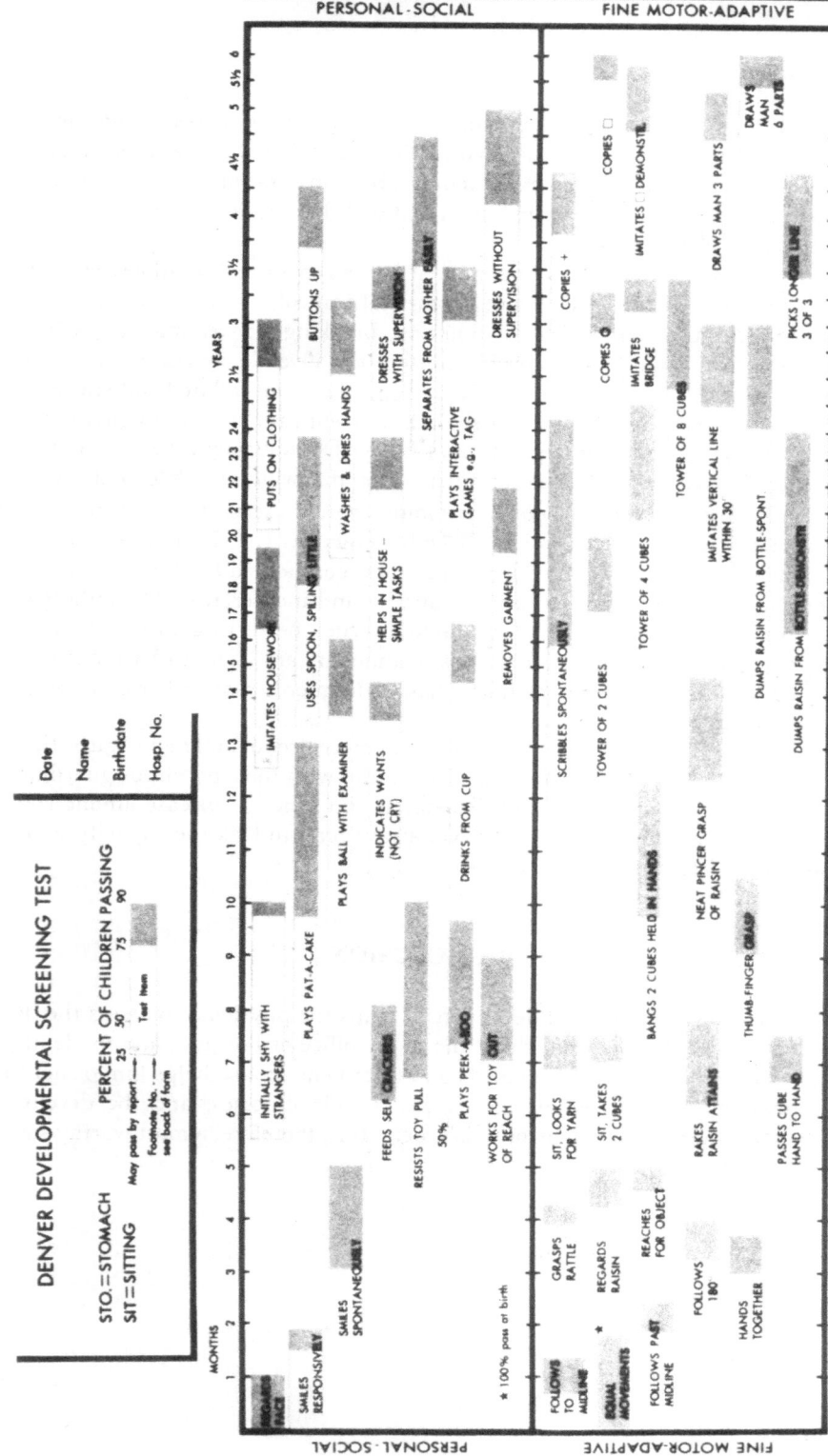

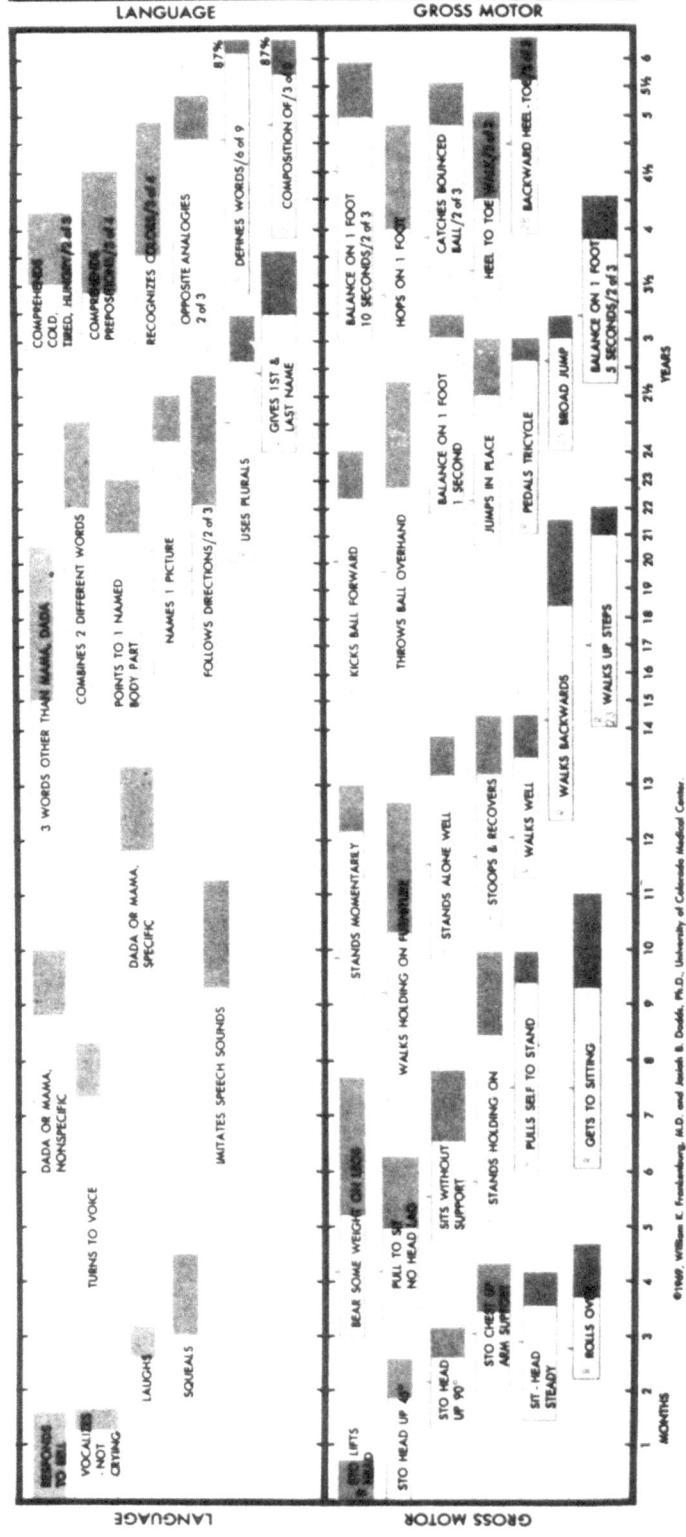

Source: Frankenburg, W.K., and Dodds, J.B.: *Denver Developmental Screening Test.* University of Colorado Medical Center (1969), with permission.

REFERENCES

1. Freedman, D. An ethological approach to the genetic study of human behavior, in *Methods and Goals in Human Behavior Genetics*. S. Vandenberg, ed. Academic, New York (1965).
2. Scarr, S. Social introversion as a heritable response. *Child Dev.* 40:823-832 (1969).
3. Bronfenbrenner, U. *Influences on Human Development*. Dryden, Hinsdale, Ill. (1972).
4. Tanner, J. *Education and Physical Growth*. London Univ., London (1961).
5. Singer, J., Westphal, M., and Niswander, K. Sex differences in the incidence of neonatal abnormalities and abnormal performance in early childhood. *Child Dev.* 39:103-112 (1968).
6. Friedman, R., Richart, R., and Van De Wiele, R. (eds.). *Sex Differences in Behavior*. Wiley, New York (1974).
7. Yalom, I., Green, R., and Fisk, N. Prenatal exposure to female hormones. Effect on psychosexual development of boys. *Arch. Gen. Psychiatry* 28:554-561 (1973).
8. Ziai, M., Janeway, C., and Cooke, R. *Pediatrics*. Little, Brown, Boston (1969).
9. Ouelette, E., Rosett, H., Rosman, N., and Weiner, L. Adverse effects on offspring of maternal alcohol abuse during pregnancy. *N. Engl. J. Med.* 297:528 (1977).
10. Sontag, L. The significance of fetal environment differences. *Am. J. Obstet. Gynecol.* 42:996-1003 (1941).
11. Ernhart, C., Graham, F., and Thurston, D. Relationship of neonatal apnea to development at 3 years. *Arch. Neurol.* 2:504-510 (1960).
12. Barnet, J. (ed.). *Pediatrics, 15th ed.* Appleton-Century-Crofts, New York (1972).
13. Koch, H. Some emotional attitudes of the young child in relation to characteristics of his siblings. *Child Dev.* 27:393-426 (1956).
14. Altus, W. Birth order and its sequelae. *Science* 151:44-49 (1966).
15. Mussen, P., Conger, J., and Kagan, J. *Child Development and Personality*, 4th ed. Harper and Row, New York (1974).
16. Cicirelli, V. Family structure and interaction—Sibling effects on socialization, in *Child Psychiatry—Treatment and Research*. M. McMillan and S. Henao, eds. Brunner/Mazel, New York (1977).
17. Sutton-Smith, B., and Rosenberg, B. *The Sibling*. Holt, Rinehart and Winston, New York (1970).
18. Cravioto, J., Delicardie, E., and Birch, H. Nutrition, growth and neurointegrative development. *Pediatrics* 38:319-372 (1966).
19. Herrington, B. Children of lesbians developmentally typical. *Psychiatr. News* (Oct. 19):20-22 (1979).
20. Wolfe, P. Maturational factors in behavioral development, in *Child Psychiatry—Treatment and Research*. M. McMillan and S. Henao, eds. Brunner/Mazel, New York (1977).
21. Harlow, H., and Harlow, M. Learning to love. *Am. Sci.* 54:244-272 (1966).
22. Rutter, M. Why are London children so disturbed? *Proc. R. Soc. Med.* 66:1221-1225 (1973).
23. Werner, E., Bierman, J., and French, F. *The Children of Kanai*. Univ. Hawaii, Honolulu (1971).
24. Hubel, D., and Wiesel, T. The period of susceptibility to the physiological effects of unilateral eye closure in kittens. *J. Physiol.* 206:419-436 (1970).
25. Harlow, H., in *Sex and Behavior*. F. Beach, ed. Wiley, New York (1965).
26. Rheingold, H. The modification of social responsiveness in institutional babies. Monographs of the Society for Research in Child Development. Volume 21, No. 2, Serial No. 63. Child Development Publications, Lafayette, Indiana (1956).
27. Spitz, R. *The First Year of Life*. Int. Univ., New York (1965).
28. Provence, S., and Lipton, R. *Infants in Institutions*. Int. Univ., New York (1965).

29. Thomas, A., Chess, S., and Birch, H. The origin of personality. *Sci. Am.* 223:102-109 (1970).
30. Kenny, T., and Clemmens, R. *Behavioral Pediatric and Child Development; A handbook.* Williams and Wilkins, Baltimore (1965).
31. Frankenburg, W. *Denver Development Screening Test—Reference Manual.* Univ. Colorado Med. C., Denver (1975).
32. Bloom, B. *Stability and Change in Human Characteristics.* Wiley, New York (1964).
33. Kagan, J., et al. Personality and I.Q. change. *J. Abnorm. Soc. Psychol.* 56:261-266 (1958).
34. Sontag, L., Baker, C., and Nelson, V. Mental growth and personality. A longitudinal study. *Monographs of the Society for Research in Child Development*, Vol. 23, No. 2, Serial No. 68. Child Development Publications, Lafayette, Indiana (1958).
35. Eagle, D., and Brazelton, T. Infants at risk—Assessment and implications for intervention, *Child Psychiatry—Treatment and Research.* M. McMillan and S. Henao, eds. Brunner/Mazel, New York (1977).
36. Spitz, R. *The First Year of Life.* Int. Univ., New York (1965).
37. Winnicott, D. *Through Pediatrics to Psychoanalysis.* Basic Books, New York (1975).
38. Piaget, J. *The Construction of Reality in the Child.* Basic Books, New York (1954).
39. Barker, P. *Basic Child Psychiatry, 2nd Ed.* Univ. Park Press, Baltimore (1976).
40. Erikson, E. *Childhood and Society.* Norton, New York (1950).
41. Galenson, E., and Roiphe, H. The emergence of genital awareness during the second year of life, in *Sex Differences in Behavior.* R. Friedman, R. Richart, and R. Vandewiele, eds. Knieger, Huntington, N.Y. (1978).
42. Chodoff, P. A critique of Freud's theory of infantile sexuality. *Am. J. Psychiatry* 123:507-518 (1966).
43. Ammons, R., and Ammons, H. Parent preferences in young children's doll play interviews. *J. Abnorm. Soc. Psychol.* 44:490-505 (1949).
44. Lapouse, R., and Monk, M. Fears and worries in a representative sample of children. *Am. J. Orthopsychiatry* 29:803 (1959).
45. Kanner, L. *Child Psychiatry*, 4th ed. Thomas, Springfield, Ill. (1972).
46. Levine, M. Children with encopresis. A descriptive analysis. *Pediatrics* 56:412-416 (1975).
47. Davidson, M., Kugler, M., and Bauer, C. Diagnosis and management in children with protracted constipation. *J. Pediatr.* 62:261-275 (1963).
48. Wright, L. Handling the encopretic child. *Prof. Psychol.* 4:137-144 (1973).
49. Marshall, W., and Tanner, J. Variations in the pattern of pubertal changes in boys. *Arch. Dis. Childh.* 45:13-23 (1970).
50. Lewis, M. *Clinical Aspects of Child Development.* Lea and Febiger, Philadelphia (1971).
51. Piaget, J. *The Moral Judgment of the Child.* Rontledge and Kegan Paul, London (1932).
52. Peters, J., Romine, J., and Dykman, R. A special neurological examination of children with learning disabilities. *Dev. Med. Child Neurol.* 17:63-78 (1975).
53. Piaget, J., and Inhelder, B. *The Psychology of the Child.* Basic Books, New York (1969).
54. Rutter, M., Tizard, J., and Whitmore, K. (eds.) *Education, Health and Behavior.* Longman, London (1970).
55. Forfar, J. The role of the pediatrician in adoption in medical practice. *Lancet* 1:1201-1203 (1969).
56. Rutter, M., and Hersov, L. *Child Psychiatry: Modern Approaches.* Blackwell, London (1977).
57. Kadushin, A. *Adopting Older Children.* Columbia, New York (1970).
58. Humphrey, M., and Ounsted, C. Adoptive families referred for psychiatric advice I. The children. *Br. J. Psychiatry* 109:599-608 (1963).
59. Humphrey, M., and Ounsted, C. Adoptive families referred for psychiatric advice II. The parents. *Br. J. Psychiatry* 110:549-555 (1964).

60. Bohman, M. *Adopted Children and Their Families*. Proprins, Stockholm (1970).

61. Vaughan, V., and McKay, R. (eds.). *Nelson Textbook of Pediatrics*, 10th ed. Saunders, Philadelphia (1975).

62. Blos, P. *The Psychoanalytic Study of the Child*, The second individuation process of adolescence, in Vol. 22. Int. Univ., New York (1967), pp. 162-186.

63. Freud, A. Adolescence, in *Psychoanalytic Study of the Child*, Vol. 13. R. Eissler, A. Freud, H. Hartmann, and E. Kris, eds. Int. Univ., New York (1958).

64. Offer, D., Marcus, D., and Offer, J. A longitudinal study of normal adolescent boys. *Am. J. Psychiatry* 126:917-924 (1970).

65. Mussen, P., and Jones, M. Self-conceptions, motivations and interpersonal attitudes of late and early maturing boys. *Child Dev.* 28:243-256 (1957).

66. Weatherley, D. Self-perceived rate of physical maturation and personality in late adolescence. *Child Dev.* 35:1197-1210 (1964).

67. Madison, A. *Runaway Teens*. Elsevier, New York (1979).

20

Mental Retardation

MICHAEL EGGER

INTRODUCTION

The syndrome of mental retardation presents a unique challenge to the affected child or adult, to his family, and to the physician who seeks to enhance his habilitation potential. It is the most common serious disorder of childhood, and it is a major social and economic problem. Yet in our country, major interest in the mentally retarded has developed only within the last three decades. Two events, the establishment in 1950 of a citizen advocacy group called the National Association for Retarded Citizens, and President Kennedy's 1963 federal mandate on mental retardation, were benchmarks for our nation's modern era of care of its retarded citizens.

The 1973 manual on terminology and classification of the American Association on Mental Deficiency (AAMD) defines mental retardation as "significantly subaverage intellectual functioning existing concurrently with deficits in adaptive behavior and manifest during the developmental period." About 3% of the nation's citizens are diagnosed at some time in their lives as mentally retarded. This figure is somewhat arbitrary and is arrived at in the following way: In intelligence tests, two standard deviations below the mean is a score of 70. By definition, almost 3% of those tested are two standard deviations below the mean, and are defined a priori as mentally retarded. However, to fit the definition, the malfunction in intellectual and adaptive skills must be noted during the development period, which traditionally means during childhood and early adolescence. Interestingly, while somewhat more than 3% of children are identified as retarded, considerably fewer than 3% are so diagnosed in adulthood. Upon reaching adulthood, the mentally retarded seem to "disappear" into the general population and are lost to followup, suggesting that their adaptive skills are sufficient for them to live in the community.

Retarded people can be categorized on the basis of the severity of the retardation. Those with intelligence quotients (IQs) of 70-89 are referred to as borderline or low normal but are not usually listed as retarded for statistical purposes. Those with IQs below 35 are considered severely retarded, are most likely to have the most severe physical anomalies, and frequently require institutional care. Table 1 lists the degrees of retardation, the IQ ranges upon which each category is based, and the percentage of retardation comprising each category. Fortunately, the more severe the retardation, the less common it is.

When a retarded child will first be identified as retarded depends on the severity of the retardation. The severely and profoundly retarded are usually identified in infancy or early childhood. The moderately retarded usually come to medical attention when their parents see delays in reaching developmental milestones such as walking, speaking, handling blocks, and identifying colors. The mildly retarded will not usually be noticed until they reach school age, when their teachers observe that they are beginning to fall behind their classmates in various skills.

With the availability of excellent treatment and educational facilities, the mildly retarded can be expected to attain about a third-grade reading level, can handle money and perform most basic tasks of daily living, and can thus live and work independently. Those who are moderately retarded can achieve about a first- or second-grade reading level, can care for their basic day-to-day needs, and can live and work in sheltered, supervised settings. The severely and profoundly retarded will usually require institutional care because of the degree of retardation, as well as the often-associated problems requiring specialized nursing care.

The causes of most cases of mental retardation are largely unknown.

Table 1   Prevalence of Mental Retardation in the Population According to Degree and IQ Range

Degree of retardation	IQ range	Approximate percentage of the retarded population
Borderline and low normal	70-89	—*
Mild	50-69	85
Moderate	35-49	12
Severe and profound	Severe = under 35 Profound = under 20	3

*Not included statistically.

Most research on genetic and biochemical causes of mental retardation has been done in the past 20 years. Today, over 2,500 defects known to produce mental retardation have been identified. The vast majority of these defects, most of which are called "inborn errors of metabolism," result from single-gene, usually autosomal recessive, inheritance. Several hundred disorders of multigene inheritance, and about 20 major chromosome disorders, have been identified as well. By and large, the genetic and biochemical disorders produce moderate to severe mental retardation. A notable exception to this is Down's syndrome, which usually produces mild to moderate retardation. Fortunately, these conditions are relatively infrequent. Taken together, the 2,500 or more known conditions account for only about 15% of cases of mental retardation. The etiologies of retardation in the other 85% are still matters of speculation. Of this 85%, neonatal hypoxia and sociocultural deprivation are commonly listed causes.

SPECIFIC SYNDROMES ASSOCIATED WITH MENTAL RETARDATION

Following is a discussion of some of the best-known syndromes associated with mental retardation. Each is a prototype for a category of disorders associated with retardation. It is important to be aware that some of them, while very well known, are rare. Sometimes only a few dozen cases have been reported, although most have variations so that partially affected individuals are seen.

Down's Syndrome

Down's syndrome is an autosomal aberration characterized by the presence of three rather than two no. 21 chromosomes in the G group It was first described by Seguin in the 19th century, and was called "furfuraceous idiocy." Later in the 19th century, Sir John Langdon Down introduced the term "mongolism." He felt that the peculiar epicanthal fold the children possessed caused them to resemble orientals. Interestingly, the condition was also known in the orient, where a term meaning "caucasian" was used to describe these children, since oriental physicians viewed them as resembling westerners. It was not until 1959 that Lejeune and Turpin delineated the specific chromosomal anomaly. The condition occurs in 1 out of 500-700 live births. Advanced maternal age is associated with increased risk: A woman under 29 has about one chance in 1,500 of having an affected child; whereas a woman in her late 40s has about one chance in 40.

Having one affected child is associated with an increased risk of having a second affected child, by about a 3:1 ratio as compared with the general population. With the exception of Down's syndrome due to translocation, most cases are isolated events in otherwise normal families.

There are several classic clinical features of the disorder. The children are almost always mentally retarded to a mild or moderate degree. They are usually hypotonic. The head tends to be small, with a rather flattened face and occiput, and there is usually a short, broad neck with rather lax skin at the sides of the neck. The eyes are small and slanted superolaterally, and there is an epicanthal fold on the nasal side of the eyes. The nose is rather small and short, and has a flattened bridge. The mouth is small and the tongue is thick and protruding. About one-fourth of these children have heart abnormalities, usually valvular or septal defects. The extremities are short, and the hands and feet tend to be broad, flat, and square. The fifth finger is small and curves inward (clinodactyly). The genitals are poorly developed, and secondary sex characteristics are usually delayed and incompletely developed. The hair on the head is dry, while pubic hair is straight and silky. The skin is coarse and dry. Distinctive patterns of finger, hand, and toe prints are noted, most prominently the "simian line," a deep, transverse crease crossing the entire palm. No specific pathological changes are noted in the central nervous system except that the brain in general, its gyri, and the cerebellum are smaller than normal. The cortex has fewer than normal nerve cells in each of its layers.

There is an increased frequency of leukemia and of Alzheimer's-senile brain disease. There is no known treatment for the condition per se. Current treatment focuses on maximizing the child's development potential.

Trisomy-D Syndrome (Patau's Syndrome, 13-Trisomy)

This is a chromosomal aberration in which there is a third chromosome in the D group (13-15). Although widely mentioned, there are only a few hundred documented cases. The incidence is about 1 in 4,600 births, and the etiology is unknown. As for Down's syndrome, the risk is higher if the mother is older. The children are severely retarded. Males have undescended testes. Seizures are frequent, and hypertonia, microcephaly, microphthalmia, and harelip and cleft palate are frequently noted. The children usually have a flexion deformity of the fingers and double-jointed thumbs. A characteristic footprint pattern is noted in most cases. There is no treatment for the condition at the present time, and the children usually die within 3-4 months after birth.

Trisomy-E (Edward's Syndrome, 18-Trisomy)

This is a trisomy condition involving the E group (16-18). The incidence is about 1 in 6,500 births, and only a few hundred cases have been described. Again, the etiology is unknown and again the risk increases with maternal age. The children are retarded, and have hypertonia in most cases. They usually have elongated skulls, low-set, malformed ears, and a poorly developed lower jaw. About 90% have a flat, protruding chest and most have hernias of the navel or groin. Flexion deformity of the fingers almost always occurs, and a short, upturned great toe with a turned heel deformity known as the "rocker bottom" is typical. Most have cardiac defects. Like Trisomy-13 syndrome, it is much more severe than Down's syndrome, and there is no specific treatment available. Death occurs in infancy.

Cri-du-Chat Syndrome

Cri-du-chat syndrome is characterized by a deletion of the distal end of the short arm of the fifth chromosome. This disorder derives its name because the infant's cry sounds like the mewing of a cat. The exact incidence of the disorder is unknown. The children are severely retarded and have microcephaly. Some have abnormally shaped, low-set ears, a moon face, and an epicanthal fold on the nasal aspect of each eye. No specific treatment is known, and the children usually die in infancy.

Turner's Syndrome

This is a sex chromosome disorder with the individual having a chromosome configuration of X0 rather than possessing a second X chromosome. The incidence is estimated at 1 in 3,000 live births, and it occurs only in females. While anomalies may be detected at birth, the most prominent findings for which the syndrome is noted occur at puberty, when the girls fail to develop secondary sex characteristics. Although pubic and underarm hair is usually present, menstruation does not occur. The girls are usually short, attaining an adult height which rarely exceeds 5 feet. The short build is accentuated by a wide chest and broadly spaced nipples. Webbing of the neck occurs, as do low-set ears, a low hairline, and a rather small lower jaw. Kidney and heart abnormalities are also common. Some children with Turner's syndrome are not retarded. Treatment is based on estrogen replacement therapy for lack of gonadal function. Although this permits development of secondary sex characteristics in most of the patients, they are usually sterile.

Klinefelter's Syndrome

Klinefelter's syndrome is a form of primary male hypogonadism. These individuals have a chromosome constitution of XXY. The syndrome occurs about once in every 400 live male births. They are at increased risk for leukemia and asthma. The disorder usually becomes noticed or obvious in adolescence, and the patients tend to be rather tall and nonmasculine in appearance. Small testes, feminine development of breast tissue, and sparse pubic hair are noted. The testes may or may not be functional. If the testes are functional, there are reduced numbers of sperm. Treatment consists of testosterone replacement, which will further the development of secondary sex characteristics but will not produce sperm. There are a variety of similar disorders with varying numbers of X and Y chromosomes. As a rule of thumb, the more extra chromosomes present, the more likely that the individual will be retarded, and the more severe the retardation.

Phenylketonuria

Phenylketonuria (PKU) is an autosomal recessive hereditary disorder which used to be called phenylpyruvic oligophrenia. The incidence of this disorder is about 1 in 10,000 births. It is most common among individuals of northern European stock, and least common among blacks and Jews. It has received considerable publicity and medical attention because it was the first inborn error of metabolism to be described, it is comparatively easy to diagnose, and early diagnosis can prevent retardation. Biochemically, the disorder is due to failure of the amino acid phenylalanine to be metabolized into tyrosine because of the absence of the enzyme phenylalanine hydroxylase. The children are normal at birth, but rapidly become retarded if they are not treated. They are usually light-haired and blue-eyed. Seizures occur frequently. Urine screening tests, while simple, have a high margin of error. The Guthrie and fluorometric tests requiring a few drops of blood are much more accurate. Phenylketonuria is one of only a handful of conditions producing mental retardation where treatment is specific.

The diet should be very low in phenylalanine. Since virtually all infant foods contain substantial quantities of phenylalanine, the children have to be maintained on a synthetic diet which is rather unpleasant and monotonous. However, if the diet is instituted within weeks of birth, little or no brain damage will occur and the children will develop normally. At one time it was assumed that the diet had to be continued for a lifetime. Some centers have reported that in most cases it can be discontinued in middle childhood, perhaps because myelinization has approached completion.

Maple Syrup Urine Disease

This is a potentially fatal hereditary disorder involving a block in amino acid metabolism. It is characterized by progressive cerebral dysfunction and unusual "maple syrup" odor in the urine. Like virtually all of the inborn errors of metabolism, it is caused by an autosomal recessive gene. This leads to failure to metabolize the branched chain amino acids leucine, isoleucine, and valine. Marked spongy degeneration of the brain and lack of development of myelin sheaths are noted. The children fail to thrive and manifest vomiting, severe mental retardation, hypertonia, and severe hypoglycemia. Sometimes the disease develops within a week of birth. If it is suspected, simple screening tests of the urine may be done. Recent evidence suggests that a diet very low in the three branched chain amino acids may prevent severe symptoms of the disorder. A synthetic diet similar to that used for phenylketonuria is required.

Wilson's Disease

Wilson's disease is due to a failure of copper metabolism secondary to a deficiency of ceruloplasmin. It is an autosomal recessive condition occurring once in about 4 million live births. The failure of development of plasma ceruloplasmin permits increase in intestinal absorption of copper and deposition of direct-reacting albumin-bound copper in the tissues of the body. The most prominent sites of deposition include the brain stem and liver. The disorder is characterized by involuntary movements and tremors, difficulty with swallowing, failure to thrive, seizures, and a brown or gray-green ring (the famous Kaiser-Fleisher ring) on the outer edge of the cornea of the eye. If recognized very early, the condition is treatable. A diet severely restricting copper may be instituted, and British antilewisite (BAL) may be used to increase copper excretion in the urine.

Homocystinuria

Homocystinuria is an autosomal recessive inborn error of metabolism characterized by a deficiency of cystathionine synthetase, which is necessary to metabolize homocystine into cystathionine. Only about 100 cases have been described, and the incidence is about 1 in 10,000. Clinically the children have flushed cheeks, osteoporosis, enlarged liver, severe mental retardation, bone deformities, abnormal blood clotting, and dislocated lenses and cataracts of the eyes. Most of the children are mildly retarded, although as the disorder progresses severe retardation ensues. A few have normal intelligence. Current treatment includes restriction of methionine and homocystine in the diet, with dietary supplements of cystathionine. The diet is synthetic and not very tasty. As an alternative the infant may be breastfed, since human breast milk is normally low in methionine and high in cystathionine.

Galactosemia

This is a hereditary disorder of carbohydrate metabolism. Its incidence is about 1 in every 25,000-50,000 births. These infants are unable to properly metabolize lactose and utilize glucose and galactose because of a deficiency in galactose-1-phosphouridyl transferase. This deficiency results in galactose accumulation in cells throughout the body. Clinically, the children fail to thrive; they vomit, have diarrhea, are listless, and experience hypoglycemic convulsions. Hyperbilirubinemia occurs. They also manifest weight loss, cataracts, a tendency to bleed, and mental retardation. If the condition is diagnosed early by urine and blood tests, the children should be placed on a galactose-free diet, and should remain on the diet for at least 3 years. If the diet is begun in the early years of life, there is a chance that all of the symptoms will be reversed or prevented. If treatment is delayed, the symptoms may be permanent, to varying degrees. As the children get older it is easier to design a balanced diet for them.

Amaurotic Familial Idiocy (Sphingolipidosis, Gangliosidosis)

There are three basic forms of this disorder: Tay-Sachs disease (the early infantile form), Bielschowsky-Jansky disease (the early juvenile form), and Spielmeyer-Vogt disease (the late juvenile form).

Tay-Sachs disease   This is a familial disease affecting children approximately 6 months after birth. It is the most commonly encountered of the three forms of amaurotic familial idiocy. It is transmitted by an autosomal recessive gene and is most frequently seen in Jews, particularly Ashkenazic Jews. It is due to a deficiency of B-d-N-acetyl-hexosaminidase, which leads to an accumulation of a ganglioside throughout the body. The first symptom is irritability, and there is a gradual deterioration. The child's vision worsens and eventually becomes blind. A "cherry-red" spot can be seen in the macula of the eye. When the child is about 3 years old he experiences rapidly developing muscular hypertonia, loses weight, and develops respiratory problems. The central nervous system of the child shows severe degeneration with deposition of ganglioside in the neurons. There is no effective treatment. For many years, only three forms of the disorder were known; there are now several dozen variants undergoing research.

Neiman-Pick Disease

This is a rare, fatal, genetic disorder of lipid metabolism. It has been reported all over the world, most commonly in Jewish infants of northeastern European ancestry. The incidence is considerably less than 1 in 10,000 births. It is characterized by deposition of lipids in many cells of the body, apparently due to a defect in the interconversion of ceramide and sphingomyelin. The disease has an early onset with rapid mental and general physical deterioration terminating in death between 6 months and 2 years of age. Within a few months of birth, the infants show reduced vitality, and a gradual paralysis of arms and legs. The skin is waxy and may be abnormally pigmented. Excessive vomiting occurs, with consequent dehydration and emaciation. The abdomen is enlarged and there is jaundice. Vision deteriorates and the child becomes blind. A cherry-red spot on the retina, similar to that of Tay-Sachs disease, is seen. The children are usually severely anemic and have abnormal white blood cells. A few cases with no involvement of the central nervous system are known. The outstanding characteristic of the disorder is the presence of large, foamy, lipid-laden cells throughout the body, particularly in the reticuloendothelial system. Clinically, the disorder is quite similar to Tay-Sachs disease. However, Tay-Sachs disease shows no lipid-laden cell infiltration. There is no effective treatment.

Marfan's Syndrome

This is a skeletal and connective tissue disorder, resulting in a tall and angular body with posture disturbances; a narrow, elongated face; long extremities; and long, spidery fingers. It was first described over a century ago, and more than 500 cases have been reported. This is one of the few inborn errors of metabolism inherited as an autosomal dominant. It occurs in at least 3 of every 200,000 births. Mental retardation occurs occasionally, but no firm figures on its frequency are available. Skeletal deformities are noted in at least three-fourths of the people with this disorder. A striking feature is the excessively tall and thin body profile, with the lower part of the body being disproportionately longer than the upper. Looseness of the connective tissue and spinal column leads to increased spinal curvature and a progressively stooping posture. The disproportion of the body parts can be demonstrated by comparing the individual height with the span of his horizontally outstretched arms. In all cases of the syndrome, arm span is greater than body height. Fingers and toes are long and wiry; frequently they are described as "spiderlike" (arachnodactyly). The muscles are slender and weak. The head is long and narrow, with the eyes deeply set in their sockets with prominent eyebrow ridges. High, arched palates are noted. The ears are often quite large, with associated thinness of the outer edges. Dislocation of the lenses of the eyes are noted in three-fourths of patients, and aortic dilatation is noted in about two-thirds of patients. Laboratory studies reveal an increased amount of collagen and fragile and less abundant elastic tissue. There seems to be an increased production and destruction of collagen.

Hurler's Syndrome

This is a rare, hereditary connective tissue disorder. It is due to a deficiency of β-galactosidase producing abnormal metabolism of mucopolysaccharides. There are at least six genetically distinct groups of Hurler's syndrome: Type 1 (Hurler's), Type 2 (Hunter's), Type 3 (Sanfilippo), Type 4 (Marquio), Type 5 (Scheir), and Type 6 (Maroteaux-Laney). In Types 1, 3, 5, and 6, transmission is autosomal recessive. In Type 2 the gene is recessive, but located on a sex chromosome (X-linked), thereby affecting males.

Patient with Hurler's syndrome manifest a number of prominent signs, which include the following: short stature; mental retardation; flexed, contracted upper extremities; spinal curvature; enlarged spleen; enlarged liver; enlarged head; thick, heavy eyebrows; clouding of the cornea; a snub nose with continuous mucus discharge; thick lips, open mouth, and large tongue; excessive amounts of hair all over the body; puffy, soft skin; valvular heart defects; short, lobster-like fingers; and bulging of the skull. Rarely do all these signs occur in one patient. Several findings aid in the diagnosis: Radiologially, a wedge-shaped deformity is seen in some vertebrae, the proximal phalanges look bullet-shaped and the distal phalanges look undeveloped. The skin manifests pale, nontender nodules, giving a corrugated, worm-like texture to the affected area, which is usually the posterior aspect of the shoulders. In the complete blood count, increased numbers of white blood cells with mucopolysaccharide inclusions are noted. On examination of the precordium, diastolic murmurs, systolic murmurs, and cardiomegaly may be noted. Many of the infants (including 100% in Type 1) die in childhood; some survive into adulthood. No specific treatment is available. Like Tay-Sachs disease, Hurler's syndrome is a condition in which only a few clinical variants were initially noted. However, current research suggests that several dozen closely related syndromes exist.

Lesch-Nyhan Syndrome

Lesch-Nyhan syndrome is characterized by elevated levels of uric acid in the blood, with developmental retardation, spastic cerebral palsy, and self-mutilating behavior. The condition was described only 15 years ago, and is due to decreased activity of a specific enzyme, hypoxanthine-guanine phos-phoribosyl transferase (HGPRT), resulting in an excess of purines. It is a sex-linked recessive condition. The overall incidence is still unknown, since only a few dozen cases have been described. Clinically, the most prominent signs are spasticity, choreoathetosis, speech impairment, and frequent vomit-ing, all of which appear when the child is about 1 year of age. Mental retar-dation is variable and not always severe. Height and weight are usually far below normal. Bizarre, self-mutilating behavior is the most salient feature of the condition. It is poignant to note that the children do feel pain, and will plead with others to keep them from biting themselves. Decreased serum levels of glutamine are noted, this also occurs with maple syrup urine disease and phenylketonuria—but the significance of this is not known. No effective treatment for the disorder is known.

DIAGNOSIS AND TREATMENT

The physician may be approached with the problem of mental retarda-tion when the family first suspects that the child is falling behind his peers in developmental skills, or when the family is concerned about how to proceed once a diagnosis of mental retardation or a retardation-producing syndrome has been made. Early detection of mental retardation requires the following: (1) A sound knowledge of mental retardation; (2) a high index of suspicion whenever there are factors in the family history, pregnancy or prenatal period which places the infant "at risk"; (3) periodic conscientious observation and examination during infancy or the preschool period; (4) routine screening for the commoner metabolic disorders such as phenylketonuria and hypothy-roidism; and (5) use of the Denver Developmental Screening Test or other similar developmental tests as part of the routine assessment of all children.

Denhoff summarized the factors placing a child at risk for developing the symptom of mental retardation. These are summarized in Table 2. The physician should be aware that several of the syndromes producing mental retardation can now be diagnosed by amniocentesis. This technique is rapid-ly expanding in usefulness, and new conditions are being added almost monthly to the list. Table 3 contains a current listing.

The basic principle of the comprehensive treatment of mentally re-tarded children include the following: (1) Keep an open-minded approach to diagnosis and treatment, and reevaluate with the same inquiring attitude; (2) Engage the family through active participation in treatment; (3) Make an early descriptive diagnosis, followed by early treatment; (4) Accept each child as he is, including all aspects of his behavior. Encourage and support

Table 2   Factors That Increase the Risk of Mental Retardation in Children

Maternal factors

1. Unmarried
2. Low socioeconomic status
3. Small stature (implies contracted pelvis)
4. Maternal age (early adolescence or over 40 years)
5. Previous miscarriage or birth of a defective child
6. Maternal hypertension, toxemia, diabetes, thyroid disease, mental retardation, pelvic irradiation, or prolonged infertility
7. Vaginal bleeding after the first trimester
8. Shock
9. Excessive amniotic fluid
10. High parity (five or more pregnancies)

Factors at birth and in the neonatal period

1. Prematurity (especially of a first-born male or twins)
2. Premature detachment of the placenta
3. Perinatal hypoxia (low Apgar scores)
4. Prolonged labor or traumatic birth
5. Any physical anomaly, especially asymmetry of face and extremities
6. Jaundice; vomiting (prolonged); seizures; failure to thrive

Table 3   Conditions in Which Antenatal Diagnosis by Anmiocentesis Has Been Made

Adrenal cortical hyperplasia
Chromosomal translocations and trisomies
Down's syndrome
Fabry's disease
Galactosemia
Gaucher's disease
Glyogen-storage disease (Type II)
G_{MI} gangliosidosis, Type I
G_{MI} gangliosidosis, Type II
Hunter's syndrome
Hurler's syndrome
Krabbe's disease
Lesch-Nyhan syndrome
Lysosomal acid phosphatase deficiency
Maple syrup urine disease
Methylmalonic acidemia
Metachromatic leukodystrophy
Niemann-Pick disease
Sex determination
Tay-Sachs disease (G_{m2} gangliosidosis)

acceptance from his family as well; (5) Focus on what the child *can* do; lead him step by step toward maximum development; and (6) Coordinate the services needed by the child, for clarity and continuity of communication are of primary importance.

The discovery that a child is mentally retarded is a major crisis, not only for the child but also for his entire family. Table 4 outlines three main crises through which families will pass: The novelty shock crisis, the personal value crisis, and the reality crisis. It also lists common parental responses to each of these three crises, positive and negative ways in which the crises are frequently resolved, and the specific treatment needs of the family. In our culture, the personal value crisis is the most difficult to resolve: In our society, socioeconomic status is largely dependent upon one's job. If the diagnosis of retardation is correct, the retarded individual, even with the best treatment programs currently available, is not going to rise to positions demanding considerable intelligence. Upward mobility is perceived as a desirable goal, and the parents, correctly perceiving that the child has reduced social and voca-

Table 4   An Operational Diagnostic Treatment Approach to Crises Faced by Families of the Retarded

Type of crisis	Common response of parents	Favorble solutions	Unfavorable solutions	Treatment strategy
Novelty shock crisis	Panic, denial, guilt	Acceptance of child "as he is"	Parents' guilt incapacitating; parents deny; child institutionalized	Careful diagnostic evaluation; early supportive counseling combining realism with hope; initiation of life planning
Personal value crisis	Less mature defense mechanisms (e.g., denial, projection, reaction formation)	Resolution of dilemma of high expectations with limited prospects; acceptance	Parents sad and disappointed; parents "shop around"; child institutionalized	Psychotherapy or counseling, with goal of acceptance of child as he is
Reality crisis	Acceptance and search for treatment and other services	Effective utilization of services	Child seen as nuisance; child underachieves; child institutionalized	Effective utilization of services

Source: Modified from F. Menolascino and M. Egger. *Medical Dimensions of Mental Retardation.* Univ. Nebraska, 1978.

tional achievement potential, may experience anger, shame, guilt, and disappointment. This may be especially difficult for parents who have themselves achieved upward mobility. Other than "curing" the rare "curable" condition, finding a niche in the parental value systems which will benefit both the child and his parents is the most important contribution that the physician or counselor can make.

As mentioned earlier, only a handful of the conditions producing mental retardation can at the present time be treated in such a way as to alleviate the physical stigmata and eliminate the mental retardation. Thus, for the overwhelming majority of the retarded, treatment is aimed at maximizing what learning potential they have. A variety of community-based treatment programs are currently available throughout the United States. These vary widely in quality and quantity, depending on the area in which one is living, but they are becoming increasingly available. As a rule, maintaining the child in his home community, preferably living at home, is better than institutional placement. Institutional placement disrupts the normal patterns of child growth, development, and interaction with peers. Also, as a whole, institutional treatment programs in this country have been disappointing. For that reason, I have listed institutionalization in the previously mentioned table as a negative way of resolving the crisis the family is undergoing. For a few individuals, particularly those who are severely retarded and have multiple congenital deformities, institutional placement may be mandatory because of the nursing care required. Apart from these unfortunate few, it is usually not required. Children can do quite well living at home, or if this becomes impossible, at a community-based group home under adult supervision.

Specific teaching programs are needed for the retarded. The most important aspect of such programs is a high staff-to-pupil ratio and the development of a series of techniques known as "precision teaching." These enable the teacher to break down learning tasks (including skills) into a series of relatively simple steps. Seemingly simple skills, such as picking up a cup and drinking from it, are actually quite complicated, involving the coordination of many muscles and the timing of several separate movements. For a retarded child who has difficulty learning such skills, breaking them down into a series of subskills, each learned in sequence with extensive drill and repetition, is imperative. This requires a considerable amount of time and one-to-one teacher-student supervision. Nonetheless, it is the best way for the skill to be taught. Once simple tasks have been grasped, placing the child or adolescent in a sheltered workshop where supervised learning of specific trade skills can occur is a helpful adjunct to formal schooling. Most of the mildly retarded will be able to graduate from such programs and work independently in the community. Most of the moderately retarded will need considerable supervision throughout their work experience, but can function quite well in such settings.

There are several emotional problems that need to be considered in relation to the mentally retarded. It has become increasingly clear that there is no natural line of separation between adequate intellectual functioning and normal social functioning. The major difference between the retarded individual and his normal peer appears to be the retarded person's overt adaptive behavior, which is socially judged. Intellectual limitations interfere both with his capacity to obtain satisfaction from his own efforts and his capacity to meet demands and expectations. Since he has adaptive difficulties, the mentally retarded individual tends to need help from others. Thus, the extent to which he is surrounded by supportive adults largely determines whether he makes a satisfactory emotional adjustment.

When adults are inconsistent in their attitudes or support and are overly demanding, undependable and nonsupportive of the child's efforts, his needs become more urgent. When he finds that the demands made upon him are confusing or impossible to meet, or when his necessarily limited accomplishments aren't appreciated, his unacceptable behavior may become intensified. Such situations may develop at home or at school and become chronic, even though parents and teachers are aware of the child's retardation. Parents may intellectually accept the child's problem, but have strong emotions that stand in the way of accepting the child as he is. This problem is frequently noted in parents who place a premium on their children's achievements. Parents may see that in their mentally retarded child, their collective hopes for personal and intellectual achievement will go unfulfilled. They become increasingly upset about the child's inability to perform at the expected level for his chronological age. Some parents may react to the child with anger and withdrawal of love, and they may consider their child stubborn, ill-tempered, or lazy. Such attitudes make it more difficult for parents to accept their child and recognize his capabilities. In turn, the child may withdraw or retaliate, and events in his immediate world may lead him increasingly to view the world as threatening. This vicious cycle can literally force him to fail, which leads to further lack of responsiveness and diminished efforts on everybody's part. The child may manifest excessive dependency, free-floating anxiety, or impulsive outbursts. The retarded individual thus may have to cope not only with intellectual limitations, but also with the handicaps produced by repeated interactions with his social system.

Under any circumstances, the mentally retarded child has difficulty adapting to sudden changes in his interpersonal environment, such as meeting new people. This difficulty makes greater demands on both the retarded individual and his family. If coupled with a lack of strong family support, this lack of flexibility may create chronic maladaptive emotional responses on the part of the child. Since all behavior is aimed at finding the safest position in the social-interpersonal system, the child's reaction may be withdrawal, timidity, or apathy. An illustration of this relationship between the retarded child's needs and the nature of his support system is a situation in which a timid child is overwhelmed by an interested, but domineering teacher. In the teacher's presence this child is unable to focus his attention and assimilate what the teacher is trying to present. However, with a less-demanding teacher, a timid child is more relaxed and may be able to mobilize his attention. Thus, relief from stresses can improve the child's behavior.

In a family setting in which failure is answered with rejection, the child is continually insecure. In addition, for reasons still not fully understood, he may have anxiety attacks, develop phobias, or manifest obsessions and compulsions. These "neurotic" disorders seldom yield to manipulation of the child's environment, so formal treatment may become necessary. This may involve psychotherapy, behavior modification, or pharmacotherapy. Excessive dependency may require formal treatment as well, although drugs would not be used.

For the retarded, adolescence is more than a transitional period of testing and separation from authority figures on the road to relative self-sufficiency. Searching for sexual identity and acceptance, moving away from the family group, and preparing for personal and financial independence all challenge the adaptive capacity of even the best-endowed youngster. Superimposed upon this, retarded adolescents may be making their first concerted move toward less dependency upon parents. Heterosexual experiences are sometimes beyond the retarded child's interest or capacity. Often, adolescence is the time when the first social relationships with persons outside his family are developing. The forced dependency of the mentally retarded individual early in life, and the subsequent limitations on his mobility and range of personal-social experiences, mean that he has not had sufficient opportunities for those interactions which permit the full development of identity.

Retarded adolescents need innovative approaches which provide protection and assistance sufficient to permit them to engage in work, play and education. This combination of support and independent function is for his psychosocial development. Realistic therapeutic planning can make all these experiences possible and, as a result, the mentally retarded adolescent can achieve an altered view of himself and his potential.

Group therapy has many advantages for adolescents who are denied the opportunity to belong to meaningful social groups. It is valuable for the mildly retarded because it gives them a chance to describe feelings, share problems, and understand profound reactions to continuing failure. Therapy sessions can substitute for the peer group that is unavailable to them.

SELECTED BIBLIOGRAPHY

Amaurotic family idiocy. *Lancet* 1:469-471 (1973).

American Medical Association. Mental retardation. A handbook for the primary physician. *JAMA* 191:183-222 (1965).

Ampola, M. Phenylketonuria and other disorders of amino acid metabolism. *Pediatr. Clin. North Am.* 20:507-536 (1973).

Ando, H. Intrafamilial incidence of autism, cerebral palsy, and mongolism. *J. Autism Childh. Schizophr.* 5:267-274 (1975).

Arey, J. The lipidoses. Morphologic changes in the nervous system in Gaucher's disease, GM2 gangliosidoses and Niemann-Pick disease. *Ann. Clin. Lab. Sci.* 5:475-488 (1975).

Baughman, F., Higgins, J., Wadsworth, T., and Demaray, M. The carrying angle in sex chromosome anomalies. *JAMA* 230:718-720 (1974).

Brinkworth, R. The unfinished child. Early treatment and training for the infant with Down's syndrome. *R. Soc. Health J. (Lond.)* 95:73-78 (1975).

Carter, C. (ed.). *Medical Aspects of Mental Retardation*. Thomas, Springfield, Ill. (1965).

Chamberlin, H. Mental subnormality. General considerations, in *Pediatric Neurology*. T.W. Farmer, Ed. Harper & Row, New York (1964).

Clements, P. Variability within Down's syndrome. Emperically observed sex differences in IQ's. *Ment. Retard.* 14:30-31 (1976).

Cox, D. A genetic study of Arileon's disease. Evidence for heterogeneity. *Am. J. Hum. Genet.* 24:646-666 (1972).

Crocker, A. Families under stress. The diagnosis of Hurler's syndrome. *Postgrad. Med.* 51:223-229 (1972).

Cusworth, D., and Dent, C. Homocystinuria. *Br. Med. Bull.* 23(1):42-47 (1969).

Dacremont, G. Niemann-Pick disease. *N. Engl. J. Med.* 289:592-593 (1973).

Dalton, J., and Epstein, H. Counseling parents of mildly retarded children. *Soc. Casework* 44:523-530 (1963).

Denhoff, E. *Cerebral Palsy: The preschool years*. Thomas, Springfield, Ill. (1967).

Donnelly, P., and DiFerrante, N. Reliability of the Booth-Nadler technique for the detection of Hunter heterozygotes. *Pediatrics* 56:429-433 (1975).

Dubois, E., and Kaplan, B. Letters. S-L-E and Klinefelter's syndrome. *Lancet* 1(7950):93 (1976).

Dumanrs, K., Gaskill, D., and Kitzmiller, N. "Le Cri-du-Chat" (crying cat) syndrome. *Am. J. Dis. Child.* 108:533 (1972).

Eisen, J. Screening program for Tay-Sachs disease. *Nebr. State Med. J.* 58:166-167 (1973).

Elias, S., and Mahoney, T. Prenatal diagnosis of trisomy 13 with decision not to terminate pregnancy. *Obstet. Gynecol.* 47:75S-76S (1976).

Ellingson, R., Menolascino, F., and Eisen, J. Clinical-EEG relationships in mongoloids confirmed by karyotype. *Am. J. Ment. Def.* 74(5):645-650 (1970).

Elsas, L. Classical maple syrup urine disease. Cofactor resistance. *Metabolism* 21:929-944 (1972).

Francis, M., and Smith, R. Polymetric collagen of skin in osteogenesis imperfecta, homocystinuria, and Ehlers-Danlos and Marfan syndromes. *Birth Def.* 11:15-21 (1975).

Francone, C. My battle against Wilson's disease. *Am. J. Nurs.* 76:247-249 (1976).

Frankenburg, W., Goldstein, A., and Olson, C. Behviorial consequences of increased phenylalanine intake by phenylketonuric children. A pilot study describing a methodology. *Am. J. Ment. Def.* 77:524-532 (1973).

Fujimoto, W. Mental retardation and self-destructive behavior. Clinical and biochemical features of the Lesch-Nyhan syndrome, in *The Genetic, Metabolic, and Developmental Aspects of Mental Retardation*. R.F. Murray and P.L. Rosser, eds. Thomas, Springfield, Ill. (1972).

Garrard, S., and Richmond, J. Diagnosis in mental retardation, in *Medical Aspects of Mental Retardation*, C. Carter, ed. Thomas, Springfield, Ill. (1965).

Gordon, N. *Pediatric Neurology for the Clinician*. Spastics Int. Med. Pub. Lippincott, Philadelphia (1976).

Groll, M., and Cooper, M. Menstrual function in Turner's syndrome. *Obstet. Gynecol.* 47:225-226 (1976).

Grossman, H. (ed.). *Manual on Terminology and Classification in Mental Retardation*, rev. ed. Am. Assoc. Ment. Def., Washington, D.C. (1973).

Hill, H. Detection of inborn errors of metabolism. Galactosemia. *Science* 179:1136-1139 (1973).

Hirst, A., Jr., and Gore, I. Marfan's syndrome. A review. *Progr. Cardiovasc. Dis.* 16:187-198 (1973).

Leonard, M. Homocystinuria. A differential diagnosis of Marfan's syndrome. *Oral Surg.* 35:214-219 (1973).

Lesch, M., and Nyhan, W. A familial disorder of uric acid metabolism and functin. *J. Pediatr.* 36:561 (1964).

Levin, B., and Jacoby, N. Mucopolysaccharidosis. *Proc. R. Soc. Med.* 65:339-341 (1972).

Libert, J., Toussaint, D., and Guiselings, R. Ocular findings in Niemann-Pick disease. *Am. J. Ophthalmol.* 80:991-1002 (1975).

Machill, G., and Knopp, A. On the population genetics of phenylketonuria in the German Democratic Republic. *Hum. Genet.* (formerly Humangenetik, Berlin) 31:107-111 (1976).

McKusick, V. Concise outline of medical genetics. *Med. Times* 94:807-815 (1966).

Menolascino, F. Psychiatric aspects of mental retardation in children under eight. *Am. J. Orthopsychiatry* 35:852-861 (1965).

Menolascino, F. Changing developmental perspectives in Down's syndrome. *Child Psychiatr. Hum. Deve.* 4(4):85 (1974).

Michael, E. Studies on the biochemical basis of the Marfan syndrome. A review. *Ala. J. Med. Sci.* 13:54-58 (1976).

Michaels, J., and Schucman, H. Observations on the psychodynamics of parents of retarded children. *Am. J. Men. Def.* 66:568-573 (1962).

Milunsky, A. Prenatal diagnosis of genetic disorders. An analysis of experience with 600 cases. *JAMA* 230:232-235 (1974).

National Institute of Health. *Facts about Mongolism, for Women Over 35* (DHEW No. 74-536). U.S. Gov. Prtg. Off., Washington, D.C. (1974).

National Institute of Health. *What Are the Facts About Genetic Disease?* (DHEW No. 75-370). U.S. Gov. Prtg. Off., Washington, D.C. (1975).

O'Brien, J. Tay-Sachs disease. From enzyme to prevention. *Proc. Fed. Am. Soc. Exp. Biol.* 32:191-199 (1973).

Rockson, S., Stone, R., Van der Weyden, M., and Kelley, W. Lesch-Nyhan syndrome. Evidence for abnormal adrenergic function. *Science* 186:934-935 (1974).

Ross, A. *The Exceptional Child in the Family*. Grune & Stratton, New York (1964).

Russell, A., Statler, M., Shina, A., and Perlman, M. Proceedings. Neonatal diagnosis of maple syrup urine disease and the influence of exchange blood transfusion. *Isr. J. Med. Sci.* 11:1218-1219 (1975).

Santavuori, P. Infantile type of so-called neuronal aroid-lipofuscinosis. A clinical study of 15 patients. *J. Neurol. Sci.* 18:257-267 (1973).

Schlottman, R. Social and play behaviors of institutionalized mongoloid and nonmongoloid retarded children. *J. Psychol.* 91:201-206 (1975).

Soltan, H. PKU screening. *Can. Med. Assoc. J.* 108:961 (1973).

Stoddard, H. The relation of parental attitudes and achievements of severely mentally retarded children. *Am. J. Ment. Def.* 63:575-598 (1959).

Taylor, A. Patau's, Edwards', and Cri-du-Chat syndrome. A tabulated summary of current findings. *Dev. Med. Child Neurol.* 9:78-86 (1967).

Vannas, A., Hogan, M., Golbus, M., and Wood, I. Lens changes in galactosemic fetus. *Am. J. Ophthalmol.* 80:726-733 (1975).

Vaughn, V. Growth and development (Chap. 2), in *Nelson: Textbook of Pediatrics*, 10th ed. V.C. Vaughn and R.J. McKay, eds. Saunders, Philadelphia (1975).

Walske, J. Copper chelaton in patients with Wilson's disease. A comparison of penicillamine and triethylene tetramine dihydrochloride. *J. Med.* (Oxford 42:441-452 (1973).

Wendel, U. Rapid diagnosis of maple syrup urine disease (branched chain ketoaciduria) by microenzyme assay in leukodytes and fibroblasts. *Clin. Chim. Acta.* 45:433-440 (1973).

Wolfensberger, W. Counseling the parents of the retarded. In *Mental Retardation.* A.A. Baumeister, ed. Aldine, Chicago (1967).

21

Early and Middle Adulthood

FREDERICK SIERLES

INTRODUCTION

Throughout the centuries, people have noticed that there are stages of adulthood. Adults at one stage are different from adults in other stages in knowledge, problem-solving ability, attitudes, priorities, health, and physical capacities. Of course, this does not mean that one stage is better than another. Young adults respect the experienced, seasoned, less-harried, "mellow" qualities of some of their elders, although they appreciate their own youth when older people are cynical, insufficiently inquisitive, or forgetful. Older adults respect the idealism, vigor, good health, and inquisitiveness of their juniors, but appreciate their own age when younger adults are naive or arrogant. Although you are an adult now, you are not quite the same person that you will be years later.

Example: When I was an intern, I admitted an elderly lady who had extensive metastatic cancer with severe anemia and weakness, verging on stupor and death, to my ward. Without presenting her with any options, I told her I was going to give her a blood transfusion and she, with a weak voice, consented. I gave the transfusion, which had little effect, and several hours later she died. When I presented her history at the clinical pathological conference the next day, the chief of service asked the audience "Would you have given her the transfusion?" The medical students and interns all said "Yes," emphasizing that the transfusion was the treatment of choice for the severe anemia. The attending physicians all responded "No," pointing out that such "heroic" effects were needless for this lady who was obviously dying and who had been presented no other alternatives. Neither response is necessarily better; however, the responses, based upon age and experience, were very different.

There are abundant nonmedical references to stages of adulthood. Sources include the *Talmud* and Confucius. According to the *Talmud*, "(age) 20 (is) for seeking a livlihood, 30 for attaining full strength, 40 for understanding, 50 for giving counsel, and 60 for being an elder" [1]. Confucius said "At 30, I had planted my feet firm upon the ground. At 40, I no longer suffered from complexities. At 50, I knew what were the biddings of heaven. At 60, I heard them with docile ear" (cited in Ref. 1).

Psychiatrists have been interested in stages of life since late in the 19th century, but the Freudian and other psychoanalytic schools initially concentrated on stages of childhood. Erikson [2] described "ages of man" from infancy to senescence. He felt that for each age to unfold fully, the preceding age had to be completed; this is called the *epigenetic concept* of development. He also described *"normative crises"* for each age group, crises which had to be resolved if the individual was to develop fully. The normative crises are listed here [2]:

Infant:	Basic trust versus mistrust
Toddler:	Autonomy versus shame and doubt
Preschool child:	Initiative versus guilt
School-age child:	Industry versus inferiority
Adolescent:	Identity versus identity confusion
Young adulthood:	Intimacy versus isolation
Middle adulthood:	Generativity versus stagnation
Late adulthood:	Integrity versus despair

Identity is a sense of who one is, a sense of sameness and continuity over time. Intimacy refers to the formation of close relationships with others, as in marriage and friendship. Generativity is the capacity and proclivity to influence others in a useful way, as in the role of parent, mentor, or teacher. Integrity is a sense of fullness and meaningfulness in contemplating one's life.

Benedek [3] also contributed to the study of adult development. She discussed parenthood (and the climacterium) as a developmental phase because parents, in assisting their children in solving problems, have an opportunity to rethink and resolve issues that were problematic for themselves when they were children. While the conclusions of Erikson and Benedek were not the product of statistical studies, their work is thought-provoking and respected.

RECENT LITERATURE

More recently, Levenson [1], Gould [4,5], and Vaillant [6] completed important studies on adulthood.

Levenson, like Erikson, specified stages of adult life, which are portrayed below:

Under 17:	Childhood and adolescence
17-22:	Early adult transition
22-28:	Entering the adult world
28-33:	Age 30 transition
35-40:	Settling down
40-45:	Midlife transition
45-50:	Entering middle adulthood
50-55:	Age 50 transition
55-60:	Culmination of middle adulthood
60-65:	Late adult transition
over 65:	Late adulthood

Levenson states that the range of years in which these periods occur is fairly fixed, and that the order in which they occur is also fixed. He does not feel that these periods constitute a hierarchy with "better" or "worse" stages. He writes: "Spring is not intrinsically a better season than winter, nor is summer better than spring" [1]. His main contribution is his delineation of how adulthood is characterized by alterations between periods of consolidation and periods of transition and reevaluation. During periods of consolidation, people stabilize their relationships. The object of these periods is comfort, stability, and predictability. During periods of transition and reevaluation, people reassess the utility of gains made in the previous consolidation period. Goals, styles of work, and aspects of marriage are reevaluated and often significantly altered.

Lik Erikson and Levenson, Gould delineated stages of adult life. Like Levenson, he didn't pay much attention to late adulthood and senescence. Here are Gould's stages [4,5]:

16-22:	"Leaving our parent's world"
22-28:	"I'm nobody's baby"
28-35:	"Opening up to what's inside"
35-45:	"Midlife decade"

One of Gould's contributions was his description of shifts in priorities, concerns, and attitudes as adults move through the life cycle. Gould developed a questionnaire in which subjects were asked to rank, in order of priority for them, a series of statements about their attitudes [5]. Age-related differences in priorities, concerns, and attitudes are graphically represented in Figure 1.

Another contribution by Gould is his description of the ongoing conflicts, each of which is fairly specific to the stage of adult development, between age-appropriate, realistic perceptions and childish views. For example, there are the common "childish" beliefs of people ages 22-28 that "rewards

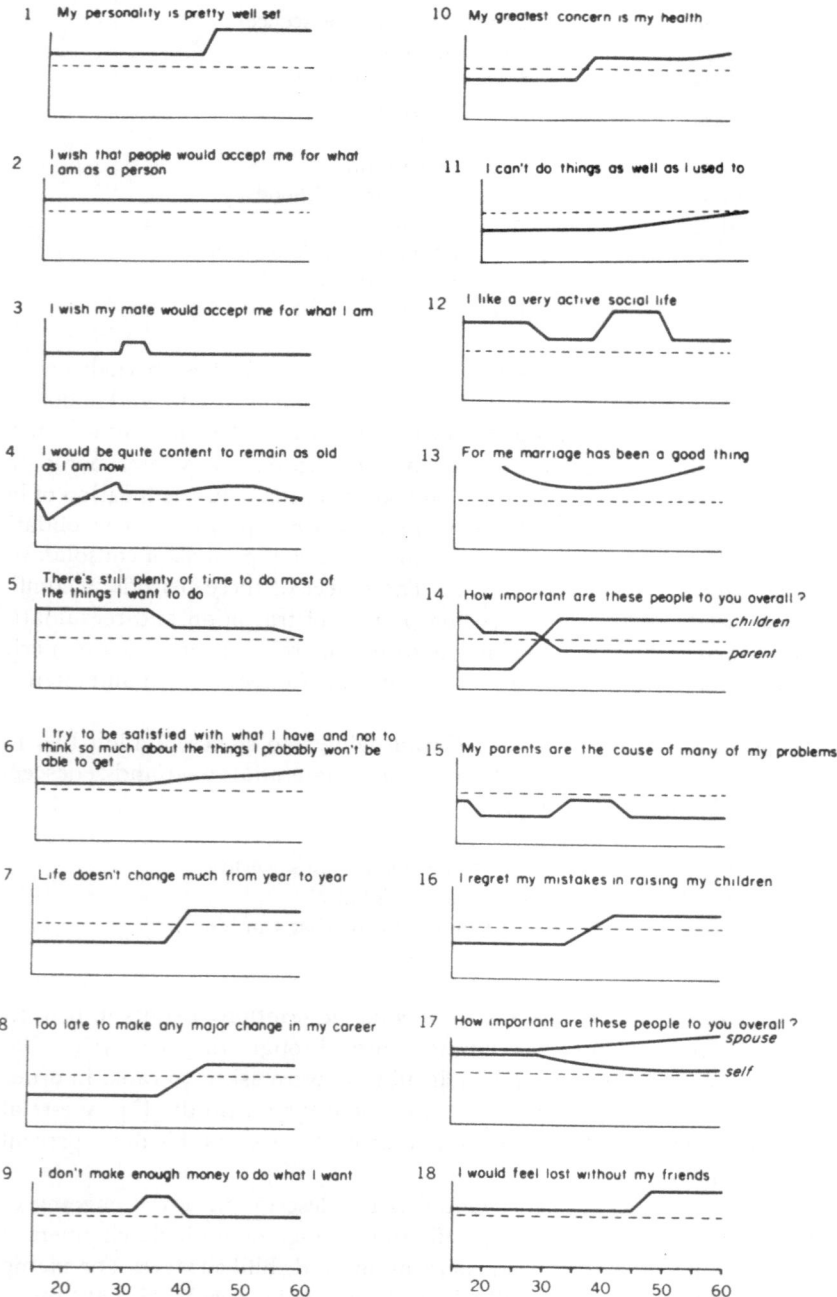

FIG. 1.   Sample curves associated with the time boundaries of the adult life span. (From R. Gould. The phases of adult life. *Am. J. Psychiatry* 129:33-53, 1972, with permission.)

will come automatically if we do what we're supposed to do," that "doing things by parents' way, with willpower and perseverance, will bring results," and that "rationality, commitment, and effort will always prevail over all other forces" [4]. While these attitudes are partially true, and may sometimes lead to success in a given area, if adhered to rigidly they will lead to disappointment and frustration some of the time. First-year residents experience many sleepless nights working on hospital wards handling night admissions, emergencies, and less-than-urgent nursing and patient requests. Although this realistically represents another step in learning a chosen vocation, and saves patients' lives, as far as most supervisors and colleagues are concerned, the first-year resident is "just another name" on an on-call roster. If a patient or relative thanks him for his efforts, it is likely that he will be the only person to do so.

The studies of Levenson and Gould are cross-sectional; that is, they studied people of different ages at the same point in time. In contrast, Vaillant [6] has made a career of doing longitudinal studies, which are studies of the *same* individuals at different phases of their own life cycles.

Vaillant demonstrated that future mental health and success are predictable to a degree. He found that a group of Harvard students, selected in 1938-1944 for certain personal attributes, performed better than their classmates during the years prior to their 25th class reunion. Their performance was significantly better in these categories: Graduated from college with honors, went on to graduate school, feels job is extremely gratifying, occupationally as or more successful than father, takes less than 2 days sick leave per year, considers current health excellent.

The attributes that Vaillant believes to be the principal determinants of success are the "adaptive (ego defense) mechanisms." The more mature a person's adaptive mechanisms, the greater the probability of future success. Vaillant's hierarchy of the maturity of the adpative mechanisms is listed in Table 1 [6].

Vaillant also shows a separate and significant relationship between each of the following and an individual's adjustment:

Warmth
Mental health of parents
Presence or absence of mental illness
General health
Taking enjoyable vacations

Curiously, Vaillant does not strongly consider the possibility that the adaptive mechanisms could be a manifestation of more fundamental determinants of good mental health, such as heredity and upbringing. He writes,

Table 1   Hierarchy of Adaptive Mechanisms

Mature mechanisms	
Altruism	Sublimation
Anticipation	Suppression
Humor	
Neurotic mechanisms	
Displacement	Reaction formation
Dissociation	Repression
Intellectualization	
Immature mechanisms	
Acting out	Passive-aggressive behavior
Fantasy	Projection
Hypochondriasis	
Psychotic mechanisms	
Delusional projection	Distortion
Denial	

Source: Modified from O. Vaillant. *Adaptation to Life.* Little, Brown, Boston, 1977, (Ref. 6).

"Man's adaptive devices are as important in determining the cause of his life as are his heredity, his upbringing, his social position and his access to psychiatric help" [6].

THE STAGES OF EARLY AND MIDDLE ADULTHOOD [1,4]

The predominant theme of development between the ages of 16 and 22 is independence from our parents. Between age 23 and 28 is a time "to explore the possibilities of adult life and to fashion a first, provisional life structure" [1]. This structure includes occupational specialization, marriage, starting a home, and parenthood. But, as Levenson writes: "No one can fully succeed in these tasks. For most . . . the life choices remain to be made, and the direction of life is uncertain or unsatisfactory" [1].

Age 28-34, which Levenson calls the "age 30 transition" and Gould associates with "opening up to what's inside," is a time of transition and re-evaluation. A series of quotes from Gould [4] elucidate some aspects of this period: "As we continue to gain greater competence in the outside world, we now listen with rapt attention to the inner strivings of our soul." "It is a time when we start to believe all the cliches we've been hearing for years, because we are starting to tune into some of the harsh realities of adult life for the first time." "We learn that life isn't fair, that sometimes no one is perfect, that sex isn't always romantic, that leopards don't change their spots, that experience and hard work do count, and that work isn't everything."

Age 35-45 is "the middle decade." Again, several quotes from Gould [4] are useful: "The sense of timelessness in our early 30's is giving way to an awareness of the pressure of time in our 40's. Whatever we do must be done now . . ." "We stand naked and exposed, toe to toe with life. Our naivete is lost forever. The illusion of our immortality is dying; in a crunch, no all-powerful hand is going to save us." "Up to this point, life was all uphill, with no thought of an end; now it is as if I am at the crown of the hill and can see the downslope for the first time. Death is a long way off, but it definitely is there." These sobering perceptions are the hallmark of this period. In view of this, the childish misconception that a promotion, or a rise in status, or an award, will make us invulnerable is both understandably common and a source of many disappointments. Another Gould insight is also noteworthy: "As we go from 35 to 45, it becomes clear, sometimes painfully clear, that we are the only, the final authority over the conduct of our own lives." Regarding the same phase, Vaillant [6] writes the following: "At 35 the men of the Grant Study could not wait to step into the driver's seat. At 50, they were far more concerned about those who worked for them and with them."

CONCLUSION

Many crucial aspects of adulthood have not been discussed here. They include marriage, parenthood, friendships, and work relationships. Although these subjects have a separate and extensive literature, each of these aspects of adulthood are colored by the themes of the stages of adulthood that we have discussed in this chapter. Although we are adults when we are 25 as well as when we are 50, and although there are constitutional and learned aspects of our characters which persist as leitmotifs throughout our lives, it is clear that we are not fully the "same people" when we are 20, 40, 60, or 80. Thus, our perceptions of ourselves and of our patients are all relative, and this may well affect the style of our patient care, and the style of our patients' responses, as our years unfold.

REFERENCES

1. Levenson, D. *The Seasons of Man's Life.* Knopf, New York (1978).
2. Erikson, E. *Childhood and Society.* Norton, New York (1950).
3. Benedek, T. *Psychoanalytic Investigations.* Quandrangle, New York (1973).

4. Gould, R. *Transformations*. Simon and Schuster, New York (1978).
5. Gould, R. The phases of adult life. A study in developmental psychology. *Am. J. Psychiatry* 129:33-43 (1972).
6. Vaillant, G. *Adaptation to Life*. Little, Brown, Boston (1977).

22

Aging

FREDERICK SIERLES

INTRODUCTION

Aging (senescence) is a gradual decline in physiological functioning as the years progress. It is debatable whether it begins with birth or in adulthood, and its causes are not known for sure. The decline in function varies in degree from individual to individual, and competence or excellence in behavior or other physiological functioning can be maintained by some at any age. For example, Slater and Roth [1] list da Vinci, Titian, Durer, Michelangelo, Voltaire, Goethe, Verdi, Renoir, and Picasso as examples of "artistic genius that continued to flower in old age."

Each year, the subject of aging becomes more important, because each year the number of elderly increases. In 1979, there were approximately 23 million people over 65, which represented 10% of the population. By the year 2030, it is expected that the elderly will comprise 20% of the population [2]. Reasons for this include the decline in birth rates, which means relatively smaller numbers of children and adolescents, and improved medical care, which enables more people to survive past the age of 65.

SOCIAL INFLUENCES

Important social influences on the elderly in America include low status, poverty, isolation, and poor accommodations. Weinberg [3] speaks of how our culture overemphasizes the future and overvalues what one "does" rather than what one "is like." In both cases, the elderly usually come out wanting, for their futures are limited and they are often retired or unemployed. Also, the elderly in contemporary America have had less formal schooling than the young [4], and the creation of trade schools has diminished the need for the elderly as teachers of trades.

Poverty is a major problem. Retirement means a 50-66% reduction in income, and pensions are fixed incomes susceptible to inflation. Only 25% of the aging are in the labor force, while in 1900, two-thirds of the elderly were employed [2]. A disproportionately large number of the elderly are agricultural workers [4]. While the aged comprise 10% of the total population in the United States, they make up 20% of our poor [2]. Over 5 million of the elderly cannot afford a telephone. The median income of older persons living alone or with nonrelatives was $3,311 per year in 1975 [2].

Isolation is a cause of loneliness. Many elderly have lost spouses and friends by death or disability. Some live alone because they are not wanted by their families; a contributing factor is the decline in existence of the multi-generation (extended) family. Others have to be alone because they are too disabled to travel by themselves to socialize. Also, the contemporary elderly are a cohort of people who are less accepting of psychiatric treatment [5]. The problem of isolation is more acute for women than for men, as there are about 138 women over 65 for every 100 men over 65 [4]. Of course, many of the elderly do not succumb to isolation; for example, there are more marriages among the elderly than ever before [6].

One in twenty of the elderly resides in an institution, usually a nursing home, and about 1 in 4 of the aged is in a nursing home at the time of his death [7]. This is a particular problem when nursing home care is substandard, as is frequently the case. Seventy-seven percent of nursing homes are run for profit [2], and many nursing home owners cut corners. Many nursing homes are understaffed and have few nurses. Eighty percent of nursing care is provided by nurses' aides and orderlies, and staff turnover rates are about 75% per year [2].

THE BIOLOGY OF AGING

Although life expectancy is increasing, it is largely the product of reducing infant and maternal death and death from infections, only modestly the result of inroads in prevention of diseases of the elderly, and probably not at all from reversal of the "aging process." Adams and Victor [8] write: "Since biblical times, when human beings were allotted three score and ten years, human life has not lengthened greatly." On reason that we have not been able to reverse the aging process is that we don't know much about it.

For example, we don't know whether aging is "programmed" into the cells and hence inevitable, whether it is the product of disease or other non-programmed events such as wear-and-tear, or some combination of both. Evidence for the programming theory comes from Hayflick and Moorhead [9], who demonstrated that human fibroblast cells, both *in vivo* and *in vitro*, underwent a fixed number of replications, regardless of environmental events (such as *in vitro* cold storage). Example of events, programmed or nonprogrammed, postulated to cause aging include DNA damage, mutation, formation of free radicals, formation of cross-linkages between molecules, wear-and-tear, accumulation of toxic metabolites, and impaired supply of nutrients [6,10].

Whatever the cause, the observable changes are clear. Shock [11] estimates anatomic and physiological decline from age 30 to 75 as shown in Table 1. Neuropathological changes associated with aging include decline in dendrites, neurofibrillary degeneration, granulovacuolar degeneration, lipofuscin accumulation, lewy bodies, hirano bodies, senile plaques, amyloid deposits, shrinkage of dendritic arbor, decrease of extracellular space, and corpora amylacea and myelin remodeling of the glia [8], as well as electroencephalogram slowing in the alpha, delta, and beta frequencies [3,6,8]. There is a decrease in the amount of rapid eye movement sleep, and stage 4 sleep almost disappears.

"Fluid intelligence" (problem-solving and reasoning when presented with new information) declines, while "crystallized intelligence" (accumulated knowledge of facts and concepts) increases until at least age 50 [12,13].

Table 1   Deterioration with Age

Physical characteristic	Percentage deterioration from age 30 to age 75
Number of taste buds	64
Power of hand grip	45
Vital capacity	44
Number of kidney glomeruli	44
Number of fibers in nerves	37
Glomerular filtration rate	31
Maximum rate of work	30
Resting cardiac output	30
Blood flow to brain	20
Total body water content	18
Basal metabolic rate	16
Body weight in men	12
Brain weight	10

Source: Modified from N. Shock. The physiology of aging. *Sci. Am.* 208:104, 1963 (Ref. 10).

In males, rapidity of achieving erection decreases, but duration of erection increases [11]. About 60% of married couples between age 60 and 74 are sexually active, although the figure drops to about 30% after age 75 [6]. Factors correlated with continuation of sex include higher socioeconomic status, better general health [6], availability of partners, and prior pregnancy and enjoyment of sex.

MEDICAL CONSIDERATIONS

Physicians treating the elderly are often faced with disease in multiple systems. This is related to the physiological changes catalogued previously, and to increased susceptibility to many categories of disease (e.g., cardiovascular disease, cancer, endocrine disease, coarse brain disease, and arthritis) [14]. The average hospital stay of an aged person is 11 days, as compared with 6 days for the rest of the population.

Despite these facts, the physician must realize that many conditions in the elderly are curable. For example, hearing loss can simply be the result of occlusion of the external auditory canals by cerumen. A number of conditions producing diffuse intellectual impairment are treatable, often with a good prognosis. These include: "depression, nonketotic hyperosmolarity diabetic syndrome; normal pressure hydrocephalus; pernicious anemia; malnutrition, often caused by the 'tea and toast' syndrome of the lonely, low-income older person; drug reactions; thyroid changes; environmental toxins; heart attacks; viral infections; anxiety; steroids; injuries, particularly head injuries due to falls; alcoholism; and brain surgery" [2]. Schuster [15] writes that the 5-year survival after cancer surgery is minimally affected by age per se, and Serpick [16] states: "From the standpoint of therapy, cancer should be regarded similarly in all age groups." And regarding psychiatric treatment, Feigenbaum [5] writes: "The evidence is that rates of improvement are of the same order as with younger age groups. What is more important is that rates of success are no worse than with the younger populations."

The elderly are more susceptible to side effects of drugs [17]. This is related to lower levels of serum albumen, decrease in renal clearance, and decreased activity of liver microsomal enzymes [17]. Physicians should routinely begin treatment of elderly patients with one-half to two-thirds of usual adult doses, monitoring plasma levels where feasible, and remaining extremely vigilant about drug side effects.

Physicians should also be aware that pain and fever are less effective warning signals of disease for the elderly. "Silent" myocardial infarctions, infections without fever, and other pathological phenomena may be missed by physicians relying too heavily on pain and fever in making diagnoses [18].

Checkups should be encouraged in these age groups, for patients and family are sometimes prone to attributing treatable disabilities to irreversible effects of age, or to withholding information about symptoms for fear that an examination will reveal something ominous [19]. Finally, attempts should be made to encourage physicians to treat and to respect the elderly, and not to practice "ageism" and what Butler [2] calls the "senile write-off." An anecdote from Butler is illustrative:

> "Consider the 101-year-old man who went to the doctor complaining that his right leg hurt. The doctor told him that hc had to expect that at this age. The man replied that his left leg was the same age as his right, but it didn't hurt [2]."

REFERENCES

1. Slater, E., and Roth, M. *Clinical Psychiatry*. Williams and Wilkins, Baltimore (1969).
2. Butler, R. Overview of aging, in *Aging: The process and the people*. G. Usdin, ed. Brunner/Mazel, New York (1978).
3. Weinberg, J. Geriatric psychiatry, in *Comprehensive Textbook of Psychiatry II*. A. Freedman, H. Kaplan, and B. Sadock, eds. Williams and Wilkins, Baltimore (1975).
4. Brotman, H. Who are the aging?, in *Mental Illness in Later Life*. E. Busse and E. Pfeiffer, eds. Am. Psychiatr. Assoc., Washington, D.C. (1973).
5. Feigenbaum, E. Ambulatory treatment of the elderly, in *Mental Illness in Later Life*. E. Busse and E. Pfeiffer, eds. Am. Psychiatr. Assoc., Washington, D.C. (1973).
6. Busse, E. Aging research. A review and critique, in *Aging: The process and the people*. G. Usdin, ed. Brunner/Mazel, New York (1978).
7. Kleh, J. When to institutionalize, in *The Geriatric Patient*. W. Reichel, ed. Hosp. Prac. Publ. Co. (1978).
8. Adams, R., and Victor, M. *Principles of Neurology*. McGraw-Hill, New York (1977).
9. Hayflick, L. and Moorhead, P. The serial cultivation of human diploid cells. *Exp. Cell Res.* 25:585-621 (1961).
10. Shock, N. Biological theories of aging, in *Handbook of the Psychology of Aging*. J. Birren, K. Schaie, and K. Warner, eds. Van Nostrand Reinhold, New York (1977).
11. Shock, N. The physiology of aging. *Sci. Am.* 206:100 (1962).
12. Horn, J., and Cattell, R. Age differences in fluid and crystallized intelligence. *Acta Psychol.* 26:107-219 (1967).
13. Eisdorfer, C. Psychophysiologic and cognitive studies in the aged in *Aging: The process and the people*. G. Usdin, ed. Brunner/Mazel, New York (1978).
14. Reichel, W. (ed). *The Geriatric Patient*. Hosp. Prac. Publ. Co., New York (1978).
15. Schuster, M. Disorders of the Aging GI system, in *The Geriatric Patient*. W. Reichel, ed. Hosp. Prac. Publ. Co., New York (1978).
16. Serpick, A. Cancer in the elderly, in *The Geriatric Patient*. W. Reichel, ed. Hosp. Prac. Publ. Co., New York (1978).
17. Lamy, P., and Vestal, R. Drug prescribing in the elderly, in *The Geriatric Patient*. W. Reischel, ed. Hosp. Prac. Publ. Co., New York (1978).

18. Reichel, W. Multiple problems in the elderly, in *The Geriatric Patient*. W. Reichel, ed. Hosp. Prac. Publ. Co., New York (1978).
19. Kornzweig, A. Visual loss in the elderly, in *The Geriatric Patient*. W. Reichel, ed. Hosp. Prac. Publ. Co., New York (1978).

23

Dying and Death

FREDERICK SIERLES

INTRODUCTION

Although death has been a subject of fascination from the beginning of recorded history, and although articles on psychology of dying have appeared sporadically in the medical literature for many years [1-5], the subject of the psychology of dying was not widely discussed or taught in medical school until the late 1960s. Kubler-Ross [6-8] and Saunders [1] are names associated with the popularization within the medical profession of the psychology of the dying. Kubler-Ross' 1969 book *On Death and Dying* [6] has reached the status of a classic. Before 1970, physicians rarely discussed the psychology of dying and often avoided treating or talking to dying patients. Today, the subject is frequently discussed and more options are considered in the treatment of dying patients. Whether physicians have become more available to dying patients is not clear.

SOMATIC DEATH AND BRAIN DEATH

Before the era of organ transplantation began in the 1960s, the diagnosis of death and the role of the physician with the dying patient were rarely subjects of controversy. Basically, death was associated with cessation of life functions and was readily "diagnosed" by a few simple diagnostic steps such as inspection for movement, assessment of the pupillary reflexes, auscultation for heart and bowel sounds, and palpation for pulses. The physician was expected to provide concerned care to the dying patient, fill out a death certificate, offer condolences, request permission for an autopsy from the relatives, and attend the autopsy.

Nowadays there are two "kinds" of deaths. The first, called "bodily" or "somatic" death, is what we have described above. The second is "brain death." This is a condition where the heart and kidneys are still functioning, and the lungs are being aerated by a mechanical ventilator, but the brain is totally nonfunctional; with brain death, bodily death is a virtual certainty within 3 months. Under such circumstances, some surgeons, with the consent of the properly designated next of kin, and employing the criteria to be presented below, will remove an organ such as a kidney for the purposes of transplantation. There are two sets of criteria for brain death, each of which has been employed in clinical settings. The Harvard criteria [9] will be quoted in detail. The Collaborative Study Criteria [9] will only be mentioned.

The Harvard Criteria for Brian Death [9]

1. *Unreceptivity and unresponsivity.* "Even the most intensely painful stimuli evoke no vocal or other response . . ."

2. *No movements or breathing.* "Observation covering a period of at least one hour by physicians is adequate to satisfy the criteria of no spontaneous muscular movements or spontaneous respiration or response to stimuli . . . the total absence of spontaneous breathing may be established by turning off the respirator for three minutes and observing whether there is any effort on the part of the subject to breathe . . ."

3. *No reflexes.* "The pupil will be fixed and dilated and will not respond to a direct source of bright light . . ." "Ocular movement (to head turning and to irrigation of ears with ice water) and blinking are absent." "There is no evidence of postural activity" (decerebrate or other). "Swallowing, yawning, vocalizing are in abeyance." "Corneal and pharyngeal reflexes are absent." "As a rule the stretch and tendon reflexes cannot be elicited."

4. *Flat electroencephalogram.* "Of great confirmatory value is the flat or isoelectric electroencephalogram." (Technical guidelines including SMV/min or higher gains, absence of response to pinch or noise, and 10-minute minimum recording time are added). "All of the above tests shall be repeated at least 24 hours later with no change." Hypothermia (temperatures below 32.2°C or 90°F) and central nervous system depressants such as barbiturates must be excluded.

Criteria for Cerebral Death (Brain Death) Proposed by the Collaborative Study of Cerebral Death of the National Institute of Neurological and Communicative Disorders and Stroke [9]

Prerequisite: All appropriate diagnostic and therapeutic procedures have been performed.

Criteria (to be present for 30 minutes at least 6 hours after the onset of coma and apnea):

1. Coma with cerebral unresponsivity
2. Apnea
3. Dilated pupils
4. Absent cephalic reflexes
5. Electrocerebral silence

Confirmatory test: Absence of cerebral blood flow.

At least five studies, some involving large numbers of patients, have shown that when the Harvard criteria are applied and the patient meets criteria for brain death, bodily death is inevitable within 3 months, with the exception of a handful of cases where the brain death resulted from drug intoxication [9]. Thus, if drug intoxication can be ruled out by historical and laboratory data, the Harvard criteria for brain death are predictive of bodily death 100% of the time [9]. Despite these statistical reassurances, many experienced physicians, particularly those who have been sued, prefer not to be involved in situations which involve the removal of organs from patients who meet criteria for brain death.

THE PSYCHOLOGY OF DYING

Kubler-Ross [6-8] wrote that all patients and their families go through progressive "stages of dying." These stages are as follows:

Denial

In denial, the patient or relative does not believe that the patient is going to die and may not even believe that he is ill, despite ample evidence to support these conclusions.

Example: A 50-year-old retired truck driver with metastatic lung cancer producing a 60-lb weight loss, and an associated progressive multifocal leukoencephalopathy producing paraplegia, states that he knows that he has lung cancer "but I'm not troubled by it. If only they'd get me to the point of walking again, I'd be all better."

Although denial may occasionally result in noncompliance with treatment or in shopping around for another doctor and another diagnosis, it is extremely common under these circumstances. If anosognosia (nonrecognition of illness) due to nondominant parietal lobe functioning can be ruled out, denial can be considered normal.

Anger

The patient realizes that he has a terminal illness, and experiences some anger in relation to the realization. The anger can be directed at himself (for not coming to the doctor soon enough, for smoking), at his family (for being able to survive him, for not suggesting medical care soon enough, for not being sufficiently understanding), at the doctors (for making the wrong diagnosis, for not being sufficiently candid or available), at life in general (for its unfairness), or at God in particular (for allowing the illness to happen).

> *Example:* A psychiatrist asks a sullen man, who has just stated that he has terminal cancer, "What are your thoughts about having the cancer?" This is a question that the psychiatrist has asked many times before with no previous problems. The patient responds with intense anger "That's a typical dumb psychiatrist's question!" and doesn't answer the question.

Bargaining

The patient takes the position that if he is on his best behavior (e.g., consents to all procedures, takes his medicine faithfully, cooperates fully with the staff), he will somehow be significantly rewarded. The expected reward is usually a longer life, but it may also be an afterlife in heaven, a cure for the illness, a peaceful or painless death, or good fortune for the survivors.

Depression

This is usually a reactive depression, associated with a sadness which is appropriate to the anticipation of dying.

> *Example:* A middle-aged man has just stated, with a somber look on his face, that he knows he is dying. When asked how he feels about this, tears well to his eyes, and he asks, plaintively, "How *could* I feel?"

Medically treatable endogenous depression must be ruled out. The patient may feel like a burden, and this is the time when suicide, if it is to occur, is most likely. However, the risk of suicide isn't much more common in dying patients than in other patients.

Acceptance

The patient accepts the idea of his impending death, and may withdraw from others in anticipation of death. He may prefer not to be visited, or not to talk when visited.

Not all patients go through all of these stages, particularly those who become seriously ill suddenly. The relatives and others close to the patient also go through these stages, although not necessarily at the same time as the patient. For this reason it is sometimes easier to be open with the patient than with a relative (or vice versa).

I believe that the majority of patients manifest features of several of the stages simultaneously. Kubler-Ross wrote that these stages often were not well circumscribed. The usefulness of this psychological "staging" is that it provides a memorable description of common psychological reactions to dying, so the physician can know what to expect. These responses are probably not unique to dying, since they occur in response to other threatening events as well. There are many classic descriptions of responses to threatening events and the descriptions overlap, as portrayed in Table 1.

THE TREATMENT OF DYING PATIENT (AND OTHER LIVING PATIENTS)

In Kubler-Ross' *Questions and Answers on Death and Dying* [7], a question is asked about why, given the limited amounts of time available to medical personel, anybody should advocate devoting more time to dying patients, at the expense of living patients. Kubler-Ross' answer, that dying patients *are* living patients, provides the crucial idea of the remainder of this chapter.

Interviewing Dying Patients

The interview principles are the same as for other patients. One of the principles is that you can ask just about anything, as long as the question is asked tactfully, is relevant, and reasonably well timed. Thus, if a patient says that he is dying, it is reasonable to ask him how he feels about dying. On the other hand, if a patient offers that he doesn't think that his condition is serious, it would be inappropriate to follow up that statement with a question about his philosophy of death. In order to assess what the patient knows about is diagnosis and prognosis, it is usually safe to ask "What kind of illness do you think you have?" or "What do you expect is going to happen to you?"

Table 1 Descriptions of Mourning Syndromes

Author	Sadness	Crying	Withdrawal	Anger	Anorexia and weight loss	Insomnia	Guilt	Identification	Motor retardation	Major Characteristics
Freud: Mourning and Melancholia (10)	✓		✓	✓			✓	✓		Sadness; decreased interest and activity; loss of libido
Lindmann: The Acute Grief Reaction (11)	✓	✓	✓	✓			✓	✓		Somatic distress; preoccupation with the image of the deceased; guilt; hostile reactions; loss of usual patterns of conduct
Spitz: Anaclitic Depression in Children (12)		✓	✓		✓	✓			✓	1. Weeping, demanding, and clinging. 2. Wailing, weight loss, and arrest of developmental quotient. 3. Lying prone, refusal of contact, insomnia, motor retardation, and susceptibility to illness
Bowlby: Mourning in Children (13)		✓	✓	✓						1. Protest 2. Despair 3. Apathy
Lifton: Survivors of Hiroshima (14)			✓	✓			✓			Imprint and activation; guilt and expiation; numbing; identification with the aggressor; explanation; scapegoating, mission
Kubler-Ross: On Death and Dying (6)	✓	✓	✓	✓			✓			1. Denial 2. Anger 3. Bargaining 4. Depression 5. Acceptance
Clayton: Normal Bereavement (15)	✓	✓	✓		✓	✓	✓			Depressed mood; sleep disturbance; crying

Giving a Diagnosis and Prognosis

The responsibility for providing a diagnosis and prognosis rests with the physician in charge of the patient's care, and it should not be relinquished or delegated under usual circumstances. Although there is no "sure-fire" formula for deciding what to tell the patient, I believe that flexibility is the watchword—the decision should be tailored to meet the needs of the situation. Let us begin by giving two examples of situations where it is logical to tell the patient his diagnosis or prognosis.

Informed Consent

Patients are entitled to know why procedures are being performed, and this usually includes provision of a diagnosis.

Example: A woman with a small breast mass is scheduled for a breast biopsy and frozen microscopic section under general anesthesia. She signs a written consent for "breast biopsy with possible radical mastectomy if the tumor is malignant," and the surgeon discusses this with her at length.

Questions From the Patient

Although there are exceptions, when people ask questions they usually want to know the answers, and the answers should be provided.

Example: A psychiatrist is called in consultation by a neurosurgeon because a patient is sad and easily annoyed. The patient has a visceral cancer, and knows it, but doesn't know that he has a brain metastasis as well. Early in the interview, the patient states that she cannot understand why her cognitive functions have decreased, and becomes insistent about being told the reason. The psychiatrist recommends to the neurosurgeon that he tell the patient about the metastasis immediately.

Anxious Patient With Precarious Cardiac Function

Here is an example where the physician might postpone giving the patient a detailed diagnosis and prognosis.

Example: A patient is admitted to an intensive care unit with an extensive myocardial infarction associated with atrial fibrillation. He appears quite anxious, talks spontaneously, knows that he is quite ill, and cooperates fully with the staff's requests, but doesn't ask for a diagnosis. During the admission interview, the physician tells him "You have heart trouble and your heart is beating irregularly," but doesn't say at that time that there is heart muscle damage or that the prognosis is guarded. He might reveal the latter to the patient if the patient were to ask.

Two studies [2,3] have been done to answer the question: "Should the patient be told?" In one [2], patients who had been told they had cancer were asked how they felt about having been told. In the other [3], the diagnosis was given to every other patient with cancer, and was withheld from the rest of the sample. The methodology of both studies was flawed, but it is worth noting that the great majority of patients in both studies, whether or not they were told the diagnosis, did not show psychiatric sequelae, thus showing a certain resiliency on the part of most of the patients regardless of what they were told. A few patients who were not told the diagnosis found out anyway and resented the withholding of information. A few patients who were given the diagnosis became noticeably upset and wished they hadn't been told, but these were exceptions.

MANAGEMENT OF COMPLICATIONS

Marks and Sachar [16], in a study of medical inpatients with pain (only some of whom had cancer or were dying), found that 37% continued to have severe distress due to pain after treatment was begun, and 41% continued to have moderate distress. They felt that most of the patients had been under-medicated wth analgesics. For example, although the pharmacologic literature records that 62-72 mg meperidine (Demerol) every 2-4 hr relieves pain in only two-thirds of cases, many of the patients in their sample who were taking meperidine were receiving doses of only 50 mg every 4 hr. In addition, they quoted reports that only 3% of addicts became addicted as a result of medical treatment, and felt that the actual figure is probably even lower.

For patient with rapidly developing brain metastatis and consequent cerebral edema and cognitive dysfunction, parenteral corticosteroids may diminish the edema and permit a several-day-long restoration of cognitive function sufficent to attend to some unfinished business.

Some less-than-traditional forms of treatment have been employed. In a double-blind crossover study, Sallan, Zinberg, and Frai [17] found that capsules of tetrahydrocannabinol were significantly better than placebo for management of nausea and vomiting secondary to cancer chemotherapy. Saunders [1], the long-term director of the St. Christopher's Hospice in London, uses Brompton's solution (a mixture of heroin, cocaine, alcohol and flavoring) for patients with intractable pain [18]. Of course, the use of heroin is illegal in the United States. Kast and Collins]19] found LSD to be an effective analgesic, but their study was not controlled.

ALTERNATIVES TO HEROIC MEASURES FOR PROLONGING LIFE

Most Americans die in the hospital, often while receiving considerable mechanical assistance from respirators, catheters, intravenous feedings, or nasogastric tubes. This is expensive and not necessary in the eyes of many, although it may be the only option or the best option in many cases. For patients, physicians, and families interested in alternatives, there are some: Patients can also choose to die at home or in a hospice. Hospices are homes for the dying in which emotional support and palliative care are the only treatment offered. The best-known of these are the St. Christopher's Hospice in London and the hospice in Fall River, Massachusetts. Unfortunately only a limited number of localities have hospices.

Other alternatives have been presented as well. Imbus and Zawacki [20] describe a choice which is given to patients admitted with burns so extensive that survival would be unprecedented. Soon after admission, these patients are told that survival would be unprecedented, and offered a choice between palliative treatment and an all-out effort to prolong life. The decision must be made at that time, because of the virtual certainty of an ensuing delirium. The authors report that most of the patients choose palliative treatment. Rabkin, Gillerman, and Rice [21] write that "orders not to resuscitate" may be written in a patint's chart, but only (1) if the illness can be expected to produce death within a year; (2) if the patient, having been properly informed while competent, has requested such orders and documented this with his signature; and (3) if the patient has not made such a request, the properly designated next-of-kin has given informed consent and documented this with his signature. Finally, there is the "living will" [22], a signed statement requesting that no heroic measures be taken once death is believed likely. The "order not to resuscitate" has been supported by the Dinnerstein decision [23] in the state of Massachusetts; however, the legal status of the living will has not yet been tested in court. Some hospitals have established special committees [24] to provide consultation to physicians faced with weighty problems relating to matters such as these.

SUICIDE AND THE RIGHT TO DIE

The precedent of patients deciding against heroic life-prolonging measures is not new and not confined to the above situations. For at least a decade, patients undergoing hemodialysis have had the option of discontinuing the hemodialysis as long as they are legally competent to do this and a reasonable effort has been made to convince the patient of the need for dialysis. Where does the refusal of heroic measures end and suicide begin? Suicide is usually the product of psychiatric illness such as endogenous depression, and usually is an active attempt to die over and above the refusal of heroic efforts in a medically hopeless case. To distinguish between the two, a complete psychiatric evaluation should be made, and the patient should be asked if he would actively try to end his life if the refusal of a medical procedure were not an option. Since suicide is usually the product of psychiatric illness, and is sometimes associated with a need on the part of a patient to control the time and mode of his death [6,7], efforts should be made to treat the psychiatric illness and prevent the suicide. This subject is discussed at length in Chapter 28.

PREDILECTION FOR DEATH AND VOODOO DEATH

These are rare phenomena which have only been anecdotally documented, but are intriguing nevertheless. In 1961, Weisman and Hackett [4] reported six cases of people who told their physician that they looked forward to dying, and that they expected to due during the surgery. They were not actively suicidal, and they were calm about what they were saying. All of them did die, either on the operating table or soon afterwards. Weisman and Hackett believed that based upon these patients' life circumstances and attitudes, death was a logical event. For example, one man's raison d'etre was in learning of the death of certain people he regarded as his enemies because they, as a group, had mistreated him when he was young. His "predilection" statement, and ensuing death, followed the death of the last member of the group of malefactors. Because of a belief in this "predilection" phenomenon, many senior surgeons postpone elective surgery on patients who calmly state that they expect to die on the operating table.

In 1942, Cannon [5] described several cases of what he called "voodoo death." In this situation, an otherwise healthy individual, believing himself to be the victim of a fatal curse, withdraws in fear, and death soon follows. Richter [25] was able to produce sudden death in rats by holding the rats over a trough. He noted that prior to their deaths, the rats manifested bradycardia, indicating to him that the voodoo death phenomenon may be the product of giving up, with its associated parasympathetic overactivity, not the result of fear with sympathetic overactivity as postulated by Cannon.

REFERENCES

1. Saunders, C. Care of the dying (6 parts). *Nurs. Times.* Oct. 9 to Nov. 13 (1959).

2. Altken-Swan, J. and Easson, E. Reactions of cancer patient on being told their diagnosis. *Br. Med. J.* 1:779-783 (1959).

3. Gerle, B., Lunden, G., and Sandblom, P. The patient with inoperable cancer from psychiatric and social standpoints. *Cancer* 13:1206-1217 (1960).

4. Weisman, A., and Hackett, T. Predilection to death. *Psychosom. Med.* 23:232-255 (1961).

5. Cannon, W. Voodoo death. *Psychosom. Med.* 19:182 (1957).

6. Kubler-Ross, E. *On Death and Dying.* MacMillan, New York (1969).

7. Kubler-Ross, E. *Questions and Answers on Death and Dying.* Macmillan, New York (1974).

8. Kubler-Ross, E. *Death: The final stage of growth.* Prentice-Hall, Englewood Cliffs, N.J. (1975).

9. Black, P. *Brain death.* N. Engl. J. Med. Aug., 299:875-878 (1978).

10. Freud, S. Mourning and melacholia, in *The Meaning of Despair.* W. Gaylin, Ed. Science, New York (1968).

11. Lindemann, E. Symptomatology and management of acute grief. *Am. J. Psychiatry* Sept. 101:141-148 (1944).

12. Spitz, R. *The First Year of Life.* Int. Univ., New York (1965).

13. Bowlby, J. Childhood mourning. *Am. J. Psychiatry* 118:481-498 (1961).

14. Lifton, R. *Death in Life: Survivors of Hiroshima.* Simon and Schuster, New York (1967).

15. Clayton, P., Halikas, J., Maurice, W., and Robins, E. Anticipatory grief and widowhood. *Br. J. Psychiatry* 122:47-56 (1973).

16. Marks, R., and Sachar, E. Undertreatment of medical inpatients with narcotic analgesics. *Ann. Intern. Med.* 78:173-181 (1973).

17. Sallen, S., Zinberg, N., and Frai, E. Antiemetic effect of THC in patients receiving cancer chemotherapy. *N. Engl. J. Med.* 293:795-797 (1975).

18. Stoddard, S. *The Hospice Movement.* Stein and Day, New York (1978).

19. Kast, E., and Collins, V. Lysergic acid diethylamide as an analgesic agent. *Anesth. Analg.* 43:285-291 (1964).

20. Imbus, S., and Zawacki, B. Autonomy for burned patients when survival is unprecedented. *N. Engl. J. Med.* 297:308-311 (1977).

21. Rabkin, M., Gillerman, G., and Rice, N. Orders not to resuscitate. *N Engl. J Med.* 295:3364-3366 (1976).

22. Bok, S. Personal directions for care at the end of life. *N. Engl. J. Med.* 295:367-369 (1976).

23. Schrom, R., Kane, J., and Roble, D. No code orders. Clarification in the aftermath of Saikewitz. *N. Engl. J. Med.* 875-878 (1978).

24. MCH Clinical Care Committee. Optimum care for hopelessly ill patients. *N. Engl. J. Med.* 295:362-364 (1976).

25. Richter, C. On the phenomenon of sudden death in animals and man. *Psychosom. Med.* 19:191 (1957).

Part V

Social Sciences, Social Problems, and
Social Systems

24

Medical Sociology

FREDERICK SIERLES

INTRODUCTION

Medical sociology is the study of how being in categories like social class, ethnic group, religion, and occupation affects the definition, incidence, prevalence, manifestations, and treatment of illness. Physicians should know about medical sociology because it contributes to understanding the multiple causes of illness and provides information about what illnesses and patient care problems to look out for. For example, although infection with the tubercle bacillus is a necessary cause of tuberculosis, tuberculosis is largely a disease of the poor and disadvantaged, who are more likely to be infected by the bacillus, are more susceptible to its effects, and are slower in reporting its symptoms to a doctor. In this chapter, I will present the core concepts of medical sociology, then catalogue correlations between social factors and the definition, incidence, manifestations, and treatment of illness, concluding with a discussion of some of the causes of these correlations.

CORE CONCEPTS

A number of definitions are in order. A *social class* is a category of people with similar economic opportunities, prestige, and power. Although most people find the notion of social classes to be undemocratic [1,2], they readily agree that certain people have better opportunities than others. Different sociologists perceive different numbers of social classes, and most think of a continuum. In this chapter, the system of Hollingshead [1] will be used; this system delineates the following five social classes:

Class 1	Upper
Class 2	
Class 3	Middle
Class 4	
Class 5	Lower

There is general agreement among sociologists about the membership of the upper class (executives of very prosperous corporations, high-ranking professionals) and the lower-lower class (chronically unemployed people or transiently employed unskilled laborers), but less agreement about the classes in between. It is generally felt that greater proportions of Americans belong to the middle class than ever before. *Socioeconomic status* is the degree of prestige associated with membership in the various social classes; it is frequently used synonymously with the term social class.

There is also variation among sociologists about criteria for social class assignment. Rainwater [2] weighs income (weighted by a factor of .57), occupation (weighted by a factor of .29), and education (weighted by a factor of 10) most heavily. Hollingshead [1,3] weighs occupation (weighted by a factor of 9), residence (weighted by a factor of 6), and education (weighted by a factor of 5) most heavily. Hollingshead has employed both a two-factor *index of social position* (occupation and education) and a three-factor index of social position (occupation, residence, and education) in his research.

Social mobility is the degree to which an individual is rising or falling in the social class hierarchy. Rising in the hierarchy is called *upward* mobility, and is often the product of obtaining education and postponing gratifications. An example is the child of a high school teacher going to medical school and becoming a physician. *Downward mobility* refers to falling in the hierarchy. Severe chronic illness sometimes results in a fall in social class; for example, patients with schizophrenia tend, as a group, to be of a lower class than that of their fathers. In the United States, there is considerably social mobility. In contrast, in a *caste system* (1940s India), the social classes are formalized and mobility between castes is prohibited.

An *ethnic group* is a group with a common national origin, religion, language, and traditions; often, there are typical external physical characteristics. *Prejudice* is the process of prejudging people without knowing what they are really like. Prejudice often diminishes an individual's opportunities, such as by exclusion from jobs or medical care. Often it affects an individual's self-esteem. Clark [4] reported that black children preferred white dolls to black dolls. When presented to the Supreme Court, this data played a part in the Court's 1954 *Brown vs. Board of Education* school integration decision. Prejudice can result in an individual functioning below his capability. Victims of prejudice are often members of highly visible minority groups, who may themselves practice self-segregation and who may themselves become prejudiced as a means of defense [5].

Adorno et al. [6] identified an authoritarian personality which is characteristic of prejudiced people. Brody [5] summarizes the authoritarian personality as follows:

> This personality type was described as one needing strong external supports, depending on conventional values, and sensitive to interpersonal status criteria and dominance . . . Related features are uncritical submission to dominant group authorities, punitive reactions to violators of conventional norms, cognitive rigidity, cynicism, tendency to projection, and unusual interest in the sexual behavior of others [5].

Segregation fosters prejudice and integration diminishes it. Prejudice may be decreased by having members of different groups participate with equal status in tasks with a common goal.

A *stereotype* is an exaggeration or caricature of characteristics believed to be associated with membership in a group. Scientific data can be misused to generate stereotypes, and stereotyping and prejudice often go hand-in-hand.

A *role* is a position or situation which has a series of rights and obligations. Most people occupy at least several roles simultaneously. For example, I am a husband, father, son, nephew, uncle, son-in-law, doctor, teacher, researcher, administrator, patient, colleague, friend, and employee. Obligations of different roles may be in conflict with each other at a given time . . . this is called *role conflict* [7], and the conflicting pressures on the individual are called *cross-pressures*. For example, physician-teachers in a medical school should be wary of—and avoid whenever possible—treating (doctor role) medical students whom they are simultaneously teaching and giving grades (administrator role) based on impressions of clinical performance. Military physicians are frequently faced with the conflict between being doctors and being military personnel; for example, what does a military physician do when a patient is homosexual, knowing that homosexuals are not permitted to serve in the armed forces? The best solution to the problem of role conflict for physicians is, wherever feasible, to assume only one of the roles, inform the patient about which role is being taken, and reject the other roles with which it is in conflict. For example, the physician-teacher can treat the student and delegate the grading responsibility to a colleague (or vice versa), or treat the homosexual and not report the homosexuality.

The rights and obligations associated with being ill (the *sick role*) were described by Parsons [8]: The person in the sick role is not held responsible for this incapacity, is excused from obligations which may exacerbate his condition, is expected to want to get better, and is expected to seek technically competent help.

Kasl and Cobb [9] have provided the following additional definitions:

> *Health behavior* is any activity undertaken by a person believing himself to be healthy, for the purpose of preventing disease or detecting it at a asymptomatic stage ... *Illness behavior* is any activity undertaken by a person who feels ill to define the state of health and to discover a suitable remedy ... *Sick role behavior* is the activity undertaken by those who consider themselves ill for the purpose of getting well [9].

A *cultural norm* is a standard of conduct. This is different from the statistical norm, which represents the statistical mean, or average. What is normal for one group is not necessarily normal for another group. For example, among poor Chicanos in San Antonio, it is acceptable to seek help from a curandera for backaches, whereas this is inappropriate behavior for a middle-class "anglo" in San Antonio.

Sociocultural integration [10] is said to occur when the basic functions of a society, such as subsistence, protection, and communications are being performed competently. *Sociocultural disintegration* is said to occur when these functions are not performed competently, and is associated with the following:

> Poverty
> Frequent migration
> Failure of communications
> Population increase
> Lack of leadership
> Broken homes
> Strikes
> Fragmentation and confusion of shared values (anomie, or normlessness)
> Rise in crime
> Maternal deprivation
> Increased stress

This in turn is associated with an increase in the incidence and prevalence of illness, especially illnesses associated with infections, accidents, malnutrition, and poor obstetrical care. As a result of the increased illness, a vicious cycle begins, with a decrease in competence of performance of the society's basic health-related functions [10].

The *family* is the basic unit of reproduction, nurturance, and the transmission of cultural norms. A *nuclear family* consists of a married couple and their children. An *extended family* consists of three or more generations living together. In America during the past several decades there has been a decreased proportion of extended families and an increased percentage of nuclear families. Some critics of our society feel that this has had a negative effect, since the extended family offers the benefits of more people sharing in family tasks, greater emotional closeness, and an increased sense of usefulness for grandparents. A *primary family* is a family where the family head is the head of the household; a *secondary family* is a family where the head is not the head of the household (*household* is a dwelling unit like an apartment or private home) [11].

Finally, there are several social sciences which need to be defined. *Ethnomedicine* is the study of how ethnic group membership influences the definition, incidence and prevalence, manifestations, treatment, and prognosis of illness; it is medical sociology applied to ethnic groups. One publication, Williams' *Textbook of Black-Related Diseases* [12] is noteworthy because it is devoted entirely to the illnesses of a single ethnic group. *Social psychiatry* is a medical sociology as it applies to the medical specialty of psychiatry. *Social psychology* is the study of how people behave in groups.

SOCIAL INFLUENCES ON THE DEFINITION, INCIDENCE, MANIFESTATIONS, AND TREATMENT OF ILLNESS

Social Factors and the Definition of Illness

What is considered a disease in one group may not be considered a disease in another: Among several South American tribes, there is a skin condition called dyschromic spirochetosis (pinta) which is considered normal and which increases the marriageability of the people who have it [13]. In our culture obesity is considered pathological, whereas it was admired in others (witness the paintings of Rubens and Renoir). Among graduate and medical students, chronic tiredness is considered normal and even a mark of diligence, whereas under certain conditions it may be a sign of a serious illness (e.g., sleep apnea). According to Mechanic [14], in some primitive cultures, some people with mental illness are chosen to be priests (but in New Hebrides, they were buried alive). Zola [15] states that among Chicanos in the Southwest, diarrhea, sweating, and coughing are considered normal, and also that low back pain is considered normal by many women of low socioeconomic status. Grier and Cobbs [16] describe a "black norm" whereby most American blacks experience chronic low-grade sadness, mistrust, and anger. Ninety percent of a supposedly "physically healthy" sample had a physical aberration or clinical disorder, raising the question Is illness the statistical norm? [15].

Low Socioeconomic Status and Illness

Of all the correlations between social categories and illness, those between lower social class and illness have been reported most extensively [1,17-20]. Compared with people of higher socioeconomic status, people of lower socioeconomic status have higher rates of parental death, separation, and divorce, more women as household heads, and greater sex role differentiation. They are less biologically sophisticated.

They are less apt to eat a balanced diet, go for health checkups for which they have to pay a fee, get free polio vaccine, go for preventive dental visits, get orthodontic care, get early prenatal care when pregnant, and get examined to see if they need eyeglasses. They have higher infant mortality rates. They are more apt to be born prematurely, to be mentally retarded, to be obese and to be chronically ill. They have a higher prevalence of sociopathy, Briquet's syndrome and schizophrenia. They are more likely to be diagnosed as psychotic than people of higher socioeconomic status.

Whether or not they are ill, they have a decreased chance of describing and reporting themselves as ill. When ill, they are more apt to be referred for medical care by a friend or relative (as opposed to being self-referred). They are more apt to have medically unattended conditions and to delay reporting cancer-revealing symptoms. They are more apt to use nonmedical personnel for the treatment of illness, and more apt to practice self-medication. When they have a psychiatric illness, the presenting symptom is more likely to be a physical one. They have more body preoccupations, are more psychologically dependent upon others, are more crisis-oriented, and are less able to plan for the future and adhere to time-bound schedules.

They they are admitted to the hospital, they are sicker and have longer hospital stays. They are more apt to be treated in wards than in private rooms, and in government-run hospitals than private hospitals. They are more likely to be treated by a "committee" [17] of house staff and medical students, and less likely to be treated by a committed [17] private doctor. They are apt to be spoken to differently by physicians. When they have psychiatric illnesses, they are more apt to be treated in a hospital and with medications (as opposed to being treated as an outpatient with psychotherapy), and are less likely to be liked by the person who is treating them. For all the above reasons, small wonder their life expectancy is shorter! Some possible causes of the above correlations will be discussed later in this chapter.

Ethnic Group and Illness

Milunsky [22] compiled a list of genetically transmitted conditions quency in blacks; this is provided in Table 1.

Mulunsky [22] compiled a list of genetically transmitted conditions associated with a number of ethnic groups; this is seen in Table 2.

Zborowski [23] wrote that Jewish-Americans and Italian-Americans tended to have a low pain threshold and low pain tolerance, as compared with Irish-Americans and white Protestant "old Americans," who tended to be stoic about pain. He felt that the Jews were more apt to be concerned about the prognostic implications of the pain (future orientation), tending not to feel relief when the doctor arrived, and to feel better only when the prognosis was felt to be good. In contrast, the Italians were annoyed about the pain the here-and-now (present orientation), and did not feel relief when the doctor came. He thought that the diminished pain threshold and pain tolerance of the Italians and Jews were learned in childhood, with the parents exhorting their children to avoid colds, fights, and injuries. He thought

Table 1   Some Conditions with an Unusually High or Low Frequency in Blacks

Frequent	*Infrequent*
Single-gene disorders	
G6PD	Cystic fibrosis
Sickle cell disease, e.g., S.S. SC, SD,	Hemophilia
SE, S thal, S Hb F	Phenylketonuria
α-Thalassemia	Wilson's disease
β-Thalassemia (African type)	Hereditary spherocytosis
Persistent Hb F	
Multifactorial disorders	
Cervical cancer	Cogenital hip disease
Esophageal cancer	Major central nervous system malformations
Hypertension	Multiple sclerosis
Polydactyly	Otosclerosis
Prehelical fissure	Osteoporosis and fracture of hip and spine
Sarcoidosis	Polycythemia vera
Systemic lupus erythematosus	Psoriasis
Tuberculosis	Skin cancer
Uterine fibroids	Pyloric stenosis
Keloids	Suicide
Lactose intolerance	Leukemia

Source: From R. Murray. Medical genetics and black-related disease, in *A Textbook of Black-Related Diseases*, R. Williams, ed. McGraw-Hill, 1975, with permission.

Table 2   Ethnically Related Genetic Disorders

Ethnic group	Disorders found with relatively high frequency
African	Hemoglobinopathies, especially Hb S, Hb C, α and β-thalassemia, persistent Hb F G6PD deficiency, African type Adult lactase deficiency
Afrikaners (South Africans)	Variegate porphyria
Armenians	Familial Mediterranean fever
Ashkenazic Jews	Abetalipoproteinemia Bloom's syndrome Dystonia musculorum deformans (recessive form) Familial dysautonomia Factor XI (PTA) deficiency Gaucher's disease (adult form) Iminoglycinuria Meckel's syndrome Niemann-Pick disease Pentosuria Spongy degeneration of brain Stub thumbs Tay-Sachs disease
Chinese	α-thalassemia G6PD deficiency, Chinese type Adult lactase deficiency
Eskimos	$E_1{}^S$ (pseudocholinesterase deficiency)
Finns	Congenital nephrosis
Irish	Neural tube defects
Japanese (Koreans)	Acatalasia Oguchi's disease Dyschromatosis universalis hereditaria
Mediterranean peoples (Italians, Greeks, Sephardic Jews)	Thalassemia (mainly β) G6PD deficiency, Mediterranean type Familial Mediterranean fever Type III glycogen storage disease
Norwegians	Cholestasis-lymphedema

Source: From A. Milunsky (ed.). The causes and prevalence of mental retardation, in *The Prevention of Genetic Disease and Mental Retardation.* Saunders, Philadelphia, 1975, with permission (Ref. 22).

that the old Americans also had a future orientation when they experienced pain, although they tended not to dramatize their suffering.

Zola [24], comparing sick role behaviors of Irish-Americans and Italian-Americans, described the following: The Irish are more apt to view themselves as sick; to have their complaints for a longer time; to have ear, nose, and throat symptoms as a chief complaint (no matter what the general symptom picture); and to have a more stoic or denial-based response to illness. In contrast, Italians were more apt to have more symptoms with a given diagnosis, to complains of more body areas being affected, to complain of more dysfunction due to the symptoms, to say the illness was more strongly affecting their personal life, and to present their symptoms more dramatically. Suchman [25] wrote that Irish-Americans are more dependent when they become ill, as compared with other groups.

Regarding ethnic group and the treatment of illness, Lieberson [26] demonstrated that physicians were more likely than others to practice medicine among members of their own ethnic group. Lieberson's study was done in 1950, and did not include members of currently disadvantaged urban minorities. But if the principle holds true, accepting more minority students into medical school by affirmative action may be a means of producing physicians for medically underserved urban minority ghettos.

Occupation and Illness

Appendix 2 lists some occupations and diseases that are statistically associated [28]. Special attention should be paid to the occupation of physician [28-30]: Physicians are more likely than the general population to get incomplete physical examinations, to be drug abusers, and to die in light plane crashes, and women physicians are more likely to commit suicide. suicide.

They are less likely to seek help for serious diseases, and less likely when hospitalized to seek help from the hospital staff. They are more likely to quit smoking. And contrary to rumor, they are no more likely to be divorced.

Social Setting and Illness

The setting in which an illness or injury occurs may influence the manifestations of that illness. Soldiers in battle [31,32] and professional and college athletes have a higher pain tolerance when injured than do people in more ordinary situations. The following is a quote from Lt. Col. Anthony Herbert on one of his Korean War experiences:

I felt the wind rush from my lungs; the force of my movement tore his rifle from his hands. It sailed past me into the rim of the hole, but it left its bayonet sticking in my side. I pounded his head into pulp, not realizing what he had done to me . . ."

"We did it, Herb, we broke out," he yelled, "come in, get the jeep and let's get the hell out of here." I got in and noticed the look on his face. "For Christ's sake, Herb, what's that in your side?" he asked. I looked down and realized for the first time what had happened. [32]

Folk Medicine

Folk medicine is the term applied to the many and varied practices outside of the medical establishment or in societies with no medical establishment. Folk medicine is practiced to a surprising extent in the United States and other industrialized countries. It reveals an "impressive array of practices" [33] that demonstrate empirical therapeutic knowledge and whose use has either been adopted by the medical profession, or independently discovered by folk healers and members of the medical profession.

These practices include "trephining; bonesetting; removal of ovaries; obstetrics, including Caesarian section, laparotomy, uvulectomy; comparative anatomy; autopsy; cautery; inoculations; baths; inhalations; laxatives; enemas; ointments; and cupping" [33]. The drugs used in folk medicine include "quinine, opium, coca, cinchona, copaiba, curare, chaulmoogra oil, ephedrine, and rauwolfia" [33].

Folk theories of the etiology of illness can be categorized as *personalistic* and *naturalistic*. In a personalistic theory of illness, sickness and health are the products of one's interpersonal relationships and relationships with deities. The concept of mal ojo, a syndrome to be discussed shortly, is a product of a personalistic system. In a naturalistic theory, there is a disharmony or imbalance of nature within one's own body. This perspective is central to Chinese acupuncture, with its theory of a balance of "yin" and "yang," and in ancient Hippocratic medicine, with its theory of a balance of four basic "humours." There are analogues of both categories in modern scientific medicine as well.

Folk medicine concerns itself with the diagnosis and treatment of disease as well as disease etiology. Members of an ethnic group or society may assign a separate diagnosis, attribute a different etiology, and provide a different treatment to a syndrome commonly recognized by the world's medical community, although there is no scientific evidence for creating a separate syndrome. Such conditions are referred to as *culture-bound disorders*. There are numerous examples. For example, among some Mexicans and Chicanos, there are the syndromes susto, mal puesto, embrujada, caida de mollera, and mal ojc [33,35]. The latter, mal ojo ("evil eye"), has counterparts in Italians and other Mediterranean Europeans, Israelis, and Arabs. In Mexico, it is commonly identified in children with chills and fever, attributed to someone looking enviously at a child, and treated by a curandera. Among Italians, it may appear as a psychosis.

Many ethnic groups have folk healers. For Chicanos, the healer is a curandera or espiritista. For American Indians, the curer is a medicine man. For blacks, folk healers include old ladies, spiritualists, or hungans (voodoo priests). Jordan [36] discusses black voodoo medicine and includes a 13-page list of illnessess and their voodoo remedies.

Alegria et al. [37] interviewed 16 Chicano curers in San Antonio. A majority were women, over 40, and retired. Their offices were located in their homes, which in turn were located in the neighborhoods in which they practiced. Their fees ranged from $3-$8 per visit. They treated culture-bound illnesses, as well as backaches, insomnia, and other common complaints. Occasionally, they would treat people for hypertension or diabetes, but only after the patient became disenchanted with conventional medical care. They were seen by Alegria and co-workers as reasonable individuals who were willing to make referrals to physicians. Although a few achieve a measure of fame, most are unknown outside of their city.

Because illness and treatment are not viewed identically in all ethnic groups and locations, it is important that medical administrators establishing a medical facility in an unfamiliar community take in account not only the incidence and prevalence of illnesses in the community, but also the belief systems of the community and the medical and folk healing resources of that community. They should include members of the community in the planning process.

POSSIBLE REASONS FOR THE RELATIONSHIP BETWEEN SOCIAL FACTORS AND ILLNESS

There are numerous explanations for the correlations be-tween social factors and illness. Certain conditions are *genetically transmitted* (see page 332), and all or many of the genes for an illness may be possessed by members of a given ethnic group. Certain occupations expose individuals to environmental *toxins* (see pages 341-355). Some communicable diseases such as tuberculosis or meningitis will spread more rapidly if large numbers of people live together under *crowded conditions*. People living in urban ghettos are more likely to be victims of *violent crimes*. *Sociocultural disintegration* (see page 328) reduces the efficiency of health-related services. Some phenomena studied by social psychologists and social psychiatrists may play a part as well, although the relationship to illness and its manifestations is less clear and less direct. These phenomena include stress due to life change, self-fulfilling prophecies, the Hawthorne effect, obedience to authority, the Stanton-Schwartz phenomenon, and diagnostic styles.

Holmes [38] and colleagues have done numerous prospective and retrospective studies which demonstrate that the more "life changes" a person experiences during a given time period, and the more stressful is each change (e.g., the death of a spouse is more stressful than going on a vacation), the more likely he or she is to develop an illness of any type subsequently. Each *life change* is weighted according to the *social readjustment rating scale* presented on page 356. People of lower socioeconomic status are more likely to "accumulate" more life change points than people of higher socioeconomic status [39]. Put simply, life for the poor is more stressful. Exactly how this translates into illness is not well understood, although there is certainly a neuroendocrine component. To minimize the effects of stress, Holmes recommend the following: (1) Know the life changes and their weighting, and bear this in mind in making a major decision, and (2) If it is still important to make the change, the patient should take especially good care of himself, pace himself, and plan ahead.

Another possibly relevant phenomenon was described by Rosenthal [40], who selected two identical groups of children matched for intelligence and prior performance. The children's teachers were told that the children in one of the groups were potentially more gifted. At intervals, all the children were given tests of cognitive function. Followup test scores of the children in the supposedly gifted group were significantly higher than those of the control group. This phenomenon, whereby people's functioning is in part determined by others' expectations, is called a *self-fulfilling prophecy*. Its medical relevance is that if physicians have expectations of low levels of functioning from certain patients, such as poor patients or minority patients, the patients may fulfill this prophecy and act noncompliant, unreliable, or incompetent. Or if a hospital department chairman has low expectations for the functioning of department members, the effectiveness of that department may be decreased.

In Chapter 12, on behavioral medicine, there is a discussion of factors contributing to patient compliance and noncompliance. Compliance is critical to the success of a treatment regimen, and potentially dangerous if the patient unthinkingly complies with an incorrect treatment. The Hawthorne effect and obedience to authority are social psychology concepts that are relevant here.

Roethslinger [41] studied the effects of orchestrated changes in working conditions of a group of employees of the Hawthorne plant of the Western

Electric Company in Chicago. He found that every single change improved worker productivity. Undoing the changes produced no decrement of productivity, unless the resulting situation was absurd, such as lighting in the plant equivalent to the lighting of moonlight. This *Hawthorne effect* was a mystery until Roethslinger realized that it wasn't the content of the change that was crucial. What was crucial was the *fact* that changes were taking place, and taking place in the context of the employees perceiving that the experimenters had their well-being at heart. This perception by the employees began at the onset of the experiment, when the experimenters consulted the employees about their needs, and solicited suggestions for change. Physicians who demonstrate concern for patients, such as by being thorough or by considering the patient's needs in making treatment decisions, are more likely to foster patient "productivity" and compliance. At my medical school, faculty-student relations improved markedly when students were included in decision-making processes by being asked to fill out course ratings and by serving as members of faculty committees.

Milgram [42] demonstrated that remarkable capacity of people for being *obedient to authority*. He recruited volunteers for a "learning experiment" in which experimental subjects were asked to administer what they believed to be electric shocks to a middle-aged "accountant" (really an experimental stooge who received no shocks) in an adjacent room whenever the accountant answered a question incorrectly. The more questions the accountant answered incorrectly, the higher the current of the electric shocks the accountant appeared to be receiving in the next room. The accountant-stooge was instructed that he should cry out in pain (and complain that he had a heart condition and couldn't take much more) when a certain "level of current" was reached. His cries usually moved the experimental subject to protest to the experimenter, but the experimenter would reply that nobody has ever been seriously injured by the shocks, and the experiment must proceed. Remarkably, all of Milgram's subjects continued obediently with the administration of the shocks. Although this experiment is flawed by the possibility that the sample of volunteer experimental subjects may have consisted of overly obedient or cruel individuals, it is fascinating nevertheless. It is conceivable that this sort of obedience played a part in the mass suicide in Jonestown. It also reveals how risky it is for patients to comply uncritically with their treatment; If the doctor prescribes the wrong treatment, the patient's condition will deteriorate.

The Stanton-Schwartz phenomenon [43] is also noteworthy. Stanton and Schwartz, studying the treatment process at Chestnut Lodge, a long-term psychoanalytically oriented psychiatric hospital, reported that a patient would manifest psychotic excitement only when two staff members were covertly in disagreement concerning the patient's treatment. This phenome-non can perhaps be extrapolatd to other medical treatment situations, where unresolved staff disagreement or staff disorganization can result in patient behavioral symptomatology.

Rosenhan [44] showed how a patient's actual disease (or lack of one) may be overshadowed by diagnostic fashion and physician misconceptions. He recruited eight apparently healthy individuals to act as patients seeking admission to one of 12 psychiatric hospitals. This *pseudopatient* group con-sisted of a pediatrician, three psychologists, a graduate student, a painter, a psychiatrist, and a housewife. They were instructed to appear in the hospital admissions office complaining of one symptom: one-word hallucinations. They were told to falsify their name, vocation, and employment, but all other aspects of their history and mental status were to be presented accurately. They were all hospitalized, with a range of 7-52 days of hospitalization and a mean of 19 days. This occurred despite the fact that they all reported to the staff on the second day that their hallucinations had disappeared!

"SOCIAL" AND "BIOLOGICAL" CAUSES OF ILLNESS

As you can see, most of this chapter was devoted to the relationship be-tween social factors and illness. It would be easy to conclude that there are clear-cut demarcations between "social" and "biological" causes of illness, but a closer look (e.g., genetic transmission, neuroendocrine regulation, alter-ation of environmental biology) reveals that this is certainly not the case. Two elegant examples show how closely the social and the biological are inter-twined.

Over a number of months, McClintock [45] recorded the day of onset of each menstrual cycle of a group of women in a college dormitory. She com-pared, in term of day of cycle onset and cycle length, groups of women who identified themselves as friends with groups of women who did not identify themselves as friends. She found that the day of onset of menstruation (a bio-logical phenomenon) became closer and closer among friends (a socioen-vironmental phenomenon) as time passed, and that the day of onset of men-struation did not become closer among women who were not friends. This phenomenon is referred to as *menstrual synchrony*.

In an animal experiment, Rosenzweig, Bennett, and Diamond [46] di-vided rats into two identical groups. He provided one group with an "en-riched" amount of stimulation, and the other group with an "impoverished" (minimal) amount of stimulation. He sacrificed some rats in each group at intervals, and found that the rats with enriched amounts of stimulation (a socioenvironmental phenomenon) had greater enlargement of the cerebral cortex (a biological phenomenon), as compared with the rats exposed to the impoverished amounts of stimulation.

REFERENCES

1. Hollingshead, A., and Redlich, F. *Social Class and Mental Illness*. Wiley, New York (1958).
2. Rainwater, L.: *Social Standing in America*. Basic Books, New York (1977).
3. Duff, S., and Hollingshead, A. *Sickness and Society*. Harper and Row, New York (1968).
4. Clark, K., and Clark, M. Racial identification and preference in Negro children, in *Readings in Social Psychology*. T. Newcomb and E. Hartley, eds. Holt, Rinehart and Winston (1947).
5. Brody, E. Psychosocial aspects of prejudice, in *American Handbook of Psychiatry*, 2nd ed., Vol. 2. S. Arieti, ed. Basic Books, New York (1974).
6. Adorno, T., Frenkel-Brunswik, E., Levinson, D., and Sanford, R. (eds.). *The Authoritarian Personality*. Harper and Row, New York (1950).
7. Horton, P., and Hunt, C. *Sociology*. McGraw-Hill, New York (1976).
8. Parsons, T. Definitions of health and illness, in the light of American values and social structure, in *Patients, Physicians and Illness*. E. Jaco, ed. Free Press, New York (1972).
9. Kasl, S., and Cobb, S. Health behavior, illness behavior and sick role behavior. *Arch. Environ. Health* 12:246-266 (1966).
10. Leighton, A. Social disintegration and mental disorder, in *American Handbook of Psychiatry*, 2nd ed., Vol. 2. S. Arieti, ed. Basic Books, New York (1974).
11. Theodorson, G., and Theodorson, A. *A Modern Dictionary of Sociology*. Barnes and Noble, New York (1969).
12. Williams, R. (ed.). *A Textbook of Black-Related Diseases*. McGraw-Hill, New York (1975).
13. Mumford, E. Culture: Life perspectives and the social meanings of illness, in *Understanding Human Behavior in Health and Illness*. R. Simons and H. Pardes, eds. Williams and Wilkins, Baltimore (1977).
14. Mechanic, D. *Medical Sociology*. Free Press, New York (1968).
15. Zola, I. Culture and symptoms. *Am. Sociol. Rev.* 31:615-630 (1966).
16. Grier, W., and Cobbs, P. *Black Rage*. Basic Books, New York (1968).
17. Duff, S., and Hollingshead, A. *Sickness and Society*. Harper and Row, New York (1968).
18. Lewis, O. *La Vida*. Random, New York (1965).
19. Rainwater, L. The lower class. health, illness and medical institutions, in *Medical Behavioral Science*. T. Millon, ed. Saunders, Philadelphia (1975).
20. U.S. Department of Health, Education and Welfare. *Health in the United States 1978* (Pub. No. PHS 78-1232). U.S. Gov't. Prtg. Off., Washington, D.C. (1978).
21. Murray, R. Medical genetics and black-related disease, in *A Textbook of Black-Related Diseases*. R. Williams, ed. McGraw-Hill, New York (1975).
22. Milunsky, A. The causes and prevalence of mental retardation, in *The Prevention of Genetic Disease and Mental Retardation*. Saunders, Philadelphia (1975).
23. Zborowski, M. Cultural components in response to pain, in *Medical Behavioral Science*. T. Millon, ed. Saunders, Philadelphia (1975).
24. Zola, I. Culture and symptoms. An analysis of patients' presenting complaints. *Am. Sociol. Rev.* 31:615-640 (1966).
25. Suchman, E. Sociomedical variations among ethnic groups. *Am. J. Sociol.* 70:319-331 (1964).

26. Lieberson, S. Ethnic groups and the practice of medicine. *Am. Sociol. Rev.* 23:542-549 (1950).

27. Occupational medicine. Health hazards of the work place. *Patient Care.* 13:183-192 (1979).

28. Schweitzer, L. The rewards and hazards of medicine as a profession, in *Understanding Human Behavior in Health and Illness.* R. Simons and H. Bardes, eds. Williams and Wilkins, Baltimore (1977).

29. Vaillant, G., Sobowall, N., and Arthur, C. Some psychologic vulnerabilities of physicians. *N. Engl. J. Med.* 287:372 (1972).

30. Pitts, F., Schuller, A., Rich, C., and Pitts, A. Suicide among U.S. women physicians. *Am. J. Psychiat.* 136:694-696 (1979).

31. Beecher, H. *Measurement of Subjective Responses.* Oxford, New York (1959).

32. Herbert, A. *Soldier.* Holt, Rinehart and Winston, New York (1973).

33. Lieban, R. The field of medical anthropology, in *Culture, Disease and Healing.* D. Landy, ed. Macmillan, New York (1977).

34. Kiev, A. *Transcultural Psychiatry.* Free Press, New York (1972).

35. Kiev, A. *Curanderismo.* Free Press, New York (1968).

36. Jordan, W. Voodoo medicine, in *A Textbook of Black-Related Diseases.* R. Williams, ed. McGraw-Hill, New York (1975).

37. Alegria, D., Guerra, E., Martinez, C., and Meyer, G. El hospital invisible. *Arch. Gen. Psychiatry* 34:1354-1357 (1977).

38. Holmes, T. Life situations, emotions and disease. *Psychosom.* 19:747-754 (1978).

39. Liem, R., and Liem, J. Social class and mental illness reconsidered. The role of economic stress and social support. *J. Health Soc. Behav.* 19:134-156 (1978).

40. Rosenthal, R., and Jacobson, L. Self-fulfilling prophecies in the classroom, in *Social and Psychologic Perspectives.* M. Deutsch, I.Katz, and A. Jensen, eds. (1968).

41. Roethslinger, F. *Management and Morale.* Harvard, Cambridge (1938).

42. Milgram, S. *Obedience to Authority.* Basic Books, New York (1973).

43. Stanton, A., and Schwartz, M. *The Mental Hospital.* Basic Books, New York (1954).

44. Rosenhan, D. On being sane in insane places. *Science* 179:250-258 (1973).

45. McClintock, M. Menstrual synchrony and suppression. *Nature (Lond.)* 229:244-245 (1971).

46. Rosenzweig, M., Bennett, E., and Diamond, M. Brain changes in response to experience. *Psychology in Progress: Readings from Scientific American.* Freeman, San Francisco (1975).

APPENDIX 1   OCCUPATIONAL HAZARDS*
Biological and Industrial Hazards

Biological Hazards

Occupation	Disease or agent
Athletes	Dermatophytosis
Bakers	Candidiasis
Bartenders	Candidiasis
Bulldozer operators	Coccidioidomycosis
Butchers	Erysipeloid
	Tularemia
Cattle breeders	Milkers' nodules
	Anthrax
	Brucellosis
	Leptospirosis
Construction workers	Rocky Mountain spotted fever
	Coccidioidomycosis (southwestern United States)
	Histoplasmosis
	Chiggers (especially southern United States)
Cooks	Tularemia
	Candidiasis
Cork workers	Farmer's lung
Cotton mill workers	Coccidioidomycosis
Dairy farmers	Milkers' nodules
	Q fever
	Anthrax
	Leptospirosis
	Aspergillosis
	Dermatophytosis
	Farmer's lung (especially handlers of hay in confined areas)
	Ticks
Delivery personnel	Rabies
Dishwashers	Candidiasis
Dockworkers	Swimmers' itch
Farmers	Rabies
	Rocky Mountain spotted fever
	Tetanus
	Plague (western United States)
	Tularemia
	Kerosene
	Aspergillosis
	Coccidioidomycosis (southwestern United States)
	Histoplasmosis

(Continued)

APPENDIX 1   OCCUPATIONAL HAZARDS (continued)

Biological Hazards (continued)

Occupation	Disease or agent
Farmers *(continued)*	Sporotrichosis Chromoblastomycosis (southern United States) Dermatophytosis Farmer's lung Chiggers (especially southern United States) Mites Ticks
Fishermen (Gulf Coast)	Mycobacterial infections
Forestry workers	Rocky Mountain spotted fever Tularemia Sporotrichosis (tree nursery workers) Ticks
Gardeners	Sporotrichosis Creeping eruption Hookworm disease Ascariasis Mites
Grain mill workers	Aspergillosis Mites Ticks
Health workers	Viral hepatitis Tuberculosis (hospital employees) Mycobacterial infections Candidiasis
Hide workers	Q fever Anthrax Dermatophytosis
Laboratory workers	Cat-scratch disease Rocky Mountain spotted fever Ornithosis Mycobacterial infections Tularemia Coccidioidomycosis Dermatophytosis
Lifeguards	Dermatophytosis Swimmers' itch Creeping eruption Hookworm disease Ascariasis
Linemen	Chiggers (especially southern United States)

(Continued)

APPENDIX 1   OCCUPATIONAL HAZARDS (continued)

Biological Hazards (continued)

Occupation	Disease or agent
Migrant workers	Coccidioidomycosis (southwestern United States)
Military personnel	Leptospirosis Coccidioidomycosis (southwestern United States)
Miners	Leptospirosis
Packinghouse workers	Candidiasis
Pet shop workers	Ornithosis Mycobacterial infections (tropical fish stores) Aspergillosis (birds) Dermatophytosis
Plumbers	Creeping eruption Hookworm disease Ascariasis
Poultry handlers	Newcastle disease Ornithosis Erysipeloid Candidiasis Aspergillosis Histoplasmosis Mites
Ranchers	Rabies Rocky Mountain spotted fever Q fever Tetanus Anthrax Brucellosis Leptospirosis Plague (western United States) Dermatophytosis Ticks
Sawmill workers	Farmer's lung
Sewer workers	Leptospirosis
Stockyard workers	Q fever Brucellosis Leptospirosis
Sugar cane workers	Leptospirosis Farmer's lung
Surveyors	Chiggers (especially southern United States)
Taxidermists	Ornithosis
Textile workers	Farmer's lung

(Continued)

APPENDIX 1 OCCUPATIONAL HAZARDS (continued)

Biological Hazards (continued)

Occupation	Disease or agent
Veterinarians	Rabies
	Cat-scratch disease
	Milkers' nodules
	Newcastle disease
	Brucellosis
	Leptospirosis
	Tularemia
	Dermatophytosis
Wool handlers	Q fever
	Anthrax
	Dermatophytosis
Workers at risk of penetrating or crush-type trauma	Tetanus
Zoo attendants	Ornithosis
	Histoplasmosis
	Dermatophytosis

Industrial Hazards

Occupation	Disease or agent
Adhesive workers	Isocyanates
	Benzene
	Styrene ethyl benzene
	Xylene hydrogen chloride
	Sulfuric acid
Agricultural workers	Calcium cyanamide
	Diphenyl
	Dinitro-o-cresol
	Arsenic
	Nitrogen oxides
Automotive workers	Gasoline
	Kerosene
	Ketones
	Trichloroethylene
	Lead, inorganic
	Nitrogen oxides

(Continued)

APPENDIX 1 OCCUPATIONAL HAZARDS (continued)

Industrial Hazards (continued)

Occupation	Disease or agent
Chemists	Carbon tetrachloride
	Chloroform
	Benzene
	Toluene
	Quinone
	Benzidine salts
	Picric acid
	Nickel and compounds
Construction workers	Portland cement
Cosmetic manufacturers	Paraffin
	Amyl alcohol
	ethyl alcohol
	Ethyl alcohol
	Ketones
	1,2-Dichloroethane
	Ethyl chloride
	Trichloroethylene
	Toluene
	Quinone
	Benzyl chloride
	Aniline
	Dimethyl sulfate
	Zinc oxide
Detergent makers	Benzene
Drug manufacturers	Turpentine
	Allyl alcohol
	Amyl alcohol
	Ethyl alcohol
	Ethylene chlorohydrin
	Ethyl ether
	Acetic acid
	Ketones
	Chloroform
	Ethyl chloride
	Methyl chloride
	Trichloroethylene
	Benzene
	Benzyl chloride
	Aniline
	Picric acid

(Continued)

APPENDIX 1   OCCUPATIONAL HAZARDS (continued)

Industrial Hazards (continued)

Occupation	Disease or agent
Drug manufacturers (*continued*)	n,n-Dimethylformamide
	Pyridine
	Dimethyl sulfate
	Bromine/hydrogen bromide
	Hydrogen chloride
	Arsenic
	Antimony
	Cobalt and compounds
	Magnesium and compounds
	Manganese and compounds
	Mercury, inorganic
	Phosgene
Dry cleaners	Naphtha
	Dichloroethyl ether
	Carbon tetrachloride
	1,2-Dichloroethane
	Propylene dichloride
	Tetrachloroethane
	1,1,1,-Trichloroethane
	Trichloroethylene
	Carbon disulfide
Dye makers	Ethyl alcohol
	Ethylene chlorohydrin
	Methyl alcohol
	Acetic acid
	Oxalic acid
	Ketones
	1,2-Dichloroethane
	Methyl and ethyl bromide
	Trichloroethylene
	Benzene
	Naphthalene
	Cresol
	Quinone
	Benzyl chloride
	Chlorodiphenyls and derivatives
	Chlorinated benzenes
	Aniline
	Benzidine salts
	Dinitrobenzene
	Dinitro-o-cresol

(Continued)

APPENDIX 1   OCCUPATIONAL HAZARDS (continued)

Industrial Hazards (continued)

Occupation	Disease or agent
Dye makers *(continued)*	Dinitrophenol
	Dinitrotoluene
	Picric acid
	n,n-Dimethylformamide
	Pyridine
	Carbon disulfide
	Dimethyl sulfate
	Bromine/hydrogen bromide
	Fluorides
	Hydrogen chloride
	Arsenic
	Magnesium and compounds
	Thallium and compounds
	Tin and compounds
	Vanadium
	Zinc chloride
	Nitrogen oxides
	Phosgene
Electrical and electronic equipment makers	Chlorodiphenyls and derivatives
	Chlorinated naphthalenes
	Picric acid
	Beryllium
	Lead, inorganic
	Magnesium and compounds
	Mercury, inorganic
	Nickel and compounds
	Platinum and compounds
	Selenium and compounds
	Graphite
Electroplaters	Hydrogen cyanide
	Carbon disulfide
	Hydrogen chloride
	Chromium and compounds
	Cobalt and compounds
	Germanium
	Platinum and compounds
	Zinc oxide
Enamel makers	Methyl alcohol
	Cresol
	Carbon disulfide
	Arsenic

(Continued)

APPENDIX 1   OCCUPATIONAL HAZARDS (continued)

Industrial Hazards (continued)

Occupation	Disease or agent
Enamel makers (continued)	Cobalt and compounds
	Lead, inorganic
	Nickel and compounds
Epoxy resin makers	Epichlorohydrin
	Ketones
Fat processors	n-Hexane
	Naphtha
	Amyl alcohol
	Dichloroethyl ether
	Ethyl ether
	Ketones
	Carbon tetrachloride
	Ethyl chloride
	Methylene chloride
	Propylene dichloride
	Trichloroethylene
	Carbon disulfide
Food preservers	Acetic acid
Food processors	Hydrogen chloride
	Sulfuric acid
Foundry workers	Methyl alcohol
	Cresol
	Chlorinated naphthalenes
	Fluorides
	Arsenic
	Beryllium
	Brass
	Cadmium and compounds
	Cobalt and compounds
	Germanium
	Lead, inorganic
	Magnesium and compounds
	Manganese and ocmpounds
	Nickel carbonyl
	Thallium and compounds
	Tin and compounds
	Zinc oxide
	Graphite
Grain workers	Carbon disulfide
	Sulfur dioxide

(Continued)

APPENDIX 1 OCCUPATIONAL HAZARDS (continued)

Industrial Hazards (continued)

Occupation	Disease or agent
Insecticide makers	1,2-Dichloroethane
	Tetrachloroethane
	Trichloroethylene
	Acrylonitrile
	Chlorinated benzenes
	Chlorinated naphthalenes
	Fluorides
	Arsenic
	Cadmium and compounds
	Lead, inorganic
	Selenium and compounds
	Phosgene
Insulation workers	Isocyanates
Lacquerers and makers	Epichlorohydrin
	Ketones
	Carbon tetrachloride
	Chloroform
	Tetrachloroethane
	Styrene/ethyl benzene
	Toluene
	Xylene
	Chlorodiphenyls and derivatives
	Chlorinated benzenes
	Zinc oxide
Laundry workers	Acetic acid
	Oxalic acid
Leather workers	Methyl alcohol
	Ketones
	Methylene chloride
	Aniline
	Arsenic
	Sulfuric acid
Lithographers	Turpentine
	Aniline
	Chromium and compounds
Match and explosive manufacturers	Picric acid
	Tetryl
	Trinitrotoluene
	Pyridine
	Arsenic

(Continued)

APPENDIX 1   OCCUPATIONAL HAZARDS (continued)

Industrial Hazards (continued)

Occupation	Disease or agent
Match and explosive manufacturers (*continued*)	Antimony Lead, inorganic Magnesium and compounds Manganese and compounds Thallium and compounds Graphite Sulfuric acid
Medical personnel	Nitrogen oxides
Metal cleaners	Kerosene Naphtha Ethylene chlorohydrin Dichloroethyl ether Dioxane Ketones Carbon tetrachloride 1,2-Dichloroethane Propylene dichloride Tetrachloroethane 1,1,1-Trichloroethane Trichloroethylene Fluorides Sulfuric acid
Millinery workers	Methyl alcohol
Oil processors	n-Hexane Naphtha Dichloroethyl ether Dioxane Ethyl ether Ketones Carbon tetrachloride Methylene chloride Propylene dichloride Tetrachloroethane Trichloroethylene Carbon disulfide
Organic chemical synthesizers	Allyl alcohol Ethyl alcohol Ethylene chlorohydrin Methyl alcohol Bis (chloromethyl) ether

(Continued)

APPENDIX 1 OCCUPATIONAL HAZARDS (continued)

Industrial Hazards (continued)

Occupation	Disease or agent
Organic chemical synthesizers (*continued*)	Epichlorohydrin
	Phthalic anhydride
	Methyl chloride
	Propylene dichloride
	Vinyl chloride
	Acrylonitrile
	Calcium cyanamide
	Hydrogen cyanide
	Isocyanates
	Diphenyl
	Styrene/ethyl benzene
	Creosote
	Quinone
	Aniline
	Penzidine salts
	Dinitrobenzene
	Dinitrophenol
	Dinitrotoluene
	n,n-Dimethylformamide
	Ethyleneimine
	Pyridine
	Dimethyl sulfate
	Bromine/hydrogen bromide
	Hydrogen chloride
	Boron hydrides
	Magnesium and compounds
	Nickel carbonyl
	Selenium and compounds
	Vanadium
	Ozone
Painters	Naphtha
	Turpentine
	Methyl alcohol
	Dioxane
	Ketones
	Isocyanates
	Arsenic
	Lead, inorganic
Paint manufacturers	Xylene
	Chlorinated benzenes
	Pyridine

(Continued)

APPENDIX 1   OCCUPATIONAL HAZARDS (continued)

Industrial Hazards (continued)

Occupation	Disease or agent
Paint manufacturers (*continued*)	Carbon disulfide
	Hydrogen chloride
	Arsenic
	Antimony
	Cadmium and compounds
	Lead, inorganic
	Manganese and compounds
	Nickel and compounds
	Graphite
Paper makers	Ethyleneimine
	Zinc chloride
	Ozone
	Sulfur dioxide
	Sulfuric acid
Photoengravers	Methyl alcohol
	Hydrogen chloride
	Chromium and compounds
	Nitrogen oxides
Photographic film developers	Quinone
	Hydrogen chloride
Pitch workers	Creosote
Plastics workers	Allyl alcohol
	Amyl alcohol
	Ethyl alcohol
	Methyl alcohol
	Acetic acid
	Phthalic anhydride
	Ketones
	Chloroform
	1,2-Dichloroethane
	Propylene dichloride
	Styrene/ethyl benzene
	Cresol
	Benzyl chloride
	Chlorodiphenyls and derivatives
	Chlorinated naphthalenes
	Aniline
	Benzidine salts
	n,n-Dimethylformamide
	Tricresyl phosphates

(*Continued*)

APPENDIX 1 OCCUPATIONAL HAZARDS (continued)

Industrial Hazards (continued)

Occupation	Disease or agent
Plastic workers (*continued*)	Carbon disulfide
	Fluorides
	Hydrogen chloride
	Boron hydrides
	Selenium and compounds
	Tin and compounds
	Zinc oxide
Potato growers	Ethylene chlorohydrin
Printers	Aniline
	Arsenic
	Antimony
	Paraffin
Refinery workers	n-Heptane
	Kerosene
	Naphtha
	Amyl alcohol
	Methyl chloride
	Benzene
	Styrene/ethyl benzene
	Toluene
	Fluorides
	Chlorinated naphthalenes
	n,n-Dimethylformamide
	Tricresyl phosphates
	Bromine/hydrogen bromide
	Boron hydrides
	Lead, inorganic
	Nickel carbonyl
	Zinc chloride
	Sulfur dioxide
Refrigeration workers	Methyl chloride
Rubber manufacturers	Turpentine
	Amyl alcohol
	Ethyl alcohol
	Ethyl ether
	Acetic acid
	Oxalic acid
	Carbon tetrachloride
	Methyl chloride
	Propylene dichloride

(Continued)

APPENDIX 1   OCCUPATIONAL HAZARDS (continued)

Industrial Hazards (continued)

Occupation	Disease or agent
Rubber manufacturers (*continued*)	Vinyl chloride
	Isocyanates
	Benzene
	Styrene/ethyl benzene
	Benzyl chloride
	Chlorodiphenyls and derivatives
	Chlorinated naphthalenes
	Aniline
	Benzidine salts
	Pyridine
	Carbon disulfide
	Hydrogen chloride
	Antimony
	Boron hydrides
	Lead, inorganic
	Selenium and compounds
	Zinc chloride
	Zinc oxide
Steel workers	Calcium cyanamide
	Hydrogen cyanide
Tannery workers	Naphthalene
	Quinone
	Picric acid
	Hydrogen chloride
	Mercury, inorganic
	Sulfur dioxide
Textile workers	Amyl alcohol
	Ethylene chlorohydrin
	Methyl alcohol
	Dioxane
	Acetic acid
	Oxalic acid
	Ketones
	Isocyanates
	Naphthalene
	Quinone
	Ethyleneimine
	Arsenic
	Antimony
	Cadmium and compounds
	Chromium and compounds

(*Continued*)

APPENDIX 1   OCCUPATIONAL HAZARDS (continued)

Industrial Hazards (continued)

Occupation	*Disease or agent*
Textile workers (*continued*)	Magnesium and compounds Mercury, inorganic Nickel and compounds Selenium and compounds Tin and compounds Zinc chloride
Upholsterers	Isocyanates
Varnish makers	Paraffin Turpentine Amyl alcohol Dichloroethyl ether Epichlorohydrin Ketones Carbon tetrachloride 1,2-Dichloroethane Tetrachloroethane Trichloroethylene Styrene/ethyl benzene Xylene Aniline Carbon disulfide Manganese and compounds Nickel and compounds
Welders	Benzene Brass Cadmium and compounds Chromium and compounds Magnesium and compounds Manganese and compounds Stibine Zinc oxide Nitrogen oxides Ozone

*From Occupational medicine. Health hazards of the work place. *Patient Care* 13:183-192, 1979, with permission.

APPENDIX 2   SOCIAL READJUSTMENT RATING SCALE
Life Change Magnitude

Life change	Magnitude
Change in eating habits	15
Change in sleeping habits	16
Change in social activities	18
Change in recreational habits	19
Change in personal habits	24
Change in working hours or conditions	20
Vacation	13
Change in family get-togethers	15
Change in financial state	38
Change in living conditions	25
Outstanding personal achievement	28
Change in responsibilities at work	29
Change in number of arguments with spouse	35
Change in residence	20
Change in health or behavior of family member	44
Change in line of work	36
Change in church activities	19
Troubles with the boss	23
Sexual difficulties	39
Son or daughter leaving home	29
Gaining a new family member	30
Personal injury or illness	53
Wife beginning or ceasing work	26
Minor violations of the law	11
Beginning or ceasing formal schooling	26
In-law troubles	29
Mortgage or loan less than $10,000	17
Marital reconciliation	45
Marital separation	65
Changing ot a new school	20
Mortgage or loan greater than $10,000	31
Major business readjustment	39
Marriage	50
Death of a close family member	63
Foreclosure of mortgage or loan	30
Death of a close friend	37
Pregnancy	40
Retirement from work	45
Being fired from work	47
Detention in jail	63
Divorce	73
Death of spouse	100

Source: Modified from Holmes, J., and Rahe, R. The Social Readjustment Rating Scale. *Journal of Psychosomatic Research* 11:213 (1967).

25

The Potentially Suicidal Patient

WILLIARD SHANKEN

INTRODUCTION

Clinicians in all specialties must be aware that suicide is the ninth leading cause of death in the United States. The history, mental status examination, and diagnosis are crucial in the evaluation of all patients with emotional problems. When you take the history, do not hesitate to ask the patient whether he is contemplating suicide. Most patients will reply honestly to this question, and enable you to estimate roughly the seriousness of the suicide risk. However, this question alone is never sufficient, and a number of historical, mental status, and diagnostic variables have to be taken into account. These variables must be viewed together; none is by itself an absolute indicator of suicide risk.

OBSERVATIONS IN THE MENTAL STATUS EXAMINATION

Hopelessness

A patient who tells you that there is *no hope* for improvement of his situation, or amelioration of his symptoms, is a significantly greater risk of suicide than one who tells you that his life might improve.

Response to the Interviewer and the Interview

If the patient is cooperative and involved with the interviewer, the risk of suicide is diminished. If the patient is withdrawn, uninvolved, or silent, he is a greater risk. A patient who has been very depressed and silent and then suddenly jumps into action (e.g., he "bolts" out of the room) is a greater suicide risk. The chance of suicide decreases if he seems more at ease as the interview progresses or if he is enthusiastic about a planned treatment program.

Depression

About 90% of people who commit suicide are depressed. The greatest risk is incurred by people with *endogenous depressions*.

Impaired Judgment or Loss of Touch with Reality

A person who can sort out the meaning of events effectively and realistically is a lesser suicide risk than one who overreacts or misinterprets events because his judgment is impaired.

Agitation

The more a patient is overtly agitated, the greater is his need to seek alleviation of his suffering by suicide.

Comfort with the Notion of Suicide

The more reassuring or comfortable the idea of suicide seems for the patient, the greater the risk. The more the patient is upset by the idea of suicide, and sees it as silly, the safer the situation.

Unexplained Lifting of Spirits

Be cautious when a previously depressed patient suddenly and unexplainably appears cheerful. It is possible that he has decided to kill himself and feels relieved by the decision.

HISTORICAL DATA

Timing of Life Events

1. *Hospital discharge:* Patients are likely to commit suicide during the month prior to hospital discharge (often while on a pass from the hospital), or within 6 months after discharge.

2. *Life stresses:* There is a higher incidence of suicide in patients who have recently lost a job or lost someone they loved.

Previous Suicide Attempts

Sixty percent of people who kill themselves have made prior suicide attempts, and 10% of people who make suicide attempts will ultimately kill themselves [1]. At the very least, a suicide attempt is a way of saying "I need help," although obviously, the implications and lethalities of attempts vary greatly.

Planned Suicide Attempts

The more deadly the suicide method chosen (e.g., a loaded gun is more deadly than antibiotic tablets), the greater the suicide risk. The less chance the potential suicide offers others to rescue him, the greater the risk; for example, one who makes a suicide attempt alone in a hotel room has a more lethal intent than one who makes an attempt while at home with a spouse or friend. Also the more specific and feasible the suicide plan, the greater the suicide risk.

Acts Anticipating Death

The suicide risk is increased if the patient has recently made out a will, or has just given away prized possessions.

Family History

If a close family member, especially a parent, has committed suicide at any time, the chances for the patient to do the same thing are much greater.

DEMOGRAPHIC DATA

Age

The risk of suicide *increases* with age. It is a rare for a person over 50 years to make an insignificant suicide attempt.

Sex

Women are more apt to make suicide *attempts*; men are more apt to actually kill themselves.

Race

American Indians are statistically more likely to commit suicide than American whites who, in turn, are more likely to commit suicide than American blacks. The white-to-black suicide ratio is about 11:2 [2]; the rates for young adults are much closer: The rate for black men between the ages of 25 and 34 is equal to that of white men. The increase in suicide risk with age does not hold for blacks: Young blacks are as likely to commit suicide as middle-aged blacks.

Religion

Protestants are more apt to commit suicide than those of the Catholic faith.

Alcoholics

Alcoholics are more prone to committing suicide than nonalcoholics.

Dialysis Patients

Dialysis patients have a suicide rate 400 times the national average[3].

Pregnant Women

Pregnant women have a low suicide rate.

MANAGEMENT OF THE SUICIDAL PATIENT

It is important to remember that most, if not all, suicidal patients have a degree of uncertainty about their intent. It is your job to attempt to shift the weight of the patient's intent towards *living*. There are a number of ways you can help the patient:

Establish a Relationship with the Patient

1. *Convey hope*: When you feel optimistic, convey this sense of optimism to the patient. Though a certain percentage of suicidal patients do commit suicide, it is well to remember that most suicidal patients don't. There is actually reason for optimism in a high percentage of patients who

initially feel suicidal. Remember, the patient may see you as his only link to life and eventual recovery.

2. *Be available*: Because of your possible role as an "island of hope," your availability becomes quite important to the patient. When you are unavailable, have a colleague on call who is well informed about the patient.

3. *Be willing to be active*: In the treatment of the suicidal patient, be willing to be active and forthright in your meetings with him, especially when he is feeling passive and overwhelmed. As the patient improves, he is often more willing and able to discuss his problems. He will also be more cooperative in taking medication.

Err on the Side of Caution

If you are concerned about the imminent possibility of suicide, hospitalize the patient. Physicians should always err on the side of hospitalization when there is serious suicidal potential. If you find that hospitalization is not needed for the patient after all, you can rectify your error. Little or no harm done! However, you cannot undo a successful suicide. It is hard to understand the reasoning of physicians who emphasize that they hardly ever hospitalize a suicidal patient.

Be Aware of Your Feelings

A patient who is suicidal invariably causes anxiety in his physician. Anxious physicians sometimes resort to ineffective mechanisms to deal with suicidal patients:

1. *"Omnipotent" denial of risk*: The physician who feels that he always can help the patient without hospitalization is denying the patient's ability to commit suicide.

2. *Anger*: A patient who is suicidal is often threatening to us. We in turn may feel angry at him for this. Be aware of this feeling and work on understanding it in yourself. Comprehending the reasons for our feeling of anger can help us to understand our patient, can help us to feel more comfortable, and can help us deal with greater equanimity with the difficult problems presented by the patient.

Be Willing to Get a Consultation

Presenting the case to a colleague, or referring your patient for a consultation visit, should be done when you begin to note denial, anger, or inadequacy within yourself, or when you do not understand what is going on with the patient. Your consultant's input may help you understand your patient as well as your own feelings. In addition, the consult is frequently a safety valve, causing a decrease in the stress you feel because you are sharing the responsibility with someone else.

Be Willing to Utilize the Patient's Immediate Family, Extended Family, and Friends

You can include any or all of these people in specific meetings or all meetings if the patient needs extra support or external control. In life-and-death emergencies, physician-patient confidentiality cannot alway be totally honored, and a relative or friend can be a vital ally to both you and the patient.

Hospitalize

Provide external controls if indicated. These include seclusion rooms, locked units, restraints, clothing searches, and one-to-one observation. Often the controls brought on by hospitalization will remove considerable anxiety from the patient and make him feel safer. These controls should be continued until the suicidal crisis appears over.

Use Medications or Electroconvulsive Therapy (ECT)

Use medications depending on the patient's primary symptoms. For seriously depressed, acutely suicidal patients, ECT is usually the preferred treatment.

REFERENCES

1. Hendin, H. Suicide, in *Comprehensive Textbook of Psychiatry 1*. A. Freedman and H. Kaplan, Williams and Wilkins, Baltimore (1967).
2. Hendin, H. *Black Suicide*. Basic Books, New York (1969).
3. Abram, H., Moore, G., and Westervelt, F. Suicidal behavior in chronic dialysis patients. *Am. J. Psychiatry* 127:1199-1204 (1971).

26

Psychiatric Aspects of Criminal Behavior

FREDERICK SIERLES

INTRODUCTION

Physicians treat criminals in penal, general hospital, and office settings. Some doctors are consultants to, or full-time employees of, penal institutions. Physicians need to know about psychiatric and general medical syndromes commonly diagnosed in criminals. And the medical profession has an obligation to do research on medical aspects of criminality. Unfortunately, despite considerable research on psychiatric syndromes associated with criminality, these contributions have thus far been of limited usefulness. One reason is that two of the commoner syndromes, sociopathy and Briquet's syndrome, have no known cure. Another is that some criminologists are not aware of the research; for example, Silberman's 1978 overview [1] of criminology makes no reference to any of the studies described below.

CORRELATES OF CRIMINALITY

Diagnosis

Guze [2] studied the relationship between diagnosis and criminality. He selected a large sample of felons and their first-degree (parents, children, and siblings) relatives, choosing every new case of a central probation office in St. Louis. Washington-St. Louis diagnostic criteria [3,4] were used, and follow-up studies were conducted 3 and 9 years later. Diagnoses included the following:

Male Felons
78% met criteria for sociopathy
43% met criteria for alcoholism
12% met criteria for anxiety neurosis
 7% had below normal intelligence
 5% were drug-dependent

Female Felons
65% met criteria for sociopathy
47% met criteria for alcoholism
41% met criteria for Briquet's syndrome
26% were drug-dependent
11% met criteria for anxiety neurosis

Thus, the overwhelming majority of felons received a psychiatric diagnosis, and many had two or more diagnoses concurrently.

Social History

Guze found that felons were more likely than the general population to be divorced or unemployed. Of course, we must note that divorce and unemployment were included in criteria for diagnosing sociopathy, and that Guze did not consider criminality itself to be an occupation.

Family Data

For the felons in Guze's study the prevalence of sociopathy, hysteria, alcoholism, and drug dependence in first-degree relatives far exceeded the prevalence of these syndromes in the general population. These were also more prevalent in spouses of felons than in the general population [2]; this nonrandom selection of marital partners is called *assortative mating*. Finally, there was an increased probability of the following [2]:

1. Being reared away from the home of biological parents (e.g., reared in orphanages, foster homes, reared by friends)
2. Having divorced or separated parents
3. Having absent or cruel parents
4. Having parents who were criminals

Hutchings and Mednick [3] found a prevalence of criminality in both biological and adoptive fathers of felons which significantly exceeded that in the general population. They also found that 16% of a sample of adoptees had criminal records, as compared with 8.9% of a nonadopted control group.

Genetic Studies

The family data are striking, but an interpretation is not immediately apparent. Criminality could conceivably result from any or all of the following:
1. Rearing in an unfavorable environment
2. Transmission of genes for sociopathy, Briquet's, alcoholism, drug abuse, or anxiety neurosis
3. Embryonic, fetal or childhood illness

Hutchings and Mednick studies a huge sample of adoptees, and found that for adopted sons (they did not study daughters) who were criminals, there was a prevalence of criminality in both biological and adoptive father which exceeded that of the general population [3]. Even when adoptive fathers were not criminal, the prevalence of criminality in the biological fathers exceeded that of the general population. Overall, the incidence of criminality in biological fathers significantly exceeded that of the adoptive fathers [3]. Table 1 shows these relationships.

Thus, the following conclusion can be drawn: "The effects of criminality of the biologic and adoptive fathers are at least partially independent" [3]. The data thus suggest both genetic and nongenetic influences. Hutchings and Mednick were careful to rule out the possibility that hidden environmental factors were "masquerading" as genetic factors; a discussion of this is beyond the scope of this chapter.

Christiansen [4] reviewed eight studies of the concordance of criminality for monozygotic twins as compared with dizygotic twins. He found that in all eight studies, the concordance was higher for monozygotic than for dizygotic twins, and in seven of the eight this difference was statistically significant. He noted that the mean concordance in large studies of criminality in monozygotic twins is about 67%. Of all the twins studied, there were only eight monozygotic twin pairs; four were concordant for criminality and four were discordant. Like the Hutchings-Mednick results, the data suggest both genetic and nongenetic influences.

Table 1   Percentage of Adopted Sons wno Are Criminals

	Criminal adoptive father	Noncriminal adoptive father
Criminal biological father	36.2%	22.0%
Noncriminal biological father	11.5%	10.5%

Source: Modified from B. Hutchings and S. Mednick. Criminality in adoptees and their adoptive and biologic parents, in *Biosocial Bases of Criminal Behavior*, S. Mednick and K. Christiansen, eds. Gardner, New York, 1977 (Ref. 3).

Concerning alcoholism and sociopathy, which are correlated with criminality, there is some evidence that genetic factors play a part. Goodwin [5] studied a group of men who had been given up for adoption by their biological parents, at least one of whom was alcoholic, while their siblings remained with these parents. Goodwin concluded: "The main finding of the study was that sons of alcoholics were no more likely to become alcoholics if they were reared by their alcoholic parent than if they were separated from their alcoholic parent soon after birth and reared by nonrelatives." Goodwin also found a similar relationship for female adoptees, but not to a statistically signlficant degree.

Schulsinger [6] studied adopted sociopaths and their relatives. Schulsinger writes: "It is immediately evident that there is a great surplus of such (sociopathic) disorders among the biological relatives of the index cases, more than 14% of whom have a psychopathic spectrum disorder compared with 5-8% among the other 3 relative groups." We must note, however, that a "spectrum disorder" is not the same as the disorder itself.

The XYY genotype has been associated with violent behavior. But there are problems with the research leading to this association; the problems include absence of controls, and retrospective case-finding among prisoners. Witkin et al. [7] studied XYY and XXY (Klinefelter) men, and found that XYY men did have an incidence of criminality significantly higher than XXY men or men in a control population, but no greater incidence of *violent* crimes than XXY men or controls.

Recidivism

Recidivism is the repetition of crime after an initial arrest or imprisonment. The problem of recidivism is enormous. In Guze's 3-year followup of male felons, he found a 68% rearrest rate (an average of 1.64 arrests per person) and a 41% reimprisonment rate (an average of .53 imprisonments per person). At 9-year followup, 85% of male felons had been rearrested at least once, and 62% had been rearrested more than once [2]. Mednick [8] views the problem from another perspective: "In a Copenhagen birth cohort of over 30,000 men, we found that. . . about 1%. . .account for more than half of the offenses."

Intelligence

Of three studies of the relationship of intelligence and criminality, two [9,10] showed that statistically, intelligence of criminals is lower than that of the general population. The third study [11] showed no significant difference.

Physiology

Some authors have postulated that sociopaths, delinquents, and habitual criminals have deficits of autonomic reactivity. When these individuals are presented with crime-related stimuli in an experimental situation, their electrodermal recovery rates (ED Rec is a measure of autonomic reactivity) are lower than those of controls [12].

Childhood Behavior

A number of longitudinal studies have related childhood behavior to adult criminality. The following were predictive of adult criminality: Rejection of teacher's authority, school failure, and discipline problems [13]; aggressiveness and inability to concentrate [14]; school failure, "playing hooky," restlessness, hyperactivity, negativism, irresponsibility, shifting in mood, and distractability [15], troublesomeness and discipline problems [16]; and aggressiveness, passivity, poor school achievement, and lower intelligence [17].

Geography

Crime rates are higher in cities than in rural areas; this correlation does not necessarily mean that city life causes crime.

Homicide

Homicide is our 10th leading cause of death. Men, especially teenagers and young adults, are more likely than women to be murderers and homicide victims. However, although women have much lower felony and homicide rates then men, homicide is among the commonest felonies committed by women. The black homicide victimization rate exceeds the rate for whites. Homicide rates are highest in areas of cities with overcrowding and high unemployment rates.

The majority of murderers know their victims, who are often relatives, colleagues, and friends; thus, the majority of homicides are intraracial. Tanay [18] postulated a "sado-masochistic" relationship between killer and victim. There is a high frequency of intoxication with alcohol or barbituates in murderers.

SUMMARY

In summary, the following factors are highly correlated with criminality: (1) Parental criminality, parental sociopathy, Briquet's, alcoholism and drug dependence, parental separation and divorce, fighting, absenteeism, deprivation, and cruelty; (2) poor school performance and deviant childhood behavior; (3) decreased autonomic responsivity, decreased intelligence; (4) diagnoses of sociopathy, Briquet's, alcoholism, drug dependence, and anxiety neurosis; (5) urban residence; (6) prior criminality; (7) criminality, sociopathy, Briquet's, and alcoholism and drug dependence in a spouse; and (8) divorce, separation, and unemployment. There is evidence for a combination of genetic and nongenetic causation of criminality, varying in weight from case to case.

REFERENCES

1. Silberman, C. *Criminal Violence, Criminal Justice.* Random, New York (1978).
2. Guze, S. *Criminality and Psychiatric Disorders.* Oxford, London (1976).
3. Hutchings, B., and Mednick, S. Criminality, in adoptees and their adoptive and biological parents. A pilot study, in *Biosocial Bases of Criminal Behavior.* S. Mednick and K. Christiansen, eds. Gardner, New York (1977).
4. Christiansen, K. (ed.). A review of studies of criminality among twins, in *Biosocial Bases of Criminal Behavior.* S. Mednick and K. Christiansen, eds. Gardner, New York (1977).
5. Goodwin, D. Family and adoption studies of alcoholism, in *Biosocial Bases of Criminal Behavior.* S. Mednick and K. Christiansen, eds. Gardner, New York (1977).
6. Schulsinger, F. Psychopathy. Heredity and environment, in *Biosocial Bases of Criminal Behavior.* S. Mednick and K. Christiansen, eds. Gardner, New York (1977).
7. Witkin, H., Mednick, S., Schulsinger, F., Bakkestrom, E., Christiansen, K., Goodenough, D., Hirschhorn, K., Lundsteen, C., Owen, D., Philip, J., Rubin, D., Stocking, M. Criminality, aggression and intelligence among XYY and XXY men, in *Biosocial Bases of Criminal Behavior.* S. Mednick and K. Christiansen, eds. Gardner, New York (1977).
8. Mednick, S. A bio-social theory of the learning of law-abiding behavior, in *Biosocial Bases of Criminal Behavior.* S. Mednick and K. Christiansen, eds. Gardner, New York (1977).
9. Blank, L. The intellectual functioning of delinquents. *J. Soc. Psychol.* 47:9-14 (1958).
10. Frost, B., and Frost, R. The pattern of WISC scores in a group of juvenile sociopaths. *J. Clin. Psychol.* 18:354-355 (1962).
11. Fields, J.G. The performance verbal IQ discrepancy in a group of sociopaths. *J. Clin. Psychol.* 16:321, 322 (1960).
12. Loeb, J., and Mednick, S. Prospective study of predictors of criminality. Electrodermal response patterns, in *Biosocial Bases of Criminal Behavior.* S. Mednick and K. Christiansen, eds. Gardner, New York (1977).
13. Robins, L. *Deviant Children Grown Up.* Williams and Wilkins, Baltimore (1966).
14. Conger, J., and Miller, W. *Personality, Social Class and Delinquency.* Wiley, New York (1966).
15. Powers, E. and Witmer, H. *An Experiment in the Prevention of Delinquency.* Columbia, New York (1951).

16. West, D. and Farrington, D. P. *Who Becomes Delinquent?* Heineman, London (1973).
17. Sorenson, L. and Mednick, S. A prospective study of predictors of criminality. school behavior, in *Biosocial Bases of Criminal Behavior*. S. Mednick and K. Christiansen, eds. Gardner, New York (1977).
18. Tanay, E. *Murderers*, Bobbs-Merrill, Indianapolis (1976).

27

Rape

FREDERICK SIERLES

INTRODUCTION

When I was in medical school, the subject of rape was not included in the curriculum. Rape is now getting some belated attention, in large part because of the feminist movement. It called attention to rape because rape victims are almost always women, and for years the legal treatment of rape victims has included innuendoes and outright statements that the woman "really wanted" the attack. Another reason for calling attention to the subject is that the frequency of rape increased during the past decade, and increased faster than other violent crimes.

Three books on the subject are noteworthy. *Against Our Will* [1] by Susan Brownmiller discusses attitudes about rape. *The Rape Victim* [2] by Elaine Hilberman includes a practical discussion of the medical evaluation and treatment of the rape victim. *Victims of Rape* [3] covers the psychology of the rape victim.

STATISTICS ON RAPE

Incidence

According to the Federal Bureau of Investigation, 46,430 women were victims of rape in 1972, and in 1974 there was an estimated total of 55,210 rapes [2]. The latter represents a 49% increase over 1969 [2]. Rape is one of the most underreported crimes, with perhaps 50-90% of rapes going unreported [2].

Characteristics of the rapist

Three-quarters of rapes involved one or two rapists (one rapist, 57%, two rapists, 16%), and group rapes constituted 27% of rapes [2]. Of all age groups, adolescents are most likely to be victims of group rape [3]. Seventy-one percent of rapes were planned in advance [2]. The rapist knew the victim 50-54% of the time [2,3]; when the victim is a child, the figure rises to 80% [3]. Physical force other than the sex acts themselves occurred 85% of the time [2]. Many of the rapists were intoxicated with alcohol. The vast majority of rapists were males under 30 [2]. The overwhelming majority of rapes are intraracial [2,3].

Characteristics of the victim

In two studies [2,3], the victims ranged in age from several months to 97 years, with the majority being between 13 and 25 years of age, and 15 being the commonest age. Most, but not all, studies show a higher rate of black than white victimization [2,3]. Eighty-two percent of the victims suffer physical injury in addition to the sex act itself, and a small percentage are murdered. However, most of the time the victim is not seriously bruised or bleeding heavily [3].

Location and timing

The majority of rapes occur at night [2,3]. More rapes occur on weekend days than on weekdays [2,3], and in warm weather rather than in cold weather [2]. Fifty-six percent of rapes occur in the victim's residence. The frequency of rape is higher in low-income areas.

THE PSYCHOLOGY OF RAPE

It would be difficult to list or discuss all of the emotional reactions experienced by victims during and after the rape. Just before the events occurs, the response can vary from overwhelming fear to disbelief. The adult or teenage victim is usually threatened with violence (a gun, a knife, a beating) [3] and must decide in a few seconds whether to physically resist or run, to "talk the assailant out of it," or to submit to the rape in preference to being killed. There is certainly no "best" response applicable to all situations.

After the rape, there are periods of numbing and disbelief, anger and sadness, guilt and shame, disgust, and fear of repetition of the crime. There are other problems such as to whom, if anyone, to tell about the rape and whether to report it to the police. These are compounded by fears about a spouse or partner treating the rape like an affair, and about defense attorneys implying that the victim "really wanted it." Additionally, there are fears of pregnancy, of venereal disease, of another rape, and of retaliation by the rapist for reporting the crime.

LEGAL ASPECTS

Legally, the woman is not required to report the rape or press charges, and is not required to come to a hospital or to accept treatment. If the case should come to court, there is a new precedent that the victim's prior sex life is not to be admitted as evidence.

TREATMENT

Depending on the circumstances, the patient may be treated by a physician in a private office, or by a rape crisis team in a hospital emergency room. Regardless of the circumstances, certain diagnostic and therapeutic activities must take place if the patient consents.

Support during the procedures

One staff member, usually but not necessarily a nurse, must remain with the patient throughout the treatment process. This person should explain the procedures, be a concerned listener, and be sure that the diagnosis and treatment are occurring with minimal delay.

The history

A physician must take a history which includes the circumstances of the rape, the presence of symptoms, the use of contraceptive techniques, the possibility of pregnancy, the existence of allergies to penicillin, the patient's general health, the means of protection against future attack, and the emotional supports available to the patient.

The patient's history of being raped must be accepted as true under usual circumstances. The physician must appreciate that the patient may feel too numb or upset to talk at length, particularly to an unfamiliar male interviewer. On the other hand, the patient must be permitted to talk at length if she wishes to do so, and the physician's awkward feelings should not impede this process.

The physical exam

The physical exam should include a careful examination for the presence of bruises and other injuries, and a clear notation of the findings. Remember that many rape victims are not bruised or bloody.

Laboratory tests

A *pregnancy test* should be done to consider pregnancy, so that a preexisting pregnancy is not subjected to abortion. A *serologic test* should be done to rule out syphilis, because the prophylactic penicillin which is to be given may render a serology negative in the presence of viable spirochetes from a preceding infection. *Slides* should be made of fluid from the endocervix and posterior fornix to detect spermatozoa. Swabs for gonorrhea should be taken from the vagina and anus. Pubic and scalp *hair combing* and fingernail clippings should be collected to obtain traces of evidence such as skin and hair from the rapist. The patient should be asked to stand on a sheet and shake off loose materials from her clothing, or else to contribute portions of her *clothing* as evidence. Special evidence collection kits, such as the *Vitullo Kit* used in Cook County, Ill., are available to facilitate the collection of evidence.

Notification of the police

At Cook County Hospital in Chicago, the police are routinely notified about all rapes. This takes the responsibility for reporting the rape from the patient to the staff, and provides police with information with no delay. The patient is informed that this is going to be done, and that she has the right not to talk to the police or to press charges. The vast majority of the patients at Cook County Hospital consent to this procedure, and don't challenge its logic. The interview by the police should be done as tactfully as the medical interview, and a staff member should be immediately available to ensure that this is the case.

Treatment

If the patient is not allergic to penicillin, she should be given 4.8 million U procaine *penicillin* intramuscularly, and 1 g *probenecid* to maintain the blood level of penicillin. If the patient is not pregnant, and the patient was not covered by contraception during the rape, she should be given 50 mg diethylstibestrol orally as a "morning after" *oral contraceptive*. Abrasions and lacerations should be treated, and tetanus toxoid should be given if needed. The patient should be encouraged to express feelings throughout the diagnostic and treatment process, and should be offered the chance to do so in the future. If there is any awkwardness about the response to the patient of an *important family member* or friend, an offer should be made to include this individual in the ensuing discussions. Printed material should be available to the patient to reinforce the explanations which are given, and the patient should be given written and verbal instructions to return if the patient experiences signs of pregnancy, mental illness, or emotional upset.

Homosexual rape

This is supposedly fairly common in prisons, and occasionally occurs elsewhere as well. The principles of treatment are basically the same as for heterosexual rape.

REFERENCES

1. Brownmiller, S. *Against Our Will: Men, women and rape.* Simon and Schuster, New York (1975).
2. Hilberman, E. *The Rape Victim.* Am. Psychiatr. Assoc., Washington, D.C. (1976).
3. National Institute of Mental Health. *Victims of Rape.* (Pub. No. 241-186/1133). U.S. Gov. Prtg. Off. Washington, D.C. (1977).

28

Forensic Medicine

FREDERICK SIERLES

INTRODUCTION

Adherence to the rules of the law has priority in the legal profession, as this quote from F. Lee Bailey reveals:

> Let's start with a hypothetical case. Two men, inmates in the same prison, write my office for help. Both have been convicted as participants in the same loan company holdup. The first man says he's innocent. He was tucked in with his girlfriend at the time of the robbery, but the jury didn't believe her. The second man doesn't deny taking part in the crime, but complains that he was never told that as an indigent he had a right to free counsel. Jailhouse lawyers have told him this is a sufficient violation of rights afforded him by the Miranda decision to win him a new trial.
>
> We write the first man: There is nothing we can do for you; innocence is not important once you're in the can. But we tell the second man he has a sixty-forty chance of winning a new trial. He writes back to say that's fine, and that a relative will be in with a retainer. "By the way," he adds, referring to the robber, "the other guy who wrote you wasn't there. I know, because I was." The revelation won't change anything. [1]

As physicians we live and work in a legal system and we have to know the rules of the law as they apply to our practice. Fortunately, these rules meet our needs and the needs of our patients most of the time, and good medicine usually coincides with good law.

> Examples: In Illinois, and in most states, a physician can treat a 15-year-old for venereal disease at the request of the 15-year-old, without the consent of his parents and without informing his parents. However, if that same 15-year-old has appendicitis, the physician could not remove his

appendix without the consent of his parent or guardian, except under special circumstances. To do such an operation without parental consent would be a serious breach of law.

This chapter will be divided into day-to-day considerations of the law in all brances of medicine; considerations related to all branches of medicine; special considerations related to all branches of medicine; and considerations relating primarily to the patient's mental status.

DAY-TO-CONSIDERATIONS

Confidentiality

A physician is expected to respect the privacy of information provided by his patient. Nurses and other medical staff working with the patient may, as "extensions" of the physician, be privy to information about the patient. A physician may be sued for failing to protect the privacy of a patient's revelations and diagnosis. A patient may give written permission to release of history and findings. There are, however, a number of exceptions to the above generalizations.

Testimony in court

If a physician is testifying in court, and the questions he is being asked are relevant to the case at hand, he can be required to testify about information which he would otherwise consider confidential.

Examples: At a commitment hearing, a consulting psychiatrist testifies that the patient threatened to drag him across the room by his tie.

Child abuse or neglect

In cases of probable or possible child abuse or neglect, the physician is required in all states to report the situation to the local child protection agency. In some states, the physician can be penalized (e.g., loss of license) if he does not report a case. If there is any evidence whatever to support his suspicions and contentions, the physician cannot be held liable for reporting the case.

Life and death emergencies

In a dire emergency, such as impending suicide or homicide, a physician may breach a patient's confidence; in fact, there are circumstances, such as potential homicide by a patient, where he may even be expected to breach the patient's confidence.

> Example: The parents of a suicidal teenager are told of the patient's suicide risk, without the patient's consent, to assure they will consent to her hospital care.

Documentations for insurance purposes

Insurance companies sometimes request portions of a patient's hospital record in order to determine whether the patient is entitled to insurance payments. If the physician makes this data available, he must get the patient's written consent and should provide the minimum amount of data necessary.

Treason

American physicians are required to report acts of treason. It should be apparent that confidentiality within the doctor-patient relationship, while vital to proper treatment, is less well respected by our legal system than the priest-penitent relationship, lawyer-client relationship, and the boss-secretary relationship.

Charting

The notes a physician makes on a medical record may be used as evidence for or against him in court, and may be the only documentation he has that he performed an indicated procedure. If I have sufficient time, I try to make notations in the chart as if the attorney for a potential litigant were sitting in the next chair. Be clear, be specific, be as thorough as possible, and give explanations and justifications for decisions.

> Example: A physician writes an order for "close observation" of a potentially suicidal patient, and does not spell out what is meant by "close observation." The patient, during a moment in which he was out of sight of the nurse, leaves the ward and commits suicide. A lawsuit follows, the central focus being the vagueness of the "close observation" order.

Informed consent

Before a medical procedure is performed, a patient should be given a thorough explanation of the reasons for, risks of, and alternatives to the procedure, so that he can make a thoughtful decision about whether to consent to the procedure. The patient must give signed consent, and the physician must document, either by a thorough note in the chart, or a copy of printed material given to the patient, that informed consent was given. There are times when a physician feels that giving an elaborate explanation might be detrimental, but if he chooses to withhold this information, he can still conceivably be sued for failure to give proper informed consent.

> Example: Before doing a videotaped teaching interview, I usually state to the patient: "I'd like to interview you in the presence of a videotape camera. The interview will last for about 25 minutes, and I'll ask you things like what brought you to the hospital, how you're doing now, and what conditions you've had in the past. This will be for teaching purposes, and will only be shown to medical students and your doctors. If there's anything you wish to withhold, you don't have to say it. It's primarily for our purposes, although you may feel more comfortable after talking about yourself. Is there anything you'd like to ask?"

Consent to psychiatric inpatient hospitalization

Patients consenting to treatment in a hospital psychiatric service must also give informed written consent, usually on a special document such as a "voluntary admission form."

Unusual circumstances

Inability to give consent

If a patient is comatose or physically unable to give consent in a life-threatening emergency, the physician may provide lifesaving treatment; it is "the better part of wisdom" to solicit the consent of the next of kin or a close relative in person or by telephone (phoned consent with a hospital telephone operator as a witness is acceptable).

Refusal to give consent

If a patient refuses treatment, and the situation is not a life-threatening emergency, the procedure should not be done at that time. If a patient refuses treatment when the situation is imminently life-threatening, and there is reason to believe the patient is incompetent to give consent, or that the refusal is a distinct suicide attempt, the physician should consider the following: he may have to act immediately and on his own because of the direness of the situation; if there is time, he should solicit the consent of, in order of priority, the spouse or a child of the patient; if there is a conflict between the wishes of the doctor and those of the patient, or between the doctor and the relative, the hospital administrator should be notified; if the hospital administrator supports the doctor's position, a judge can be petitioned to issue a court order.

Treatment of minors

For the treatment of minors (usually this refers to people under 18 years), a parent or guardian must give consent. There are some exceptions to this rule.

1. *Emancipated minors.* These are teenagers under age 18, either married, a parent, or pregnant. They may themselves consent to medical treatment.
2. *Venereal disease.* In some states, a minor may, without parent's consent, receive information about, examination for, and treatment of venereal disease.
3. *Psychiatric treatment in a public facility.* In Illinois, a teenager of 16 or 17 may voluntarily admit himself, without parent's consent, for inpatient psychiatric treatment in a public hospital. Also, a minor of 14 to 17 may receive, without parent's consent, up to five 45-min psychotherapy sessions in a community mental health center.
4. *Dire emergencies.* If no parent or guardian is available in a life-threatening emergency, the physician can render lifesaving treatment; however, the physician should have someone try to locate the parent or guardian.

SPECIAL CONSIDERATIONS

Good Samaritan laws

These laws, in existence in most states, hold that a physician rendering care to a patient in an emergency will have limited liability for his actions as long as he doesn't crudely malpractice, and as long as he doesn't abandon the patient.

Example: A physician, watching a movie in a theater, responds to a call "Is there a doctor in the house?" He examines a 55-year-old woman who has fainted and recovered from a hyperventilation episode. He accompanies the patient in an ambulance to a local hospital and reports his findings to the emergency room physician. If he were sued for malpractice, it is likely that he would not be held liable.

Testimony in court

On the witness stand, it is difficult to "rest on your laurels" as a physician. Pomposity, smugness, and the use of unfamiliar medical jargon are frowned upon by the judges and attorneys who run the courtroom and who aren't automatically impressed by doctors. Be honest, be clear, and use simple lay terms where possible.

> Example: A physician is testifying during a court martial. He uses the word "Thorazine" in a sentence without explaining it, as if he were talking to a colleague. The defense attorney interrupts, and asks, "Doctor, will you explain to the court what Thorazine is and what it does?"

Physicians and witnesses in general do not have to be experts to testify about the *facts* of a case. An *expert witness* is a person who, by virtue of particular knowledge or skills and based upon the judge's discretion, is allowed to give testimony as to his *opinions*, which can then be entered into the record as facts. At the beginning of their testimony, physicians, "expert" and "nonexpert," are asked for their training and credentials.

Lawsuits

On a statistical basis, for every four American physicians, there is one lawsuit brought against a physician *each* year (25 suits per 100 physicians per year) [2]. Of course, not all physicians are sued with equal frequency. The most frequently sued specialists are, in decreasing order: Anesthesiologists, orthopedists, surgeons in general, and obstetricians [2]. In one California study, 46 physicians (.6% of the California physician population) accounted for 10% of all claims and 30% of all awards [3]. In 1970, about 10% of malpractice claims reached trial. Of the remaining 90%, an unknown proportion was settled with compensation out of court [3]. In court, the majority of trial cases are won by the defendants [3]. In 1970, the median payment to claimants was $2,000 [3]. From 1973 to 1978, about 50% were for improper treatment and about 25% were for misdiagnosis, the latter representing a significant increase since 1970 [3]. Apparently the public is aware of the physician's increasing diagnostic capability. Making guarantees (e.g., "If you let me operate on you hand, I'll make it as good as new") leaves a physician highly vulnerable. From 1973 to 1978, only 2.5% of claims were for failure to give informed consent [3]. In psychiatry, the most common reasons for lawsuits are associated with "injuries to a person," such as those that result from faulty diagnosis, improper certification, failure to take proper suicidal precautions [including failure to give electroconvulsive therapy (ECT) indicated], injuries from drugs or ECT, or sexual intercourse with a patient. As of

1973, there were no recorded cases of successful lawsuits associated with poor psychotherapy per se or failure to commit a patient [4]. Physicians are now expected to provide optimal care to patients, not merely to keep up with the standards of the community in which they practice.

The high frequency of claims is frightening, and has contributed to the increased cost of malpractice insurance (some surgeons pay as much as $20,000 per year for malpractice insurance) and to the coining of the phrase "defensive medicine." However, Schwartz and Kamesar [5] argue that the threat of a lawsuit may be an effective deterrent to malpractice, and that actual malpractice is fairly common. These authors claim that for every six cases of actual physician malpractice, only one results in a malpractice claim.

Respondeat superior

An employer or supervisor of a person engaged in the treatment of patients may be held legally responsible for the actions of the employee or supervisee. This responsibility applies both to situations where the physician was expected to instruct the people who work under him in how to handle situation (ministrative responsibility) and to situations where the people who work under him have to make discretionary decisions (discretionary responsibility).

Example: A patient commits suicide in a hospital because of inadequate suicide precautions. The hospital, as well as the doctor, is sued and decides to settle out of court.

Res ipsa loquitor

This term means "the thing (the act) stands for itself." Before the 1960s, when a patient claimed that an injury was the result of a medical procedure, the burden of proof rested with patient, not the physician. Now, when the injury occurred at the time of the procedure the burden of proof lies with the physician, who must demonstrate that the injury was not a possibility, about which the patient had been forewarned, of a competently performed procedure.

Contingent fees

These are fees paid to attorneys; they represent a percentage of the amount a client receives for a successful lawsuit. Contingent fees have been criticized on the grounds that they are an impetus for attorneys to become overzealous in developing the client's action, and justified on the grounds that they allow poor people, or people who couldn't otherwise afford an attorney, access to high-quality legal services.

CONSIDERATIONS RELATING PRIMARILY TO A PATIENT'S MENTAL STATUS

Competence

There are different kinds of competence. In competency determinations, a final or binding decision can be made only by a court of law. However, psychiatrists or other physicians may be asked to offer tentative opinions. The key issue in competency is conformity to legal criteria, not diagnosis.

Testamentary capacity (Competence to make a will)

No matter what the diagnosis, the patient must be able to all of the following: (1) He must know he is making out a will; (2) he must know the extent of his possessions (his bounty); and (3) he must know to whom he could be logically expected to give his possessions (the natural objects of his bounty), even if he does not wish to give these possessions to any or all of these people.

Competence to stand trial

No matter what the diagnosis, the patient must be able to participate intelligently and cooperatively with his attorney in his defense.

Competence to enter into a contract (e.g., marriage, consent for surgery)

No matter what the diagnosis, the patient must comprehend the nature and consequences of the contract:

Example: A patient, who deliberately lacerated his neck with a razor blade in a suicide attempt associated with an affective disorder, reveals that he knows that he has a deep cut in his neck and that it will need to be explored and repaired under anesthesia by a surgeon. He gives his written consent for the procedure and the consulting psychiatrist writes on his chart that the patient appears to know the nature and consequence of this "contract," meaning the consent to undergo surgery.

Competence to manage funds

The consulting physician tentatively determines if the *patient* will manage his funds in a reasonable manner and not grossly hoard or squander them because of impaired judgment resulting from mental illness. If the physician (ideally a psychiatrist) feels the patient is incompetent, and the court verifies this in its proceeding, the court can appoint a guardian to manage the patient's funds.

Involuntary hospitalization

An adult patient may be involuntarily hospitalized only on the grounds of imminent dangerousness to himself or others. Criteria for dangerousness are rarely spelled out in writing, although a recent Hawaii Supreme Court ruling established that dangerousness to property does not constitute dangerousness for purposes of involuntary hospitalization. Although there is no supporting legal precedent or scientific data, I apply the following criteria to my clinical decisions:

Both 1 and 2 are required:

   1. The patient has brain dysfunction (psychiatric illness) causing one of the following three situations to exist:

    a. The patient has a suicidal tendency.

    b. The patient has a homicidal tendency.

    c. The patient has severe cognitive deficits rendering him unable to care for himself or solicit others to care for him.

   2. The severity of item 1 must such that there is at least a 1 in 10 chance that the patient or a potential victim will be dead or crippled within 2 weeks.

Admittedly, these criteria cannot be literally measured and only serve as a conceptual guideline. In most states, any physician may hospitalize a patient involuntarily for several days if the patient meets the physician's criteria for dangerousness. Statutes governing the actual involuntary hospitalization procedure vary from state to state.

Beyond several days, a patient may be detained against his will only by direction of a court as a result of a commitment hearing, in which a psychiatrist is usually asked to testify. The patient usually has the option of a bench hearing or a jury hearing.

Periods of commitment usually last for several months at a time, and are subject to frequent review. Since a commitment is a legal equivalent of an imprisonment, a commitment hearing is call a mittimus hearing. For the same reason, a committed patient may request a writ of habeas corpus, a request for release. Many courts allow commitments to be terminated with mutual agreement between the patient, the physician, and the hospital, without requiring permission of the court at the time of the release.

Insanity defense in criminal proceedings

Insanity is a legal, not a medical term. Criteria vary from state to state. A final and binding decision can be made only by a court, although psychiatrists may testify as expert witnesses. In the United States, the insanity defenses are as follows:

The M'Naghten rule

All states include this test in one form or another. It holds that a person is not guilty of a crime by virtue of insanity if, at the time of the criminal act, and due to mental illness or defect, he was *unable to comprehend the nature and quality of his act and that the act was wrong.*

Example: A patient was arrested for going AWOL from a military hospital. Later, he stated to a psychiatrist that he went AWOL because he feared he would be killed by the hospital staff. The psychiatrist stated this when testifying in the court martial and the patient was found not guilty by virtue of insanity.

The irresistable impulse rule

Some states employ this criterion. It holds that a person is not guilty by virtue of insanity if at the time of the crime he was acting under the influence of an "irresistable impulse" (uncontrollable passion).

American Law Institute model penal code

Some states employ this standard. It holds that a person is not guilty by virtue of insanity if, at the time of the offense, due to mental disease or defect, and in the absence of a record of habitual or repeated offenses, he meets M'Naghten or irresistible impulse criteria.

REFERENCES

1. Bailey, F. *The Defense Never Rests.* Stein and Day, New York (1971).
2. Waltz, J., and Inbau, F. *Medical Jurisprudence.* Macmillan, New York (1971).
3. Curran, W. Malpractice claims. New data and trends. *N. Engl. J. Med.* 300:26-27 (1979).
4. Slovenko, R. *Psychiatry and Law.* Little, Brown, Boston (1973).
5. Schwartz, W., and Kamesar, N. Doctors, damages and deterrence. *N. Engl. J. Med.* 298:1282-1290 (1979).

29

Health Care Delivery I: Quality of Our Health Care System

FREDERICK SIERLES

INTRODUCTION

One could be a competent clinician without being expert about the American health care system, just as one can be a contributing citizen without expertise on government and economics. However, knowing about the system may decrease the number of questions a physician needs to ask others on a day-to-day basis. Such questions include:

To whom should I send a bill for my treatment of this 75-year-old man?

How do my earnings compare with those of the average American physician?

What would the AMA do for me if I joined it?

To whom should I write to get a medical license in my state?

Is there an alternative to taking and passing the National Boards?

I want to do a clinical research project. Whose approval must I get?

Many physicians occupy administrative positions such as dean, department chairman, and program director. These physicians need to know additional information like: What agencies can provide my department with grant funding? How can I get my newly formed residency program accredited? How can I tell if a certain foreign-educated applicant to my staff is properly accredited?

ACCOMPLISHMENTS OF OUR HEALTH CARE SYSTEM

In general, our system has been innovative and effective in the prevention and treatment of illness, but by many indicators, it is not the best in the world, and not all Americans have access to the best care. The following advances have been made:

Children

Infant mortality decreased 33% between 1965 and 1974 [1]. In 1976, the infant mortality rate was 15.2 deaths under age 1 per 1,000 live births [2], our lowest up to that time. Between 1965 and 1974, deaths of babies from gastrointestinal diseases decreased 50%, influenza and pneumonia by 58%, and immaturity by 61% [1]. Maternal mortality has decreased by one-third [1].

Adults

In 1976, the average life expectancy from birth was 72.6 years; in 1900, the figure was 47.1 years [2]. In 1977, the crude death rate was 8.8 deaths per 1,000 population, the lowest in our history [2]. Age-adjusted death rates have declined for heart disease in general, ischemic heart disease in particular, cerebrovascular disease, accidents, influenza, pneumonia, diabetes, and arteriosclerosis [1].

The Poor

Death rates for blacks have decreased more rapidly than those for whites; death rates for Indians have decreased for a number of causes [1]. For the poor, access to medical care has also improved. Low-income families covered by government-funded health programs now receive health service at almsot the same rate as for middle-class families, and physician visits have increased [1].

Reasons

Improvement in the health of a population comes from improved *primary prevention* (prevention of disease occurrence), *secondary prevention* (detection of illness before symptoms and signs develop), and *tertiary prevention* (reduction of disability and infirmity once a symptomatic disease has been identified).

Immunizations for diphtheria, pertussis, tetanus, polio, measles, mumps, and rubella have drastically reduced the prevalence of these illnesses. Requirement of the use of lead-free gasoline has helped in the effort to control air pollution. Public health agencies and the media are encouraging people to "keep in shape" and to stop smoking. Of people between 12 and 74 years of age, 57% reported that their recreation involved "much" exercise or that they are physically quite active in their usual day at work [2]. Over 29 million people have stopped smoking [2,3], 95% of whom have done so without entering any formal program for treatment of smoking [2]. Community water fluoridation which, incidentally, costs only 10-40 cents per year per person served [2], has reduced tooth decay in children. This is particularly important since dental caries are an extremely common chronic health problem.

Screening to detect serious illness has been helpful; this has included blood pressure checks, proctoscopy and Papinicolao smears. Multiphasic (multiple tests for multiple systems) screening is being employed at some centers, and receiving government support. Sophisticated diagnostic procedures have enabled physicians to make earlier and better diagnoses; these include amniocentesis, angiography, colonoscopy, computerized axial tomography, duodenoscopy, echography, telemetry, His-bundle electrocardiography, mammography, radioisotope scanning, and thermography.

There have been major developments in the treatment process itself. Drugs that have been used extensively for the first time in the 1960s and 1970s include contraceptive hormones, cephalothin, diazepam, dolophine, droperidol, gentamycin, haloperidol, L-dopa, lithium carbonate, propranolol, Rhogam, and urokinase. Relatively new surgical procedures, which include cardiac pacemakers, cryosurgery, laser-beam surgery, and vascular bypass surgery, have made important contributions.

COMPARISONS OF EFFECTIVENESS OF HEALTH CARE

As was stated before, despite the above developments the health of Americans is not, by some indicators, the best in the world, and not all Americans have access to the best medical care. People in Sweden, France, and the Netherlands have a higher life expectancy than Americans [4]. Twelve countries have lower infant mortality rates [5]. Mortality from lung cancer and other serious respiratory diseases has been increasing, and 42% of American men and 32% of American women are smokers [2]. Twelve percent of deaths in the United States have been deemed "sentinel deaths"; that is, deaths that could have been prevented by some form of medical intervention [2].

Large numbers of children are not fully immunized against childhood diseases; for example, in 1976, 34% of children 1-4 years of age were not immunized against rubella [2]. Twenty-five percent of women who gave birth to live infants in 1976 had not seen a physician during their first trimester [2]. Ten percent of adults have never been immunized [2]. Fifty-two percent of Americans have not seen a dentist during the past year, and 20% of people over the age of 5 have not seen a dentist in the last 5 years [2].

Russia has a higher physician-patient ratio [4]. Despite our own high ratio, there is a maldistribution of physicians. Millions of people still live in doctor-shortage areas, most of which are situated in rural areas and inner cities, locations where it is difficult to attract physicians. Medical specialists and short-term general hospitals are more likely to be located in high-income sections of metropolitan areas; for example, in 1973, there were 4.8 obstetrician/gynecologists for every 10,000 women of childbearing age in metropolitan areas, compared to 1.8:10,000 in nonmetropolitan areas [2]. There is a decreased proportion of primary care physicians in contrast to the proportion that existed earlier in this century. One consequence is that emergency rooms treat many patients with nonemergency-type problems.

While birth rates have been down for the past two decades [4], our population, 217.7 million people at the beginning of 1978, continues to increase. Our population is expected to double by the year 2065, so 435.4 million people are going to require good medical care by that year [2].

REFERENCES

1. Davis, K. U.S. Health care: The road ahead. *Journal of Medical Education* 52:33-37 (1977).
2. DHEW Publications No. (PHS) 78:1232. *Health in the United States, 1978.*
3. Mausner, B. An ecologic view of cigarette smoking. *Journal of Abnormal Psychology* 81:115-126 (1974).
4. DHEW Publication No. (PHS) (HRA) 76-1233. *Health in the United States: A Chartbook, 1975.*
5. Rosser, J., and Mossberg, H. *An Analysis of Health Care Delivery.* Wiley, New York (1977).

30

Health Care Delivery II: Relationship of the Health Care System to Society in General

FREDERICK SIERLES

INTRODUCTION

Our health care system is an integral part of American society, and is vulnerable to changes in all aspects of society. In the social sphere, civil rights and changes in the doctor-patient relationship have had effects. In the economic sphere, inflation weighs heavily, and in the political arena, increased influence of the government has occurred.

THE SOCIAL SPHERE

Civil Rights

The civil rights movement was reborn in the 1950s, peaked in the late 1960s, and continues with vigor today. As a result, health care is now perceived as a right, not a privilege. The health care of many underprivileged groups has been affected.

The Poor

The poor have been helped by government programs. Medicaid (Medical care for the indigent) and Medicare (Medical care for the aged) were established by an Act of Congress in 1965. Medicare covers hemodialysis for many poor people who would have died from renal failure. Affirmative Action generated admissions of minority students to medical schools in the 1970s. In academic year 1975-1976, 8.2% of medical students were minority students [1]. Community mental health legislation led to the establishment of mental health centers in areas with large numbers of poor people.

The Elderly

A number of government and nongovernment organizations have provided assistance to the elderly. Like Medicaid, Medicare (medical care for the aged) was established by an Act of Congress in 1965. The U.S. Commission on Civil Rights stated in 1977 that medical schools, hospitals, and other employers could be sued under the Age Discrimination Act if qualified people were not hired because of age. An employment pool for emeritus professors in the health professions was established in 1977 by the Association of American Medical Colleges. Recently, the mandatory retirement age has been increased to 70 by an Act of Congress.

Women

The feminist movement, sometimes backed by government support, has successfully lobbied for an increased rate of professional school admissions for women; 20% of incoming medical school classes are now composed of women [2]. The "psychology of women" has been included in medical school curricula. There has been an increased response of the medical community to the crimes of rape and woman abuse. Legal abortions, based on a mutual decision between a woman and her physician, are now available.

Children

In cases of child abuse, the physician is required to report the situation to local authorities, and is allowed to hospitalize the child without the parents' consent; the physician is regarded as the child's, not the parent's doctor. To facilitate the treatment of veneral disease in teenagers, most states allow a physician to treat a minor without consent of the minor's parents. In some states the age at which a teenager can consent to his own admission to the psychiatric unit of a hospital has been lowered from 18 to 16.

The Handicapped

There is a federal affirmative action program concerning the hiring and life-style of the handicapped. Two highly visible examples were the appointment of a paraplegic (Max Cleland) as Chief of Veterans Affairs, and the requirement by government agencies for development of handicapped parking and bathroom facilities in public places.

The Mentally Ill

Court decisions have played a role in guaranteeing the rights of the mentally ill. In the *Rouse vs. Cameron* and *Donaldson vs. O'Connor* court decisions, a principle called "right to treatment" was established, whereby anyone committed to a mental hospital because of dangerousness or "insanity" is entitled to the same standards of treatment that are provided to any hospitalized patient.

Students

The Buckley Amendment to a 1975 Act of Congress established that students are entitled to see all documents used in evaluating them.

Research Subjects

All agencies seeking government funding for scientific research on humans must have Human Studies Committees to ensure that research subjects are participating with full knowledge of experimental conditions and possible ramifcations.

The Doctor-Patient Relationship

There have been significant changes in the doctor-patient relationship. With the increased specialization of physicians during the 1960s and 1970s, it is highly likely that a patient will be treated by a number of physicians, each of whom may know him less well than the "old-time GP." The frequency of lawsuits against physicians is on the rise. As a result, there has been an increase in malpractice insurance costs, with the passing of virtually all of these costs to the patient. Physicians and patients sometimes see themselves in an adversary role, with the term "defensive medicine" being used fairly frequently. For the first time, there are countersuits against lawyers and patients by sued physicians. As a result of the above phenomena, there is a government-backed priority for establishing primary care treatment relationships, primary care residencies, and the teaching of medical school and postgraduate courses in interviewing, empathy, and communication.

THE ECONOMIC SPHERE

In this area, the most prominent factor has been inflation, which has been massive (14% in 1979). In the late 1970s, health care costs inflated at a greater rate than costs in other industries,* with the greatest increment being in hospital costs, slightly more than half of which [3] are for personnel. Two factors contributing to the inflation of health care costs have been the proliferation of expensive technology and the increase in malpractice insurance costs. A third, and perhaps more important, factor is the fact that 67% of medical expenses are not paid by patients themselves, but by "third-party payers," which consist of the government and insurance carriers [2]. The "real" (corrected for inflation) out-of-pocket cost of medical care for the consumer has not increased since 1950 [3]. In circumstances where all or almost all coverage for a patient is by a third-party payer, there is a tendency for the physician to be less cost-conscious in ordering laboratory tests and billing, and for the patient to "get his money's worth." This is compounded by pressure by hospitals on physicians to maintain high hospital censuses.

While some increase in the cost of medical care is inevitable during times of inflation, costs can certainly be markedly influenced by the behavior of hospitals, physicians, and patients. For example, one study [2] revealed a 17-fold variation in lab test costs in a sample of hospitals. In considering inflation, it is also important to realize that the economic sphere interdigitates with the social and political spheres; if, for example, in an effort to cut costs, Medicaid and Medicare pay physicians less for medical care, physicians will be less likely to treat Medicaid and Medicare patients [3].

THE POLITICAL ARENA

In the political arena, there has been increased control over the practice of medicine by the government, by insurance carriers, and by the profession itself. As an agent for civil rights, and as the nation's largest medical bill-payer (among federal expenditures, health care costs are second only to defense spending), the government has been highly influential.

Affirmative action is backed by the threat of withholding federal funds. The National Institutes of Health and the National Institute of Mental Health have been giving progressively more grant funds for government-created research projects, and grants whose thrust coincide with government priorities. The transfer of American-born medical students from foreign medical schools to American medical schools under the Coordinated Transfer Application System (COTRANS) Program was backed by federal capitation (money "per head") funding.

Federal monies for training programs have been directed towards the

*Health care is our third largest industry after construction and agriculture.

"creation" and teaching of primary care physicians, and proportionately less federal support is being given to medical education in the specialties, education which does not relate to the above priorities, and medical education in general. As a consequence, there has been a depletion of medical school department budgets, and yearly increments of salaries of medical school faculty are not remotely competitive with the yearly inflation of salaries of industrial union members. Most medical school faculty are not union members.

Under the 1974 Health Planning and Resources Development Act, government-supported "regionalization" limits the number and type of services in a given area; for example, only certain hospitals in a locality may own a computerized axial tomographic (CAT) Scanner.

REFERENCES

1. Undergraduate Medical Education. *JAMA* 238:2767-2780 (1977).
2. Schroeder, S., Kenders, K., Cooper, J., and Peimme, T. Use of laboratory tests and pharmaceuticals: Variations among physicians and effect of cost audit on subsequent use. *JAMA* 225(8):969-973 (1973).
3. DHEW Publication No. (PHS) 78:1232. *Health in the United States, 1978.*

31

Health Care Delivery III: Third-Party Payers

FREDERICK SIERLES

INTRODUCTION

In the previous chapter, we referred to the massive costs paid by third-party payers, and we discussed the influence of third-party payers in the health care system. We will now discuss the payment mechanisms themselves.

GOVERNMENT PAYMENT

Medicare

Medicare stands for Medical Care for the Aged, a program initiated in the Kennedy Administration (1960-1963) and passed into law in 1965 by Congress in the Johnson Administration (1964-1968) as an amendment to the Social Security Act. The Medicare law has been amended somewhat since 1965. Medicare covers people over age 65; certain chronic kidney disease patients under 65; disabled people under 65 receiving railroad retirement benefits, and disabled people under 65 receiving Social Security benefits. Overall direction of Medicare rests with the Health Care Financing Administration of the United States Department of Health and Human Services. Funding for Medicare comes totally from the federal government. State governments have a minimal role; in some states, the state government may review and attest to the quality of care being provided by institutions receiving Medicare payment.

Although the overall administration of Medicare rests with the federal government, day-to-day business is managed by insurance companies such as Blue Cross/Blue Shield.

In the original Medicare law, it was stated that Medicare was not supposed to influence the methods by which a physician treated a patient; it was designed simply to pay some of the treatment costs. But by being able to grant, withhold, or limit funds for different types of treatment, there is a direct influence on medical practice. For example, Medicare will not pay for treatment in a private or state psychiatric hospital, but will pay for treatment in the psychiatric unit of a general hospital.

Medicaid

This is Medical Care for the Indigent, also initiated in the Kennedy Administration and passed into law in 1965 as an amendment to the Social Security Act. Unlike Medicare, there were government sources of payment for medical care for the indigent prior to 1965; however, the earlier programs were not as extensive as they are now. Medicaid covers all people receiving cash assistance from the government; all medically indigent aged, blind, and disabled at the discretion of each state government; and medically indigent dependent children. The financial burden of Medicaid is borne by both federal and state governments, with one exception (Arizona does not participate). The proportion that each state and the federal government pays is based upon a formula.

USHBP and CHAMPUS [1]

The military provides its own on-post free medical care for military personnel and their "dependents" (e.g., spouses, children), with the military personnsel getting first priority unless there is an emergency. The program under which this care is provided by military physicians (or private physicians under contract with the military) is called the Uniformed Services Health Benefits Program (USBHP).

When a specific medical service is not provided for dependents on a military post, the dependent may be treated by a civilian physician in a civilian facility under the Civilian Health and Medical Program of the Uniformed Services (CHAMPUS). Like Medicare and Medicaid, CHAMPUS had its origin in a 1965 Act of Congress.

PRIVATE PAYMENT

Health Maintenance Organizations (HMOs)

"An HMO is a system of organizing, financing and delivering health care services to a defined and voluntary enrolled population. The concept of an HMO is not synonymous with the prepaid group practice model, although most current HMOs are based on this model" [2]. In the HMO, the subscriber pays a fixed amount of money yearly to the multispeciality group (the HMO), and as a result most of his basic medical services are covered. In the case of one of the largest HMOs, the Health Insurance Plan (HIP) in New York, only basic outpatient services are covered, so the subscriber has to purchase his own hospitalization policy.

The patient may be treated elsewhere at any time, but the patient must pay for this himself. Besides HIP, well-known HMOs include Kaiser-Permanente, the Ross-Loos Medical Group, and the Group Health Cooperative of Puget Sound [3]. Approximately 5% of Americans are enrolled in HMOs [2], and the number is increasing, but not greatly. Reasons offered for the modest response to HMOs include: (1) Some of these organizations may be perceived by patients as large, forbiding institutions; (2) HMO offices are not always located near a patient's home, and there may be no HMO in a given locality; and (3) the American Medical Association has not been vigorous in supporting HMOs.

Blue Cross/Blue Shield and Private Insurance Carriers

Large numbers of Americans are enrolled in private health insurance plans or in Blue Cross/Blue Shield. The former are profit-making and the latter is a tax-exampt, nonprofit organization. For both, the subscriber pays a fixed amount of money, and is then free to choose any physician or hospital for his care, as long as the care is medically indicated and the medical procedure is covered by the insurance plan. Subscribers can subscribe individually or as part of a group coverage program. There are two types of coverage, basic and major medical coverage, the latter usually serving as a supplement to the former. To give examples to basic and major medical coverage, I will quote from the Blue Cross/Blue Shield policy formerly held by faculty at my medical school [4].

I   Hospitalization benefits (*Basic*):
    A. Days of care per illness or accident: 365
    B. Room:
        1. Semi-private or ward paid in full
        2. Private room partial coverage
        3. Intensive care unit paid in full
    C. Hospital extras such as drugs, x-rays, operating room paid in full
    D. Outpatient emergency and emergency medical care for the initial visit only within 72 hours.

E. Outpatient surgery initial visit only, paid in full.

F. Maternity paid in full after 270 days of membership

II   Doctors medical-surgical benefits (basic):

A. Usual and customary surgical benefits

B. In-hospital medical care for 365 days, each accident of illness.

C. Maternity benefits for Doctor's delivery charge

III   *Major Medical* supplement to above Basic Benefits after the benefits of the basic plan outlined above . . . and after you experience $100 out-of-pocket expenses . . . This Major Medical Plan will pay 80% of all additional covered medical expenses up to a combined maximum of $50,000 for hospital-related expenses and doctor-related expenses (exception: outpatient mental health care is covered by 50% up to a lifetime maximum of $5,000).

IV   Dependent coverage: unmarried dependent children are covered up to their 23rd birthday.

In 1973, 73.5 million people were enrolled in Blue Cross/Blue Shield, about 82% having group contracts. Virtually all people over age 65 have good hospital coverage through Medicare. However, 11% of our population does not have government, Blue Cross/Blue Shield or private coverage [5], and are vulnerable to a financial catastrophe if they become seriously ill. This problem is considerable in rural areas (where 26% of nonfarmers and 39% of farm employees have no form of health insurance), and among people recently laid off from jobs, in between jobs, or on maternity leave [5].

REFERENCES

1. Navy Rights and Benefits. *All Hands* (1979).
2. Rosser, J., and Mossberg, M. *An Analysis of Health Care Delivery*. Wiley, New York (1977).
3. Shindell, S., Salloway, J., and Oberempt, C. *A Coursebook in Health Care Delivery*. Appleton-Century-Crofts, New York (1976).
4. Blue Cross/Blue Shield Publications EB-890. *Your Health Care Program* (1976). Blue Cross/Blue Shield, 233 N. Michigan, Chicago, Ill. 60610.
5. DHEW Publications No. (PHS) 78:1232. *Health in the United States, 1978.* ·

32

Health Care Delivery IV: Influential Organizations

FREDERICK SIERLES

A discussion of the American health care delivery system must include the organizations which control it.

THE UNITED STATES DEPARTMENT OF HEALTH AND HUMAN SERVICES

This is the most powerful health care agency in America; its secretary is a member of the President's cabinet. Its agencies include the following:

1. The Social Security Administration
2. The United States Public Health Service (USPHS)
   a. The Center for Disease Control (CDC)
   b. The Food and Drug Administration (FDA)
   c. The Health Services Administration (HSA)
   d. The Health Resources Administration (HRA)
   e. The National Institute of Health (NIH)
   f. The Alcohol, Drug Abuse and Mental Health Administration (ADAMHA)
      (1) The National Institue of Mental Health (NIMH)
3. The Health Care Financing Administration
   a. Medicare and Medicaid
4. The Office of Human Development Services
5. The Office of Child Support Enforcement
6. Regional Offices

THE VETERANS ADMINISTRATION (VA)

Among other things, this organization is responsible for administering the nation's VA hospitals and for giving pensions for medical disability incurred during active duty in the military ("service-connected" disability). Large numbers of patients are treated in VA hospitals, and large numbers of VA hospitals have medical school affiliations.

STATE AND CITY DEPARTMENTS OF HEALTH

These agencies are responsible for running state and city hospitals, for inspecting hospitals, and for setting safety and health standards. If separate from state departments of health, state departments of mental health serve similar functions in the mental health sphere.

STATE DEPARTMENTS OF EDUCATION AND REGISTRATION

These agencies are responsible for the licensing of physicians to practice within a state.

THE AMERICAN MEDICAL ASSOCIATION (AMA)

This organization, founded in 1847, is the most influential professional organization for physicians. It is supported primarily by membership fees and journal advertising. It provides a number of services, including the following [12]:

1. Lobbying on behalf of the medical profession
2. Presenting medical conferences
3. Publication of the *Journal of the American Medical Association* and many specialty journals such as the *Archives of Internal Medicine* and *Archives of Psychiatry;* publication of the newspaper *American Medical News,* and the lay magazine *Today's Health*
4. Overseeing local medical societies
5. Running the AMA *Joint Commission for Accreditation of Hospitals (JCAH),* which inspects hospitals every 2 years
6. Giving the *Physicians Recognition Award* for efforts in continuing medical education (CME) for physicians
7. Answering questions from physicians concerning medicolegal issues, and providing pamphlets about medicolegal subjects
8. Providing loan guarantee services for some medical students

THE NATIONAL MEDICAL ASSOCIATION (NMA)

This organization provides, for black physicians, some of the same services that the AMA provides for its members. Members of the NMA may also be members of AMA. Services offered by the NMA includes lobbying; publication of the *Journal of the National Medical Association;* support of the *Student National Medical Association* (SNMA); presentation of national conferences; and provision of tutoring, counseling and legal services for black medical students.

THE ASSOCIATION OF AMERICAN MEDICAL COLLEGES (AAMC)

It publishes the *Journal of Medical Education (JME)*, has national conferences, provides workshops for medical school faculties, publishes a weekly news report, and does on-site accreditation inspections for the Liaison Committee on Medical Education (LCME). It has three departments working under its Board of Directors: These are the Council of Teaching Hospitals, the Council of Academic Societies, and the Council of Deans.

THE NATIONAL BOARD OF MEDICAL EXAMINERS (NBME)

This is an independent organization that produces national certifying (accrediting) examinations for medical students who have completed basic sciences (Part I), clerkships (Part II), and the first year of postgraduate medical training (Part III).

Full NBME certification, based on passing Parts 1-3, is accepted for accreditation by most American states as long as it is taken and passed within a requisite number of years prior to application for a state medical license. The NBME also produces the Federation Licensing Examination (FLEX), a certifying examination taken by American or foreign medical school graduates who have not taken, or not passed, Parts 1-3 of the National Boards. Finally, the NBME gives assistance to some specialty boards in the production and grading of their certifying examinations.

THE EDUCATIONAL COUNCIL FOR FOREIGN MEDICAL GRADUATES (ECFMG)

This agency arose as a committee representing the AAMC, the American Hospital Association (AHA), the AMA, and the Federation of State

Medical Boards (FSMB). It devised what it beleived would be "an effective mechanism for measuring educational attainment in the absence of intimate knowledge of the educational background of foreign physicians." To satisfy this mandate, this organization performs three functions: (1) it verifies that a foreign medical school is of acceptable quality; (2) it verifies that a foreign medical graduate has in fact attended the acceptable medical school; and (3) it verifies by the ECFMG examinations that a foreign medical graduate has sufficient knowledge to practice medicine competently. All foreign medical school graduates must meet ECFMG standards before being allowed to practice in an American hospital.

THE AMERICAN HOSPITAL ASSOCIATION

This is an organization which represents the interests of hospital administrators throughout the country. Among other things, it has produced the *Patient Bill of Rights* [2], and it lobbies for the interests of hospitals.

PEER SERVICE REVIEW ORGANIZATIONS (PSRO)

This attained formal legal status in 1970 as the Bennett Amendment to the Social Security Law. Based on the medical profession's resistance to socialized medicine, and a civil rights-consumerism push for better policing of medical care, one compromise was for the medical profession to establish formal treatment guidelines with review by colleagues (peer review). The PSRO laws stated that the medical profession must have a formal PSRO system by 1974. At present, PSRO is still in an early state of development.

THE COORDINATING COMMITTEE ON MEDICAL EDUCATION (CCME)

This is an influential nongovernment agency which is controlled by the medical profession itself. It consists of representatives of the Association of American Medical Colleges, the American Medical Association, the American Hospital Association, the American Board of Medical Specialties (ABMS), and the Council of Medical Specialty Societies (CMSS). The CCME in turn consists of four branches which serve a number of significant functions.

The *Liaison Committee on Medical Education (LCME)* is responsible for accrediting medical schools, with AAMC personnel doing much of the on-site inspection of medical schools.

The *Liaison Committee on Graduate Medical Education (LCGME)*. This body has a review board which accredits residency training programs.

The *Liaison Committee on Continuing Medical Education (LCCME)* plays a supervisory role in continuing medical education.

The *Liaison Committee on Allied Health Education (LCAHE)* has a supervisory role in education in the allied health services.

REFERENCES

1. American Medical Association. *What Do You Get For Your Dues?* (pamphlet), undated A.M.A., 535 North Dearborn Street, Chicago, Illinois 60610.
2. Rosser, J., and Mossberg, M. *An Analysis of Health Care Delivery*. Wiley, New York (1977).

33

Health Care Delivery V: Providers of Health Care

FREDERICK SIERLES

INTRODUCTION

This chapter will touch upon some data concerning institutions and individuals providing health care.

Medical practice can be divided into primary care, secondary care, and tertiary care [1]. *Primary care* is the treatment of common conditions on an outpatient basis. *Secondary care* is the care of somewhat more complex or serious conditions in local community hospitals. *Tertiary care* is highly specialized intensive care, as practiced in large academic hospitals. Of 1,000 randomly selected members of a typical population in one year, "an average of 720 people visited a physician in a ambulatory setting at least once, 100 were admitted to a hospital at least once, and only 10 were admitted to a university hospital at least once" [2].

In 1976, there were 404,338 physicians in the United States, an increase of 23% since 1970 [3]. Excluding physicians working for the federal government, 213,117 physicians provided predominantly office-based care, and 79,035 provided predominantly hospital-based care [3]. From 1970 to 1976, there was an increase of 39% in the number of physicians in internal medicine, a 26% increase in pediatrics, and a 4% decrease in general practice [3]. In 1973, there were more physicians in surgical specialties and medical specialties than family physicians [4]. The 1973 figures are as follows:

Surgical specialties	99,497
Medical specialties	77,598
General practice	65,069

Internal medicine	44,806
General surgery	29,665
Psychiatry and neurology	24,912
Obstetrics and gynecology	19,530
Pediatrics	18,864
Opthalmology	10,158
Other specialties	28,191
Total	333,330

There are more physicians in solo practice than there are physicians in partnership, and more physicians in partnerships than in group practice [3]. But there is a trend in the direction of group practice: in 1969, 18% of physicians were in group practice; in 1975, the figure had increased to 24%. More surgery is being done than ever before. Between 1965 and 1966 and 1975 and 1976, there was a 25% increase in the number of operations performed per unit population [3]. Physicians work long hours and put in more hours per day when they are self-employed than when they are salaried [3]. In 1974, the average annual net income (income after taxes) of an American physician in office-based practice was about $52,000 [1].

OTHER HEALTH CARE OCCUPATIONS

Here is a list, based on 1973 figures, of numbers of people in different health care occupations [4]:

Occupation	Number
Nursing aides, orderlies and attendants	910,000
Registered nurses	815,000
Practical nurses	459,000
Physicians (MD)	333,330
Pharmacists	132,900
Dental assistants	116,000
Dentists	105,400
Radiological technologists	100,000
Dietetic and nutritional services	68,000
Dental hygienests	21,000
Physicians (DO)	12,000

HOSPITALS

In 1976, about half the hospitals in the United States were owned by nonprofit organizations [3]. Another 36% were government-owned, and only 14% were owned by profit-making organizations [3]. Eighty-six percent of hospitals are "general medical and surgical" in nature, and only 14% of hospitals are specialty hospitals, such as ear, nose, and throat hospitals or psychiatric hospitals [3]. The average hospital bed capacity is about 225 [5]. The mean hospital occupancy rate is about 80% nationally.

PSYCHIATRIC HOSPITALS AND CLINICS

Since the mid-1960s, there has been a radical shift in the locations of care of psychiatric patients. The patient populations, and average length of stay, of state psychiatric hospitals have declined markedly. Visits to outpatient clinics, most prominently to community mental health centers, have increased, as have admissions to psychiatric units of general medical and surgical hospitals. There have been a number of state psychiatric hospital closings as a result.

Reasons for these changes include improved diagnosis and treatment, and the *community psychiatry* (application of public health principles to psychiatry) movement, which advocates care of patients in their own locality as opposed to care in geographically remote facilities (like many of the state psychiatric hospitals). The process whereby the responsibility for care shifts from state hospitals and nursing homes to community clinics is called *deinstitutionalization*. This process has not been entirely successful, of course; because of the severity of their illness, because of weak family supports, and because of poor psychiatric care, large numbers of chronically ill psychiatric patients function poorly while out of the hospital, and need frequent (usually brief) readmissions. This problem has been likened to a "revolving door," and its solution is currently a government funding priority.

NURSING HOMES

During the past decade, there has been a large increase in the numbers of nursing homes, an increase in the employee/patient ratio in nursing homes, and an increase in the amount of money spent for nursing home care. During the partial "clearing out" of state psychiatric hospitals during the late 1960s and early 1970s, many chronically ill patients were transferred to nursing homes and sheltered care homes, the latter designed for people who are partially disabled but still capable of a modicum of self-care. In 1977, there were about 18,300 nursing homes serving about 1,287,400 residents [3]. Seventy-one percent were female, 85% were over age 65, 58% were widowed, and 92% were white [3]. Their mean age was 78 years and mean length of stay 2.7 years [3].

REFERENCES

1. Rosser, J., and Mossberg, M. *An Analysis of Health Care Delivery*. Wiley, New York (1977).
2. White, K. Life and death in medicine. *Scientific American* 229:30 (1973).
3. DHEW Publications No (PHS) 78:1232. *Health in the United States, 1978*.
4. DHEW Publication No (PHS) (HRA) 76-1233. *Health in the United States: A Chartbook* (1975).
5. Shindell, S., Salloway, J., and Oberempt, C. *A Coursebook in Health Care Delivery*. Appleton-Century-Crofts, New York (1976).

34

Biostatistics

FREDERICK SIERLES

INTRODUCTION

Medical students and physicians are bombarded with claims, conclusions, and generalizations about research, clinical diagnoses, and treatments. Because people tend to trust what they see in print, medical students or physicians may accept these conclusions at face value. This is sometimes a mistake, as many conclusions, upon which many diagnoses and treatments are based, are incorrect. The consequences for the health of many patients can be disastrous. One example is the overdiagnosis of schizophrenia in the United States (described by Rosenhan [1] and Taylor and Abrams [2]), and the consequent mismedication of healthy, depressed, or manic patients with neuroleptic drugs.

A knowledge of biostatistics is a means of establishing whether data you gather is reliable and valid, and whether the data or claims of others are reliable and valid. Of course statistics are no substitute for hard work or clear thought, and certainly statistics can be "fudged" or misused.

THE CORE EXAMPLE

To make this subject more understandable, we will repeatedly use this core example of a behavioral sciences course given to 12 students in a small medical school class. In this course, evaluation was based upon a proficiency examination (a pretest to establish competence before taking the course) and a final examination. Attendance was voluntary.

Of the 12 registered students in the class, only eight took the proficiency exam. On the proficiency exam the students scores were 67, 69, 75, 77, 78, 80, 81, and 86 questions correct. On the final examination, the scores were 72, 73, 77, 80, 80, 80, 84, 84, 86, 90, 91, and 96 questions correct. The percentage of classes attended by each student were 4, 50, 50, 68, 72, 76, 84, 84, 84, 88, 100, and 100%. The students graded the instructors and rated the instructors' performance on a rating scale.

Raw scores are the number of correct answers that an examinee gets on a test.

In the core example, are the student's scores on the proficiency exam and final exam raw scores? (*Answer:* Yes.)

Variables are things that can be measured and which can vary. Examples of variables are pulse, blood pressure, exam scores, and psychiatric rating scale scores.

In the core example, what is the frequency of students who got a score of 80 on the final examination (*Answer:* 3).

Is the instructor's level of enthusiasm a variable? (*Answer:* Yes, if students are rating the instructor's level of enthusiasm on a rating scale.)

Frequency is the number of times that a certain value of variable appears.

In the core example, what is the frequency of students who got a score of 80 on the final examination (*Answer:* 3).

A distribution is a set of values arranged in order.

In the core example, what is the distribution of scores on the proficiency examination? (*Answer:* 67, 69, 75, 77, 79, 80, 81, and 86.)

In a *frequency distribution*, the number of times that each value appears is listed next to each value.

Make a frequency distribution for the final examination. *Answer:*

Exam Grade	Frequency
72	1
73	1
77	1
80	3
84	2
86	1
90	1
91	1
96	1

Graphs are a way of picturing the relationships between two or more variables. two types of graphs are frequency polygons and histograms. *Frequency polygons* employ points connected by lines. *Histograms* are rectangles to portray what is needed. A frequency polygon is pictured in Figure 1. A histogram is pictured in Figure 2.

Using data from the core example, draw (1) a frequency polygon for the percentage of classes attended, and (2) a histogram for the scores on the final examination (*Answer:* The correct answers are portrayed in Figs. 3 and 4.)

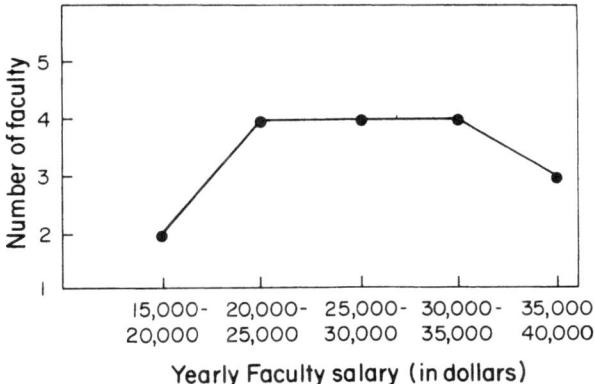

FIG. 1. A frequency polygon showing salary ranges of members of a hypothetical medical school department faculty.

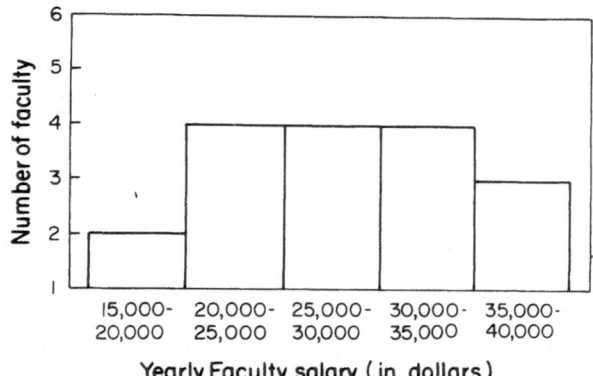

Yearly Faculty salary (in dollars)

FIG. 2. A histogram showing salary ranges of a hypothetical medical school department faculty.

A normal curve is the frequency polygon or histogram that would be approximated if infinite numbers of people were measured on a biological variable which was multifactorially determined, such as blood pressure, pulse, respiratory rate, height, weight, and intelligence quotient (IQ). Characteristics of such a curve include the shape of a bell and perfect mirror-image symmetry. Also, the mean, mode, and median, to be discussed later, are identical. When the sample of people is large but not infinite, the frequency polygon is also bell-shaped ("bell-shaped curve"), but not perfectly so. For didactic purposes, the normal and the bell-shaped curve will be considered synonymous. Figure 5 portrays a bell-shaped curve.

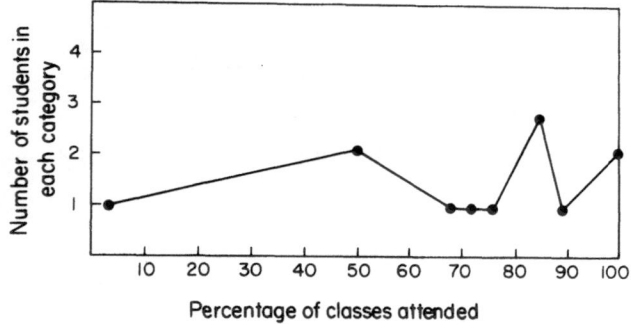

Percentage of classes attended

FIG. 3. A frequency polygon for the percentage of classes attended in the core example.

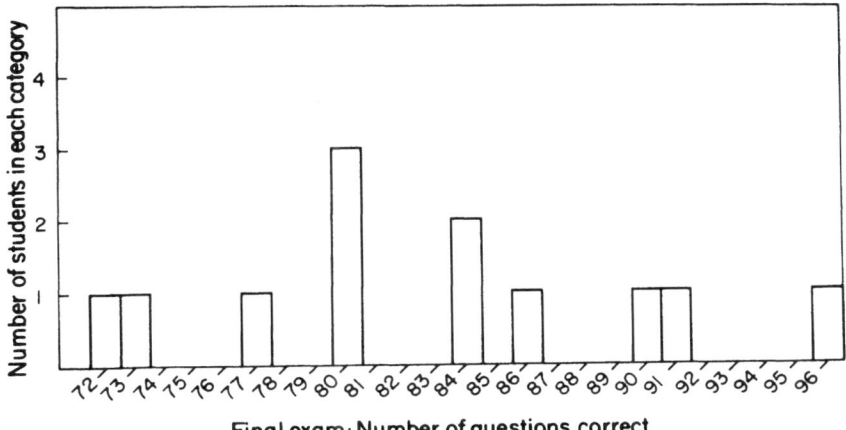

FIG. 4. A histogram for the percentage of classes attended in the core example.

Central tendency is the term that applies to the most characteristic points of a frequency distribution. As can be seen form the bell-shaped curve in Figure 5 the largest number of values cluster around the middle of a curve; thus, central tendency tells us more about the sample as a whole than measurements at the opposite ends of the sample (*deviant values*). Of course, statistically deviant members of a sample may stand out, and this can result in an inaccurate sterotyping of the sample by a nonscientific observer. Many statistical calculations require some measure of central tendency.

The measures of central tendency are the mean, the mode, and the median. The *mean* is the average value; it is obtained by adding all the values and dividing the sum by the number of measurements.

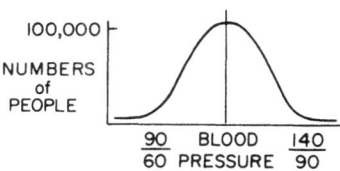

FIG. 5. A bell-shaped curve for the blood pressures of people in a population.

In the core example, the mean score for the final exam is calculated as follows:

$$
\begin{array}{r}
72 \\
73 \\
77 \\
80 \\
80 \\
80 \\
84 \\
84 \\
86 \\
90 \\
91 \\
\underline{96} \\
993
\end{array}
$$

$993 \div 12 = 82.75$. The mean score for the final exam is therefore 82.75.

In the core example, what is the mean score for the proficiency exam? (*Answer:* 76.6.)

The *mode* is the most frequently observed value in a sample.

In the core example, the mode for the percentage of classes attended was 84%, based on the fact that three people attended 84% of the classes. The closest competitors for the mode of the percentage of classes attended were 50% (two students) and 100% (two students). Now ascertain the mode (modal score) for the final examination. (*Answer:* 80.)

When two or more of the most common observations are made with approximately equal frequency, although clearly distant from each other on the polygon, the curve is called bimodal (or multimodal). Figure 6 is an example of a bimodal distribution.

The *median* is the measurement above which half of the measurements fall and below which the other half fall. For the measurements 4, 5, 9, 13, and 18, the median is 9. In the above case, where the number of measurements is

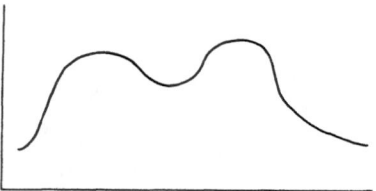

FIG. 6.   Shape of a bimodal distribution.

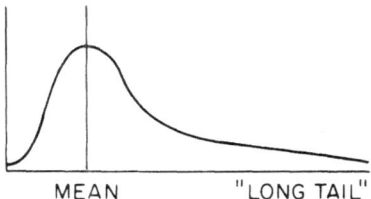

MEAN   "LONG TAIL"

FIG. 7. A positively skewed curve with the long tail on the right.

odd, detecting the median is easy. When the number of measurements is even, the average of the two middle measurements is the median.

In the core example, the median for the final exam was $80 + 84/2 = 82$. Now compute the median score for the proficiency exam. (*Answer:* $77 + 78 \div 2 = 77.5$.)

When the "observation in the middle" occurs several times in an asymmetrical fashion, such as in the distribution 2, 4, 4, 4, 8, 9, 10, a special calculation (which will not be discussed here) is needed to establish the median. When the sample is not large enough to produce a bell-shaped curve, the graph may be asymmetrical, or *skewed*. Skewed graphs have a "long tail" on one side and the mean on the other, as portrayed in Figures 7 and 8. When the mean lies to the left, and the long tail to the right, as in Figure 7, the curve is called *"positively skewed."* When the mean lies to the right, and the long tail to the left, the curve is called "negatively skewed."

In the core example, in what way is the curve for the percentage of classes attendes skewed? (*Answer:* Negatively skewed.)

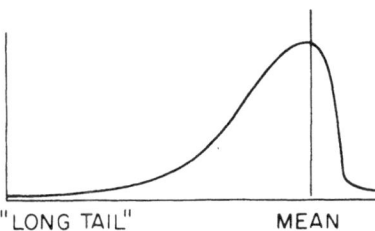

"LONG TAIL"   MEAN

FIG. 8. A negatively skewed curve with the long tail on the left.

The mean is the most frequently used measure of central tendency. But a problem in using the mean occurs when the sample is small and when one value is extremely deviant ("out of kilter") from the others—the mean is "vulnerable" to being overinfluenced by this extreme value. For example, in the sample 3, 7, 9, 11, 13, 196, the mean (39.83) does not give a true picture of central tendency. In cases like this, the median should be used instead of the mean.

In addition to knowing the central tendency of a group, it is also important to know about variability within the group. Central tendency tells you about the most characteristic observations. *Variability* adds additional information; it tells you to what extent the observations in the sample tend to stray, deviate, or vary from the center. Thus, variability tells you to what extent the central tendency truly characterizes, or is typical of, the group as a whole. For example, in the sample 4, 5, 5, 6, the mean of 5 is more typical or characteristic of the sample than the mean of 5 is typical or characteristic of the sample 1, 1, 2, 5, 16; thus, the former sample is less variable than the latter.

> In the core example, which is more variable, the percentage of classes attended or the final examination scores? (*Answer:* The percentage of classes attended.)

Variability is measured by the range, the variance, and the standard deviation. The *range* can be stated either as the lowest and the highest score or as the difference between the two.

> In the core example, the range of scores in the proficiency exam is 67-86, or 19. What is the range for the final exam scores? (*Answer:* 72-96, or 24.)

In a manner analogous to the mean of a small sample being strongly influenced by extremely high and extremely low values, the range, by definition, is determined only by two (highest and lowest) values. Thus, range is not a highly accurate, stable reflection of the variability of the sample as a whole. More stable measures of variability are the *variance* and the *standard deviation*. The variance is the average of the squared deviations of each of the values from the mean. The standard deviation is the square foot of the variance; it is thus measured by the formula

$$\sigma = \sqrt{\Sigma x^2 / N}$$

where x is the difference between each value and the mean value, x^2 is the sum of the squares of the differences between each value and the mean value, and N is the number of scores or measurements. An even more accurate formula for standard deviation, especially when the sample is small, is

$$\sigma = \sqrt{\Sigma\, x^2\, /\, N\text{-}1}$$

for reasons which we will not discuss here.

In the core example, the standard deviation of the proficiency exam raw scores is computed as follows:

The mean of the proficiency exam raw scores is 76.63.

The difference between each score and the mean is as follows:

        76.63 − 67 = 9.63
        76.63 − 69 = 7.63
        76.63 − 75 = 1.63
        76.63 − 77 = 0.37
        76.63 − 79 = 2.37
        76.63 − 80 = 3.37
        76.63 − 81 = 4.37
        76.63 − 86 = 9.37

The square of each difference is as follows:

        9.63^2 = 92.74
        7.63^2 = 58.22
        1.63^2 = 2.66
        0.37^2 = 0.14
        2.37^2 = 5.62
        3.37^2 = 11.36
        4.37^2 = 19.10
        9.37^2 = 87.80

The sum of the squares of the difference is as follows:

        92.74
        58.22
         2.66
         0.14
         5.62
        11.36
        19.10
        87.80
        _____
       277.64

The sum of the squares of the difference divided by the number of values minus 1 is 277.64 ÷ 7 = 39.66. This is because N, the number of proficiency exam scores, is 8, and $N - 1 = 7$.

The square root of the sum of the squares of the difference divided by the number of values minus one is 6.30.

The standard deviation is 6.30. This is much less than the standard deviation for the percentage of classes attended, which is 27, and less than the range of proficiency exam raw scores, which is $86 - 67 = 19$.

There is an important relationship between the standard deviation and the normal curve. In the normal curve, 68% of values fall within 1 standard deviation, plus and minus, from the mean, 34% of values are between the mean and plus (or minus) 1 standard deviation from the mean; 94% of values are within 2 standard deviations, plus and minus, from the mean; and 99.7% of values are within 3 standard deviations, plus and minus, from the mean.

If the mean raw score on an exam for a medical school class is 92 points, and the standard deviation is 7, what percentage of the class scores between 85 and 99 points? The answer is 68%.

Example: The mean raw score for a medical school class on an examination is 60 points. 95% of the students scored between 50 and 70 points. What is the standard deviation for the exam scores? (*Answer:* 5.)

Another connection between the standard deviation and a normal curve is that the standard deviation occurs at the inflection point (the point where the curve goes from convex to concave) of the curve, as portrayed in Figure 9.

As you can see from the preceding calculations on a "finite" medical school class, despite the fact that the abovementioned percentages (34%, 68%, 94%, and 99.7%) apply exactly to the normal curve only, the standard deviation is used in many computations in which there is no normal or bell-shaped curve.

A *correlation* is a way of assessing the relationship between two variables, and answers the questions "What happens to one variable as the other changes in value?" Correlation is not synonymous with cause: If two variables are correlated, they may or may not be causally related to each other. A *positive correlation* occurs when, as one variable increases, the other increases. This also means that as one decreases, the other decreases. A nega-

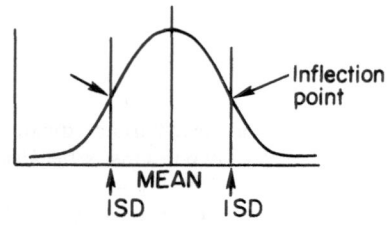

FIG. 9. The standard deviation is located at inflation points on the curve.

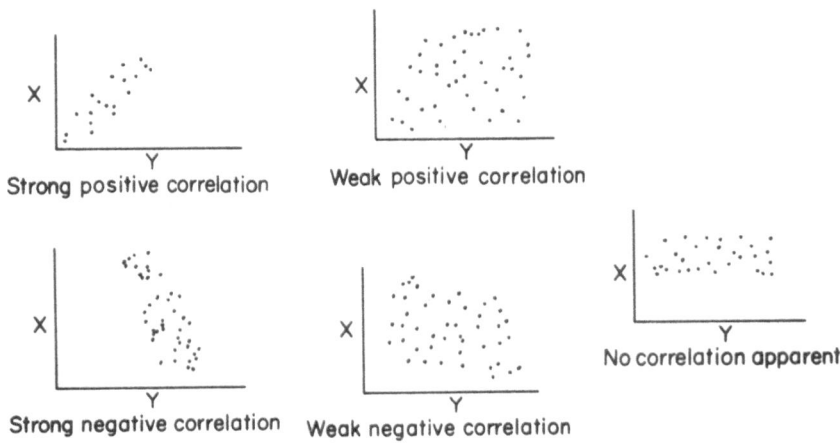

FIG. 10. Types of correlations.

tive correlation occurs when, as one variable increases, the other decreases. The maximum positive correlation is +1.0, and the maximum negative correlation is −1.0. The higher the *correlation coefficient* (which is sometimes measured as the *Spearman product-moment correlation coefficient*) the stronger the magnitude of the correlation, regardless of whether there is a plus or a minus sign before the coefficient. For example, a correlation of −0.65 is of a stronger magnitude than a correlation of = 0.45. Figure 10 portrays different types of correlations. The r is the symbol for correlation coefficient. An r of 0.2-0.4, plus or minus, is a weak correlation. An r of 0.7-1.0 is a strong correlation.

In our core example, the correlation between percentage of classes attended and final exam scores is −0.47. Is this a weak medium or strong correlation? (*Answer:* Medium.)

The correlation between proficiency exam scores and final examination scores is = 0.23. Is this a weak, medium, or strong correlation? (*Answer:* Weak.)

Does this mean that a good attendance record is causally related to a high grade on the final exam? (*Answer:* It may or may not be.)

There is at least one other factor which may be involved: Motivation. Highly motivated students are more likely to attend classes and to get higher grades. Also, by attending classes, they are more likely to learn information that appears on the final. More sophisticated statistical techniques (e.g., *regression analysis*) could help to clarify the matter further.

Now let us assess what we have just done. We have stated that, for the semester in question, there is a weak positive correlation between proficiency and final exam scores, and a medium positive correlation between percentage of classes attended and final exam scores.

Are we to accept these as real, true, or significant relationships, or could these relationships have occurred by chance, accident, or coincidence? To make an analogy, let us use another example. Suppose a 5-year-old tosses a coin 10 times, and gets 2 heads and 8 tails. Then a 12-year-old tosses the coin, gets 9 heads and 1 tail. There is a strong positive correlation between age and obtaining heads by a coin toss. Could this positive correlation have occurred by chance, accident or coincidence? Obviously.

Tests of the *statistical significance* of a correlation (the probability that a correlation was not accidental or coincidental) begin with the statistician-scientist making a hypothesis called the null hypothesis, which states that the correlation could have occurred by chance. For a relationship to be considered significant, the statistician-scientist must *reject the null hypothesis*.

Without discussing the formulas used to compute the statistical significance of a correlation and the coefficient of correlation itself, the results of doing this computation with the data in our core example are the following: The significance (P) of the correlation between percentage of classes attended and the final exam score is $P = <0.05$. This means that the chances of this correlation occurring by chance are less than 5 out of 100. The significance (P) of the correlation between proficiency exam score and final exam score is $P = <0.10$ and >0.05. This means that the chances of this correlation occurring by chance are between 5 and 10 out of 100. Traditionally, the cut-off level for statistical significance is $P = <0.05$, or less than 5 chances out of 100. Therefore, the 0.47 correlation between percentage of classes attended and final exam score is statistically significant. Is the $+0.23$ correlation between proficiency exam score and final exam score statistically significant by traditional standards? (*Answer:* No.)

Assessment of statistical significance does not apply only to the significance of a correlation. We are also interested in the significance of many other types of relationships. The traditional cut-off point for statistical significance of $P = <0.05$ holds for other relationships as well, but the tests for significance vary depending on the relationship to be measured. The *t test* is used to assess the significance of the difference between means.

In the core example, the *t* test could be used to assess the significance of the difference between the mean scores on the final exam of the students who did and didn't take the proficiency exam. The *chi square* (χ^2) test is used to assess the significance of the difference between ratios or proportions. Suppose the students were asked to grade two instructors' teaching performance using grades of A, B, C, and F. Also suppose the results were as follows:

	A	B	C	F	N
Instructor 1	1	4	6	1	12
Instructor 2	7	5	0	0	12

The significance of this table, which includes ratios of grades for each instructor, would be measured by a *chi square test*.

Now let us move to validity and reliability. *Validity* answers the question, "Does this test measure what it's supposed to measure?" There are several kinds of validity. *Content validity* is the degree to which a test measures behaviors in the same proportions as they are valued. This concept is very important in school test situations. If a medical school course teaches two subjects in a certain proportion, then examination should test the two subjects in the same proportion. For example, if a behavioral sciences course devotes 3% of its allotted time to biostatistics and 3% of its allotted time to medical sociology, then the exam, to have content validity, should devote 3% of its questions to biostatistics and 3% to medical sociology.

Predictive validity applies to the degree to which a test score is correlated with some kind of performance in the future. To determine if the final exam in the core example is a valid predictor of future performance in psychiatry, it would be helpful to know the correlation between the behavioral sciences final exam scores and the students' clerkship grades in psychiatry. *Concurrent validity* is the degree to which a test is correlated with simultaneous performance in other, related tasks.

In our core example, it would be interesting to note the correlation between observed (by the instructor) knowledge of behavioral sciences based upon classroom performance compared with the final exam's measurement of knowledge of behavioral sciences.

Reliability answers the questions "Would the results or conclusions have been the same if the evaluation was repeated at a different time, using the same test?" and "Are the results reproducible?"

For school examinations, psychological tests, and research questionnaires, there are three ways of assessing the instrument's reliability. In *test-retest-reliability*, the identical test is repeated on the same subjects on a second occasion. In *alternate form reliability*, comparable versions of a test are given to the same subjects on a second occasion. In *split-half reliability*, a single test is divided into comparable halves, and the results are compared. In assessing the reliability of clinical observations of patients or of diagnoses made on patients, *interrater reliability* is employed. This is measured by correlation coefficients for ratings by pairs of examiners, by the percentage of agreements between examiners, or by *weighted Kappa* (see Chap. 8).

Most educators believe that the reliability of written exams is greater than that for oral exams, especially if the oral exam is given by different examiners to different students using different case examples. This is why different raters on oral exams, or in clinical research, must get together beforehand to be sure they're using the same rating criteria. This is also why the use of uniform criteria for psychiatric diagnosis has been a boon to psychiatric research. Reliability values of 0.7 or above are considered acceptable.

> The reliability of the proficiency exam in our core example was 0.78. The reliability of the final exam was 0.70. Was this an acceptable degree of reliability? (*Answer:* Yes.)

Finally, we must discuss the biomedical research in general. Biomedical researchers should organize their research by preparing a *protocal*, which should include the following [3]:

1. Importance of the study
2. *Literature review*
3. Design and methodology, including:
   Data-gathering procedure
   Data-assessment procedure
   Dealing with the issue of risk to the study subjects
   Pilot study
   Revision based upon pilot study
4. Data collection
5. Data analysis
6. Preparation of material for publication

Experienced biomedical researchers commonly offer the following advice in doing research [3,4]: Study topics in which you are truly interested, and ask questions you truly want answered. In reviewing the literature, you will often be surprised to learn how little is known about your area of interest; don't let a weakness in statistics deter you from following up on a creative idea. There are usually others who can provide statistical assistance; be sure to solicit other opinions in preparing an article for publication. Use the preferred style of the journal to which the article is being submitted; do not be deterred by initial rejections.

There are other important concepts which need to be discussed. A *pro-*

spective study is one in which the study is planned out before the data is gathered. *A retrospective* study is one which analyzes data gathered in the past. In theory, prospective studies are preferable, but huge numbers of research studies are retrospective.

A *cohort* is a group of people with a given characteristic, such as people born in 1942, who are followed up at successive points in time. The term for a prospective study that employs regular followups of a cohort of people is a *longitudinal* study. Cohort studies are an excellent way of studying the course of a disease, and often very helpful in learning about the causes of a disease. But they are usually very time-consuming and expensive.

An experiment is a prospective study in which the researcher does something to influence or change the research subject, such as exposing him to mosquito bites (the classic yellow fever experiment of Walter Reed) or treating his manic episode with lithium. Experiments should include a *matched control* group (subjects who have characteristics similar to those of the subjects receiving the procedure) for whom the protocol is the same in all respects except for the procedure being tested. Experiments are an excellent way of determining cause and effect, but carry the risk of injury to the subject, as well as the risk of depriving the control subject of the benefits of the procedure under study. Ideally, experiments should be *"double-blind,"* with neither the subject nor the rater knowing whether a given subject is the recipient of the procedure or is a control subject. Double-blind studies are designed to minimize the bias of the experimenter.

A *sample* is a limited number of people who are being studied in lieu of studying the entire *population*, which would be studied if conditions were ideal. Samples are used instead of entire populations because it is rare to be able to properly study entire populations. For example, in order to study the frequency of cheating among all American medical students (the population) it would be necessary to distribute thousands of questionnaires in all states with medical schools. It would be more practical to distribute questionnaires to a sample of students in several representative medical schools, and then use this sample to generalize about the American medical student population as a whole.

REFERENCES

1. Rosenhan, D. On being sane in insane places. *Science* 179:250-258 (1973).
2. Taylor, M., and Abrams, R. The phenomenology of mania. A new look at some old patients. *Arch. Gen. Psychiatry* 29:520-522 (1973).
3. Friedman, G. *A Primer of Epidemiology*. McGraw-Hill, New York (1974).
4. Sainsbury, P., and Kreitman, N. *Methods of Psychiatric Research*. Oxford, London (1975).

Index

427